U0294899

中医
临床

The plant shown on the cover is *Cornus officinalis*. In Chinese medicine, its dried ripe fruit is known as shān zhū yú (山茱萸 , *Fructus Corni*), more commonly known as the asiatic cornelian cherry fruit. shān zhū yú acts to replenish the liver and kidney, while also displaying astringent and consolidating effects. This medicinal is widely used in the clinical treatment of both male and female infertility.

Project Editors: Liu Shui, Rao Hong-mei & Zeng Chun
Copy Editor: Rao Hong-mei
Book Designer: Li Xi
Cover Designer: Li Xi
Typesetter: Wei Hong-bo

The Clinical Practice of Chinese Medicine

Male & Female Infertility

中医
临床

The Clinical Practice of Chinese Medicine

Male & Female Infertility

Chen Zhi-qiang

Professor of Chinese External Medicine,
Director of the Department of Surgery,
Vice President of the Second Teaching
Hospital of Guangzhou University of CM

Li Li-yun

Guangdong Province Entitled Famous Chinese
Medicine Physician, Professor of Chinese
Medicine Gynecology, the Second Teaching
Hospital of Guangzhou University of CM

With Co-authors (From the Second Teaching Hospital of Guangzhou University of CM)
Dai Rui-xin, M.S. TCM, Resident   **Xu Min**, Ph.D. TCM, Associate Chief Physician

With Contributors (From the Second Teaching Hospital of Guangzhou University of CM)
Wang Shu-sheng, Chief Physician   **Bai Zun-guang**, M.S. TCM, Associate Chief Physician

Translated by
Zhao Yan,
Ph.D. TCM

Guan-hu Yang,
M.D., Ph.D., L.Ac., Prof.

Liu Yong,
M.D.& Ph.D. ER

Edited by   **Harry F. Lardner**, Dipl.Ac.

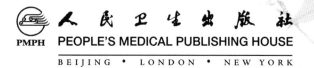

人民卫生出版社
PMPH PEOPLE'S MEDICAL PUBLISHING HOUSE
BEIJING • LONDON • NEW YORK

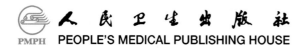

PMPH PEOPLE'S MEDICAL PUBLISHING HOUSE

Website: http://www.pmph.com

Book Title: The Clinical Practice of Chinese Medicine:
Male & Female Infertility
中医临床实用系列：男性不育与女性不孕

Contact address: No. 19, Pan Jia Yuan Nan Li, Chaoyang District, Beijing 100021, P.R. China, phone: 8610 5978 7340, E-mail: zzg@pmph.com

First published: 2008
ISBN: 978-7-117-10024-3/R · 10025

Cataloguing in Publication Data:
A catalog record for this book is available from the CIP-Database China.

Printed in The People's Republic of China

ISBN 978-7-117-10024-3

9 787117 100243 >

Members of Translators and English Editors

For Male Infertility

Translators:

Guan-hu Yang, M.D., Ph.D., L.Ac., Prof.

Yong-tao Liu, M.D.

Jia-xiu Zhuang, M.D., L.Ac.

Xu Hou, M.D., L.Ac.

Liu Yong, M.D.&Ph.D. ER

Jin Shi-hui, M.D. GP

Zui Fang, M.D., L.Ac.

Yun-peng Luo, M.D., L.Ac.

David Wang, M.D., L.Ac.

Bin Yang

English Editors:

C. Fritz Froehlich, M.S., L.Ac.

Aletha Tippett, M.D.

Kare Froendhoff, M.S.

For Female Infertility

Translators:

Zhao Yan, Ph.D. TCM

Huang Min, M.S. TCM

Li Hong-Lei, M.S. TCM

Zheng Qi

English Editors:

Guan-hu Yang, M.D., Ph.D., L.Ac., Prof.

C. Fritz Froehlich, M.S., L.Ac.

III

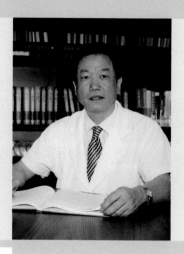

陈志强　教授

Professor **Chen Zhi-qiang** was born in 1957, and is today a chief physician, professor, and doctoral advisor at the Second Clinical Medicine College of Guangzhou University of Chinese Medicine. He also serves as vice-president and director of the surgical teaching and research department. Professor Chen excels in the integrative treatment of stubborn and critical diseases, and also achieves fine therapeutic effects in the treatment of urinary and prostate conditions. He has supervised 6 research projects at both ministerial and provincial levels, and has been also distinguished with 5 provincial awards. He has published over 30 academic papers, serving as chief director of 4 monographs including Clinical Diagnosis and Treatment in Andriatrics with Chinese Medicine (published by People's Medical Publishing House) and Integrative Surgery. He is also responsible for overseeing the national continuing education program. Professor Chen serves as the Director of the Specialty Board of the Chinese Association of Integrative Medicine, Vice-director of the Special Andriatrics Board of the Chinese Association of Traditional Chinese Medicine, Vice-director of the Specialty Surgery Board of the Chinese Association of Traditional Chinese Medicine, and is also a standing council member of the Chinese Medicine Specialty Board of the China Sexology Association.

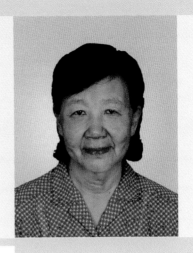

李丽芸　教授

Professor **Li Li-yun** is a master's level advisor at the Second Clinical Medicine College of Guangzhou University of Chinese Medicine. She previously served as Director of Gynecology at the Guangdong Provincial Hospital of Chinese Medicine. She has accumulated an abundance of clinical experience in her nearly 50 years of clinical teaching and research work. She specializes in the integrative treatment of menstrual disorders, female infertility, and female genital inflammation. Professor Li has developed multiple approaches in the treatment of gynecological disease, and is highly respected for her contributions to the field. She is a highly sought-after physician, especially by patients suffering with infertility. Professor Li was entitled Renowned Physician of Chinese Medicine in Guangdong Province, also winning 2 provincial awards. She was further recognized as Master Physician in the National Master and Apprentice Education Program. She currently serves as a council member of the Guangdong Promotional Committee of Chinese Medicine, and Advisor of the Gynecology Specialty Board of the Guangdong Provincial Association of Chinese Medicine.

Foreword

Chinese medicine is a broad and profound art of healing. It is a well-established and comprehensive system of medicine with an ancient origin and a long rich history. Throughout the ages, it has made a significant contribution to the prosperity of the Chinese civilization. The system of pattern differentiation and treatment fully reflects the Chinese medical view of health and disease as a holistic concept, the emphasis on the body's ability to regulate itself and adapt to the environment, and the need for individualized treatment. The integration of diseases and syndromes is the consummation of treatment based on pattern differentiation; it fully displays the superior characteristic of this discipline, and has an extensive influence on the development of the art of Chinese medicine.

The intention of this series of books is to introduce accurate Chinese medical diagnosis and treatment of various diseases to overseas readers.

The Chinese edition of *The Clinical Practice of Chinese Medicine* was edited by the Second Teaching Hospital of Guangzhou University of CM (also known as Guangdong Provincial Hospital of TCM), and published by People's Medical Publishing House. When the series was published in 2000, it was widely accepted in clinical practice due to its originality, distinguishing features, richness in content, completeness, accuracy, and outstanding emphases. This series has become a trademark of standard in the eyes of Chinese and integrative medical practitioners. During the second printing of this series of books, Professor Deng Tie-tao praised, "For a series to be printed a multiple number of times, shows that it is highly regarded and has received excellent reviews." In order to keep up with the constant development of medical science, this series was revised and re-published in 2004 by People's Medical Publishing House. Due to its popularity, it has been reprinted numerous times since.

The English edition of this series of books includes 20 volumes:

- ✧ *COPD & Asthma*
- ✧ *Coronary Artery Disease & Hyperlipidemia*
- ✧ *Stroke & Parkinson's Disease*
- ✧ *Chronic Gastritis & Irritable Bowel Syndrome*
- ✧ *Diabetes & Obesity*
- ✧ *Gout & Rheumatoid Arthritis*
- ✧ *Menstrual Disorders I: Dysfunctional Uterine Bleeding & Amenorrhea*
- ✧ *Menstrual Disorders II: Premenstrual Syndrome, Dysmenorrhea & Perimenopause*
- ✧ *Endometriosis & Uterine Fibroids*
- ✧ *Pelvic Inflammatory Disease & Miscarriage*
- ✧ *Postpartum Hypogalactia & Breast Hyperplasia*
- ✧ *Male & Female Infertility*
- ✧ *Urticaria*
- ✧ *Eczema & Atopic Dermatitis*
- ✧ *Lupus Erythematosus*
- ✧ *Scleroderma & Dermatomyositis*
- ✧ *Diseases of the Accessory Organs of the Skin*
- ✧ *Psoriasis & Cutaneous Pruritus*
- ✧ *Herpes Zoster & Fungal Skin Infections*
- ✧ *Chloasma & Vitiligo*

Clinical application varies by individual and by location; when this is combined with the rapid development of medical science, the treatment methods and medicinal dosages may also vary accordingly. When using these books as a reference guide, overseas readers should confirm the formulas and dosages of medicinals according to the individual health condition of the patient, as well as take into account the origin of the Chinese medicinals.

The quotes in these books were taken from various medical literature during the compilation process. We have deleted some of the contents of the original texts for the purpose of uniformity and ease in readability. We ask for the reader's forgiveness and express our respect and gratitude toward the original authors.

Due to the complicated nature of the diagnoses and treatments covered in these books, and the wide range of topics they touch upon, it is inevitable that one may encounter errors while reading through them. We respectively welcome constructive criticism and corrections from our readers.

The clinical practice of medicine changes with the constant development of medical science. The books in this series will be revised regularly to continuously adapt to the development of traditional Chinese medicine.

Editorial Board for the English edition of
The Clinical Practice of Chinese Medicine **series**
March, 2008

Wu Xian-zhong

Specialist of Integrative Medicine, Academician of Chinese Academy of Engineering, Professor, Tianjin Medical University, Chairman of Tianjin Institute of Acute Abdomen Research on Integrative Medicine

Wang Yong-yan

Specialist of Chinese Internal Medicine, Academician of Chinese Academy of Engineering, Professor and former President of Beijing University of CM, and Honorary President of China Academy of Chinese Medical Science

Chen Ke-ji

Specialist of Cardiovascular & Aging Diseases, Academician of Chinese Academy of Science, Professor of Medicine, Xiyuan Hospital, and Institute of Aging Medicine, China Academy of Chinese Medical Science, Consultant on Traditional Medicine, WHO

GENERAL COORDINATOR

Lü Yu-bo

Professor & Vice President, Guangzhou University of CM, President, the Second Teaching Hospital of Guangzhou University of CM

EDITORS-IN-CHIEF

Luo Yun-jian

Guangdong Province Entitled Famous Chinese Medicine Physician, Professor of Chinese Internal Medicine, & former Vice President of the Second Teaching Hospital of Guangzhou University of CM

Liu Mao-cai

Guangdong Province Entitled Famous Chinese Medicine Physician, Professor of Chinese Internal Medicine, & former Vice President of the Second Teaching Hospital of Guangzhou University of CM, Former Chairman of Institute for Aging Cerebral Diseases, Guangzhou University of CM

MEMBERS (Listed alphabetically by name)

Deng Zhao-zhi

Professor of Chinese Internal Medicine, Guangzhou University of CM

Fan Guan-jie

Professor of Chinese Internal Medicine, Director of Department of Education, the Second Teaching Hospital of Guangzhou University of CM

Fan Rui-qiang

Professor of Chinese External Medicine, Director of Department of Dermatology, the Second Teaching Hospital of Guangzhou University of CM

Huang Jian-ling

Professor of Chinese Medicine Gynecology, Director of the First Department of Gynecology, the Second Teaching Hospital of Guangzhou University of CM

Huang Pei-xin

Professor of Chinese Internal Medicine, the Second Teaching Hospital of Guangzhou University of CM, Head of the Research Project of Cerebral Disease Treatment on Chinese Internal Medicine, Sponsored by SATCM China

Huang Sui-ping

Professor of Chinese Internal Medicine, Director of Department of Digestion, the Second Teaching Hospital of Guangzhou University of CM

Li Li-yun

Guangdong Province Entitled Famous Chinese Medicine Physician, Professor of Chinese Medicine Gynecology, the Second Teaching Hospital of Guangzhou University of CM

Liang Xue-fang

Professor of Chinese Medicine Gynecology, Director of the Third Department of Gynecology, the Second Teaching Hospital of Guangzhou University of CM

Lin Lin

Professor of Chinese Internal Medicine, Director of Department of Respiratory, the Second Teaching Hospital of Guangzhou University of CM

Liu Wei-sheng

Master of the National Master and Apprentice Education Program, Professor of Chinese Internal Medicine, the Second Teaching Hospital of Guangzhou University of CM

Wang Xiao-yun

Professor of Chinese Medicine Gynecology, Director of Department of Gynecology, Head of Teaching Division of Gynecology, the Second Teaching Hospital of Guangzhou University of CM

Lin Yi

Professor of Mastopathy in Chinese Medicine, the Second Teaching Hospital of Guangzhou University of CM, Head of the National Key Subject –Mastopathy in Chinese Medicine

Si-tu Yi

Professor of Chinese Medicine Gynecology, the Second Teaching Hospital of Guangzhou University of CM, Head of the National Key Subject – Chinese Medicine Gynecology

SPONSORED BY

The Second Teaching Hospital of Guangzhou University of CM, also known as **Guangdong Provincial Hospital of TCM**

Preface

Infertility is a health condition that seriously impacts the quality of life for many of families today. WHO statistics show that the incidence rate of infertility has reached 5%~15% over the world, appearing even higher in western countries. Nearly 1 in 5 couples suffer from infertility, affecting 50~80 million people. Moreover, this number is increasing by 2 million each year. In recent years, advances in assisted reproductive technique (ART), intracytoplasmic sperm injection (ICSI) and in vitro fertilization (IVF) have made a significant difference. However, the field of reproductive medicine also faces various problems, such as relatively low pregnancy rates along with high multiple pregnancy and abortion rates. The cost of treatment is also often prohibitively expensive.

The practices of Chinese medicine, integrative gynecology, and andriatrics all display distinct therapeutic effects in the treatment of all types of infertility. In China, assisted reproductive technologies are often combined with Chinese medicinal therapies or acupuncture to improve the conception rates and reduce side effects. In cases of male infertility, the causes are often associated with low sperm quality, quantity, and motility. In this respect, Chinese medicine displays a unique superiority.

The authors of this book are all Chinese medical doctors who possess abundant clinical knowledge due to their years of practicing gynecology and andriatrics. During this compilation process, we have consulted with a variety of specialists to collect advice and suggestions and to also summarize their experience with a collection of effective treatments. We have also referenced a large number of national and international documents that analyze and explore the subject based on current research results. This book is a comprehensive summarization and refinement of the clinical treatment of infertility with Chinese medicine. It is also our thorough reflection on the most salient points and challenges of this subject.

In this book, both female infertility and male infertility are fully addressed. Readers will find an organized and thorough presentation of each disease, including a brief overview followed by sections covering etiologies and pathomechanisms, treatment modalities, prognosis, preventive healthcare, clinical experiences of renowned Chinese physicians, perspectives of integrative medicine, quotes from classical texts, and relevant modern research.

In order to ensure a better understanding of the contents of this Chinese medical book series, we have recognized that different readers have different needs and desires.

First, medical professionals, practitioners, and students can read this series for professional study and application, and should have a solid background in the basic theories of Chinese medicine. Prior to reading this book, they should also understand the properties and proper dosages of Chinese medicinal, and their contraindications when combined. It is most essential to have a clear understanding of both their functions and incompatibilities.

Second, interested general readers should pay attention to the characteristics and advantages of Chinese medicine, and the special methods of Chinese medicine in the areas of prognosis and preventive healthcare. In terms of application, Chinese medicinals should be prescribed only under the guidance of professional Chinese medical physicians.

We hope that these books will prove to be useful and valuable to all of those involved in the field of Chinese medicine, including practitioners, students, teachers, patients, medical doctors who are interested in Chinese medicine and anyone who may be seeking answers to their questions about the efficacy of Chinese medicine.

Hopefully, this book will help our readers gain a deeper understanding of Chinese medical diagnosis and treatment in the field reproductive medicine. We also aim to bridge the gap between the methods of Chinese medicine and modern biomedicine through the discussion of integrative treatment approaches.

Due to the advancing nature of clinical medicine, we apologize for any out-dated or incorrect information that may appear in these books. We hope that readers will not hesitate to offer their comments and suggestions on how to improve the content of this material.

Chen Zhi-qiang & Li Li-yun
Guangzhou, China
March, 2008

Contents

Female Infertility

Male Infertility

by **Chen Zhi-qiang**,

Professor & Chief Physician of Chinese External Medicine;
Director of the Department of Surgery

Dai Rui-xin,

M.S. TCM, Resident Physician of Chinese External Medicine

Wang Shu-sheng,

Chief Physician of Chinese External Medicine

Bai Zun-guang,

M.S. TCM, Associate Chief Physician of Chinese External Medicine

OVERVIEW

Infertility may be diagnosed when a couple has been unable to conceive following one year of unprotected sexual intercourse. When resulting due to dysfunction in the male, the condition is referred to as male infertility. According to WHO statistics, infertility afflicts nearly one in seven couples, with 20% of cases resulting directly from male dysfunction. An additional 30% involves problems with both parties, so male infertility is a factor in about half of all cases.

Early Chinese medical literature records a number of specific disease names which also describe this condition.

CHINESE MEDICAL ETIOLOGY AND PATHOMECHANISM

In Chinese medicine, this condition usually involves several internal organs, generally including the kidney, liver, heart, and spleen. However, this disorder is mainly associated with the kidney because of its function of storing essence and governing reproduction. When kidney qi is exuberant and the genuine yin is also sufficient, *tiangui* will arrive. If a healthy man and woman have sexual intercourse at this time, conception will occur.

Congenital deficiency, kidney qi deficiency, and depletion of the life gate fire often result in male sexual dysfunction. Impotence, insufficient erection, or weak ejaculation often occurs due to deficiency of yang qi. Sexual intemperance damages the kidney, often resulting in thin semen with low sperm counts. Prolonged or untreated illnesses can damage yin and exhaust both essence and blood. Hyperactivity of fire due to yin deficiency leads to seminal emission, night sweats, and thick sticky semen. All of these patterns can eventually lead to male infertility.

Emotional disorders may lead to impotence when the liver fails to maintain the free flow of qi. Liver qi stagnation may also transform into hyperactivity of liver fire which then consumes kidney water. When kidney water fails to nourish liver wood, the genitals become malnourished, and the passage of semen may also become inhibited.

Overthinking and taxation may damage the heart, causing deficiencies of heart qi and heart blood. The resulting deficiencies of blood and original qi may also lead to seminal weakness and deficiency.

Splenic transportation and transformation failure leads to the formation of phlegm-damp. Retention of phlegm-damp can transform into heat, resulting in retention of damp-heat in the lower burner which blocks the life gate fire. This can cause seminal emission, premature ejaculation, and impotence.

External contraction of pathogenic damp-heat and damp-heat pouring downwards leads to obstruction, dead sperm, and static blood. There may be distending pain of the lower abdomen, non-liquefaction of semen, and failure of ejaculation.

Emerging patterns that manifest with lassitude and fatigue can also contribute to impotence and infertility, particularly those associated with constitutional deficiency.

The etiology and pathogenesis of male infertility can be summarized within six main patterns.

(1) Deficiency of Essential Qi due to Congenital Deficiency

The kidney stores essence and also governs reproduction. Kidney essence includes both congenital essence and acquired essence. Originating from the parents, congenital essence thus forms the material basis for reproduction and growth. Essence can also transform into qi. When kidney qi becomes abundant, *tiangui* arrives to enter the penetrating and conception vessels. Essence is able to mature only when these two vessels become abundant. Women will then begin to menstruate, and men will produce seminal fluid. Sexual intercourse can result in conception at this time.

However, reproductive disorders often occur due to congenital essence deficiency. Congenital factors are known to affect children born to parents who marry too early or bear too many children, especially when the parents are close relatives. Reproductive disorders appear in a considerable proportion of these individuals after they mature.

(2) Essential Qi Deficiency Cold due to Debilitation of Life Gate Fire

Excessive sexual activity consumes essence and qi, even during adolescence. Over a period of time, this leads to deficiency of kidney qi and debilitation of life gate fire. Without the warmth and nourishment of the life gate fire, the essential qi becomes cold and deficient. This pattern is known as essential qi deficiency cold, which results in a decline of both sperm production and sexual function.

(3) Phlegm Turbidity and Blood Stasis Obstructing Semen

Excessive consumption of alcohol and greasy foods damages the function of the spleen and stomach, especially in the overweight and obese. When foods are not properly transformed, phlegm may form and begin to brew internally. As phlegm flows downward, it can inhibit the production and transformation of semen, and also obstruct its orifice. Blockage of the seminal passage directly affects reproductive function.

Indirect causes include prolonged illness affecting the collaterals, and physical injury that results in blood statis. When static blood remains in the kidney or obstructs the seminal passage, the normal production of semen may also decrease. In some cases, ejaculation may become inhibited and the seminal fluid will accumulate internally.

(4) Damp-heat Pouring Downward due to Improper Diet

Excessive consumption of alcohol or greasy and spicy foods can damage the spleen and stomach, leading to the formation of damp-heat and phlegm. Damp-heat and phlegm-fire pouring downward can affect the quality of the seminal fluid, often resulting in male infertility. Individuals presenting constitutional hyperactivity of yang qi are especially affected.

(5) Liver Stagnation due to Emotional Disorders

Damage by the seven affects often leads to stagnation of liver qi and the disruption of its function of free coursing. Disharmony of visceral qi and debilitation of ancestral qi may also result. In their early stages, conditions associated with emotional disorders mainly manifest as disorders of the qi dynamic. Later on, pathological changes of essence and blood are inevitable because the viscera have become affected. In cases where kidney essence becomes stagnant, infertility may result. Regarding the emotions, excessive sadness most often leads to sexual dysfunction. Sexual frustration is often followed by a libidinal decline that can eventually cause impotence. In fact, any of the seven affects in excess (joy, anger, anxiety, thought, sorrow, fear, and fright) can adversely affect sexual function.

(6) Qi and Blood Deficiency due to Prolonged Illness or Taxation

Both qi and blood may become deficient due to insufficient spleen qi, spleen and stomach damage due to taxation, constitutional deficiency, or an incomplete recovery from a prolonged illness. All lead to failure of qi and blood engendering and transformation. Essence and blood are closely related, because essence is derived from blood. So, the engendering of essence is also affected when the spleen becomes deficient. The resulting essence and blood deficiency may also manifest as infertility.

The pathogenesis of male infertility can be quite complex. It may be associated with patterns of deficiency, excess, cold, heat, phlegm, stasis, or constraint. The organ mainly affected is the kidney, which is also directly related to the proper functioning the liver, spleen and heart.

Essentially, infertility results from kidney qi deficiency with a failure of yin essence transformation. However, failure of transportation due to spleen deficiency also causes essence deficiency and infertility. Upward flaming of heart fire often results in non-interaction between the heart and kidney, which can lead to sexual dysfunction. Qi and blood disharmonies associated with patterns of liver constraint are also contributing factors, and especially the resulting failure of free coursing. Other associated patterns include heat in the liver channel, hyperactivity of ministerial fire, and phlegm obstructing the ancestral sinews. Whether the syndrome is spleen deficiency, blood deficiency, phlegm-damp, static blood, liver cold, damp-heat or liver constraint, all of these patterns eventually result in kidney essence deficiency when male infertility appears as a result.

CHINESE MEDICAL TREATMENT

Before treatment begins, it is necessary to clearly differentiate the presenting patterns. Male infertility may be associated with deficiency or excess, cold or heat, disorders of qi and blood, or imbalances of yin and yang. Proper treatment naturally follows accurate pattern and disease differentiation. The key to this disease lies in the kidney, which is also closely related to liver, spleen, and heart function. The general approach to treatment involves tonifying the kidney while also nourishing essence. Specific treatments may be applied to regulate kidney yin and yang, nourish kidney essence, and course the passage of kidney essence.

This disorder generally presents with deficiency at the root and excess at the branch. Treatment of the root condition mainly involves the kidney and spleen. Kidney tonification methods include nourishing yin, replenishing essence, and invigorating yang. Treatment of the branch involves methods that invigorate blood, transform stasis, clear heat, disinhibit dampness, transform phlegm, and dissipate binding.

Bitter medicinals are generally contraindicated, as well as those excessively cold or hot in nature. The excessive use of bitter flavors may damage the stomach, causing stomach duct pain, nausea and vomiting. They may also damage yang and cause declined sexual desire, decreased seminal quality, and impotence. Excessive warming of the kidney while invigorating kidney yang often leads to congestion and edema of the reproductive tract. This can aggravate inflammation, consume yin essence, and reduce the quantity and quality of seminal fluid.

Pattern Differentiation and Treatment

(1) Kidney Yin Deficiency

【Syndrome Characteristics】

Main manifestations include scant seminal fluid, low sperm count, poor sperm liquefaction, and relatively high numbers of abnormal sperm. Symptoms and signs include weak knees and lumbar pain, dizziness, tinnitus, seminal emission and premature ejaculation. Other manifestations include abnormal erection, disorders of ejaculation, insomnia, forgetfulness, vexing heat in the five hearts, night sweating, dry mouth and throat, emaciation, pain in the heels, and dry stools. The tongue appears red with little or no coating. Pulses are thready and rapid.

This pattern is often seen in males with excessive sexual desire and intemperate sexuality.

【Treatment Principle】

Nourish yin, tonify kidney, and replenish essence.

【Commonly Used Medicinals】

To tonify the kidney and replenish essence, select *gǒu qǐ zǐ* (Fructus Lycii), *shú dì huáng* (Radix Rehmanniae Praeparata), *huáng jīng* (Rhizoma Polygonati), *hé shǒu wū* (Radix Polygoni Multiflori), *tù sī zǐ* (Semen

Cuscutae), *shān zhū yú* (Fructus Corni), *fù pén zǐ* (Fructus Rubi) and *ròu cōng róng* (Herba Cistanches).

【Representative Formula】

Wǔ Zǐ Yǎn Zōng Wán (五子衍宗丸) modified with *Zuǒ Guī Yǐn* (左归饮).

【Ingredients】

菟丝子	*tù sī zǐ*	15g	Semen Cuscutae
枸杞子	*gǒu qǐ zǐ*	15g	Fructus Lycii
覆盆子	*fù pén zǐ*	15g	Fructus Rubi
熟地黄	*shú dì huáng*	15g	Radix Rehmanniae Praeparata
山茱萸	*shān zhū yú*	10g	Fructus Corni
五味子	*wǔ wèi zǐ*	10g	Fructus Schisandrae Chinensis
山药	*shān yào*	10g	Rhizoma Dioscoreae
茯苓	*fú líng*	10g	Poria
车前子	*chē qián zǐ*	20g	Semen Plantaginis
甘草	*gān cǎo*	3g	Radix et Rhizoma Glycyrrhizae

【Formula Analysis】

Tù sī zǐ (Semen Cuscutae), *gǒu qǐ zǐ* (Fructus Lycii), *fù pén zǐ* (Fructus Rubi), and *shú dì huáng* (Radix Rehmanniae Praeparata) act to tonify the kidney, nourish yin, replenish essence, and benefit marrow. *shān zhū yú* (Fructus Corni) and *wǔ wèi zǐ* (Fructus Schisandrae Chinensis) tonify the kidney and secure essence. *Shān yào* (Rhizoma Dioscoreae) fortifies the spleen and secures essence. *Chē qián zǐ* (Semen Plantaginis) disinhibits dampness and frees the passage of semen, being astringent in nature. *Wǔ wèi zǐ* (Fructus Schisandrae Chinensis) is both astringing and discharging. *Fú líng* (Poria) and *gān cǎo* (Radix et Rhizoma Glycyrrhizae) benefit the source of engendering and transformation by nourishing the spleen and stomach.

This formula acts to tonify the kidney and replenish essence. It is applicable for most infertility patients because it supplements without excessive warming, and nourishes without cloying.

【Modifications】

➤ With seminal emission or premature ejaculation, add *mǔ lì* (Concha Ostreae) 15g, *lóng gǔ* (Os Draconis) 15g, *wǔ wèi zǐ* (Fructus Schisandrae Chinensis) 10g and *qiàn shí* (Semen Euryales) 10g to astringe and secure the essence and qi.

➤ With low sperm count and low survival rates, add *dǎng shēn* (Radix Codonopsis) 15g, *mài mén dōng* (Radix Ophiopogonis) 15g and *hé shǒu wū* (Radix Polygoni Multiflori) 10g to fortify the spleen, tonify the kidney, and invigorate the essence and qi.

➤ With high numbers of non-viable sperm, combine the formula with *Chén Shì Bǔ Shèn Huó Jīng Tāng* (陈氏补肾活精汤) to tonify the kidney and replenish essence.

The formula contains the following medicinals.

熟地黄	*shú dì huáng*	10g	Radix Rehmanniae Praeparata
肉苁蓉	*ròu cōng róng*	10g	Herba Cistanches
淫羊藿	*yín yáng huò*	10g	Herba Epimedii
仙茅	*xiān máo*	10g	Rhizoma Curculiginis
何首乌	*hé shǒu wū*	10g	Radix Polygoni Multiflori
枸杞子	*gǒu qǐ zǐ*	15g	Fructus Lycii

➤ With non-liquefaction of sperm, combine the formula with *Chén Shì Bǔ Shèn Huó Jīng Tāng* (陈氏补肾活精汤) to tonify the kidney and promote sperm generation.

The formula contains the following medicinals.

玄参	*xuán shēn*	10g	Radix Scrophulariae
麦门冬	*mài mén dōng*	10g	Radix Ophiopogonis
天门冬	*tiān mén dōng*	10g	Radix Asparagi
生地黄	*shēng dì huáng*	10g	Radix Rehmanniae Recens
熟地黄	*shú dì huáng*	10g	Radix Rehmanniae Praeparata
枸杞子	*gǒu qǐ zǐ*	15g	Fructus Lycii
知母	*zhī mǔ*	10g	Rhizoma Anemarrhenae
泽泻	*zé xiè*	10g	Rhizoma Alismatis

➤ With effulgent fire due to yin deficiency, add *zhī mǔ* (Rhizoma Anemarrhenae) 10g, *huáng bǎi* (Cortex Phellodendri Chinensis) 10g, *hàn lián cǎo* (Herba Ecliptae) 10g, and *mǔ dān pí* (Cortex Moutan) 10g to nourish yin and clear heat.

➤ With obvious kidney essence depletion, add *huáng jīng* (Rhizoma Polygonati) 15g, *lù jiǎo jiāo* (Colla Cornus Cervi) 5g, and *zǐ hé chē* (Placenta Hominis) 10g to strongly tonify original yin.

➤ With kidney yin insufficiency accompanied with damp-heat, apply *Zhī Bǎi Dì Huáng Wán* (知柏地黃丸), *cāng zhú* (Rhizoma Atractylodis) 10g, *chē qián zǐ* (Semen Plantaginis) 10g, *bì xiè* (Rhizoma Dioscoreae Hypoglaucae) 10g, and *tǔ fú líng* (Rhizoma Smilacis Glabrae) 10g to tonify the kidney, replenish essence, clear heat, and disinhibit dampness.

➤ With blood in the semen due to effulgent fire scorching the vessels with yin deficiency, apply *Zhī Bǎi Dì Huáng Wán* (知柏地黃丸), *bái máo gēn* (Rhizoma Imperatae) 10g, and *dì yú tàn* (Radix Sanguisorbae) 10g to nourish yin, purge fire, cool blood, and stanch bleeding.

(2) Kidney Yang Insufficiency

【Syndrome Characteristics】

Cold clear semen, low sperm count with poor motility, weak ejaculation, declined sexual desire, premature ejaculation, and impotence. Other manifestations include cold pain of the lumbus and knees, lassitude, fatigue, bright white facial complexion, shortness of breath after movement, cold limbs, cold and damp sensations of the genital region, long voidings of urine, and profuse nighttime urination. The tongue appears pale and swollen with a thin white and moist coating. Pulses are deep thready and weak, especially at the *chi* position.

【Treatment Principle】

Tonify kidney, warm yang, and nourish essence.

【Commonly Used Medicinals】

Select *ròu cōng róng* (Herba Cistanches), *xiān máo* (Rhizoma Curculiginis), *yín yáng huò* (Herba Epimedii), *bā jǐ tiān* (Radix Morindae Officinalis), *fù pén zǐ* (Fructus Rubi), *tù sī zǐ* (Semen Cuscutae), *shú fù zǐ* (Radix Aconiti Lateralis Praeparata), *ròu guì* (Cortex Cinnamomi), and *lù fēng fáng* (Nidus Vespae).

【Representative Formula】

Jīn Guì Shèn Qì Wán (金匮肾气丸) modified with *Wǔ Zǐ Yǎn Zōng Wán* (五子衍宗丸).

【Ingredients】

肉苁蓉	*ròu cōng róng*	10g	Herba Cistanches
仙茅	*xiān máo*	10g	Rhizoma Curculiginis
淫羊藿	*yín yáng huò*	10g	Herba Epimedii
熟附子	*shú fù zǐ*	10g	Radix Aconiti Lateralis Praeparata
肉桂	*ròu guì*	10g	Cortex Cinnamomi
山茱萸	*shān zhū yú*	10g	Fructus Corni
山药	*shān yào*	10g	Rhizoma Dioscoreae
五味子	*wǔ wèi zǐ*	10g	Fructus Schisandrae Chinensis
覆盆子	*fù pén zǐ*	10g	Fructus Rubi
熟地黄	*shú dì huáng*	15g	Radix Rehmanniae Praeparata
菟丝子	*tù sī zǐ*	15g	Semen Cuscutae
枸杞子	*gǒu qǐ zǐ*	15g	Fructus Lycii

Decoct in 500 ml water until 100 ml remains. Take 50 ml warm, twice daily.

【Formula Analysis】

Ròu cōng róng (Herba Cistanches), *xiān máo* (Rhizoma Curculiginis), *xiān líng pí* (Herba Epimedii), *fù zǐ* (Radix Aconiti Lateralis Praeparata) and *ròu guì* (Cortex Cinnamomi) act to warm the kidney and invigorate yang. *Shú dì* (Radix Rehmanniae Glutinosae Conquitae), *tù sī zǐ* (Semen Cuscutae), *gǒu qǐ zǐ* (Fructus Lycii) and *shān zhū yú* (Fructus Corni) nourish yin, tonify the kidney, and replenish essence and marrow.

Shān yào (Rhizoma Dioscoreae) tonifies the spleen and secures essence, promotes the engendering and transformation of essence, and so assists the root of later heaven. *Wǔ wèi zǐ* (Fructus Schisandrae Chinensis) and *fù pén zǐ* (Fructus Rubi) tonify the kidney, secure essence, and astringe essential qi. This formula acts to tonify yang within yin. As Zhang Jing-yue pointed out: "Those who excel at tonifying yang always seek yang within yin. When yang is assisted by yin, its generation and transformation become endless."

【Modifications】

➢ With impotence, declined sexual desire, or thin semen, add *yáng qǐ shí* (Actinolitum) 15g and *jiǔ cài zǐ* (Semen Allii Tuberosi) 10g to tonify the kidney and invigorate yang.

➢ With low sperm survival rates (below 50%), add *Chén Shì Wēn Shèn Huó Jīng Tāng* (陈氏温肾活精汤) to tonify the kidney and engender essence. The formula contains the following medicinals.

鹿鞭	*lù biān*	10g	Cervi Testis et Penis
枸杞子	*gǒu qǐ zǐ*	15g	Fructus Lycii
淫羊藿	*yín yáng huò*	10g	Herba Epimedii
巴戟天	*bā jǐ tiān*	10g	Radix Morindae Officinalis
熟附子	*shú fù zǐ*	10g	Radix Aconiti Lateralis Praeparata
肉桂	*ròu guì*	3g	Cortex Cinnamomi

➢ With non-liquefaction of semen, add *gān jiāng* (Rhizoma Zingiberis) 5g and *ròu guì* (Cortex Cinnamomi) 3g to warm the kidney and promote qi transformation.

➢ With white blood cells in the seminal fluid, add *chūn gēn pí* (Cortex Ailanthi) 10g and *Bì Yù Sǎn* (碧玉散) to clear heat.

Bì Yù Sǎn (碧玉散) contains the following medicinals.

石膏	*shí gāo*	20g	Gypsum Fibrosum
甘草	*gān cǎo*	5g	Radix et Rhizoma Glycyrrhizae
青黛	*qīng dài*	10g	Indigo Naturalis

➢ With seminal emission and premature ejaculation, add *lián xū* (Stamen Nelumbinis) 10g, *lóng gǔ* (Os Draconis) 15g, and *qiàn shí* (Semen Euryales) 10g to secure the storage of essence.

➢ With ejaculation failure, add *zǐ shí yīng* (Fluoritum) 10g and *wáng bù liú xíng* (Semen Vaccariae) 10g to invigorate blood and downbear counterflow.

➢ With cold lumbar pain, add *bǔ gǔ zhī* (Fructus Psoraleae) 10g and *xù duàn* (Radix Dipsaci) 10g to tonify the liver and kidney and strengthen sinews and bones.

➢ With fifth-watch diarrhea, add *ròu dòu kòu* (Semen Myristicae) 10g, *bǔ gǔ zhī* (Fructus Psoraleae) 15g, and *wú zhū yú* (Fructus Evodiae) 15g to tonify the kidney and check diarrhea.

Modern pharmacological research has revealed that medicinals that tonify the kidney and invigorate yang possess functions similar to male hormones. These include *shé chuáng zǐ* (Fructus Cnidii), *yín yáng huò* (Herba Epimedii), *xiān máo* (Rhizoma Curculiginis), *bǔ gǔ zhī* (Fructus Psoraleae), *gǒu qǐ zǐ* (Fructus Lycii), *shān yào* (Rhizoma Dioscoreae), *bā jǐ tiān* (Radix Morindae Officinalis), and *lù fēng fáng* (Nidus Vespae). These medicinals act to support the function of the sexual organs and also promote the engendering of sperm.

(3) Qi and Blood Dual Deficiency

【Syndrome Characteristics】

Thin semen, low sperm count, declined sexual desire, impotence or premature ejaculation, lusterless complexion, weak constitution, lassitude of the spirit, fatigue, palpitations, poor sleep, profuse dreaming, forgetfulness, dizziness, blurred vision, poor appetite, torpid intake, shortness of breath with no desire to speak, and pale nails. The tongue appears pale with little coating. Pulses are deep and thready.

【Treatment Principle】

Tonify qi, fortify the spleen, nourish blood, and engender sperm.

【Commonly Used Medicinals】

To tonify qi and fortify the spleen, select *rén shēn* (Radix et Rhizoma Ginseng), *dǎng shēn* (Radix Codonopsis), *bái zhú* (Rhizoma Atractylodis Macrocephalae), *fú líng* (Poria), and *huáng qí* (Radix Astragali).

To tonify blood, select *shú dì huáng* (Radix Rehmanniae Praeparata), *dāng guī* (Radix Angelicae Sinensis), *bái sháo* (Radix Paeoniae Alba), and *ē jiāo* (Colla Corii Asini).

【Representative Formula】

Modified *Bā Zhēn Shēng Jīng Tāng* (八珍生精汤).

【Ingredients】

党参	*dǎng shēn*	10g	Radix Codonopsis
白术	*bái zhú*	10g	Rhizoma Atractylodis Macrocephalae
茯苓	*fú líng*	10g	Poria
白芍	*bái sháo*	10g	Radix Paeoniae Alba
当归	*dāng guī*	10g	Radix Angelicae Sinensis
阿胶	*ē jiāo*	10g	Colla Corii Asini
黄芪	*huáng qí*	15g	Radix Astragali
熟地黄	*shú dì huáng*	15g	Radix Rehmanniae Praeparata
菟丝子	*tù sī zǐ*	15g	Semen Cuscutae
枸杞子	*gǒu qǐ zǐ*	15g	Fructus Lycii
黄精	*huáng jīng*	15g	Rhizoma Polygonati
紫河车	*zǐ hé chē*	15g	Placenta Hominis
甘草	*gān cǎo*	3g	Radix et Rhizoma Glycyrrhizae

Decoct in 500 ml water until 100 ml remains. Take 50 ml warm, twice daily.

【Formula Analysis】

Dǎng shēn (Radix Codonopsis), *bái zhú* (Rhizoma Atractylodis Macrocephalae), *fú líng* (Poria), *gān cǎo* (Radix et Rhizoma Glycyrrhizae), and *huáng qí* (Radix Astragali) act to tonify qi and fortify the spleen. *Shú dì* (Radix Remanniae Glutinosiae), *bái sháo* (Radix Paeoniae Alba), *dāng guī* (Radix Angelicae Sinensis), and *ē jiāo* (Colla Corii Asini) nourish blood and calm the heart. *Tù sī zǐ* (Semen Cuscutae), *gǒu qǐ zǐ* (Fructus Lycii), *huáng jīng* (Rhizoma Polygonati), and *zǐ hé chē* (Placenta Hominis) tonify the kidney and promote the engendering of sperm.

【Modifications】

➢ With low sperm motility, add *yín yáng huò* (Herba Epimedii) 10g and *bā jǐ tiān* (Radix Morindae Officinalis) 10g to tonify kidney yang.

➢ With thin semen, add *huáng qí* (Radix Astragali) 15g, *bái zhú* (Rhizoma Atractylodis Macrocephalae) 10g, and *hóng shēn* (Radix et Rhizoma Ginseng Rubra) 5g to tonify qi and promote the engendering of sperm.

➢ With scant semen and low sperm count, add *shān yào* (Rhizoma Dioscoreae) 15g, *hé shǒu wū* (Radix Polygoni Multiflori) 10g, and *nǚ zhēn zǐ* (Fructus Ligustri Lucidi) 10g to tonify the kidney and promote the engendering of sperm.

➢ With ejaculation failure, add *shí chāng pú* (Rhizoma Acori Tatarinowii) 15g, *yuǎn zhì* (Radix Polygalae) 10g, *fú shén* (Poria cum Pini Radice) 10g, and *wú gōng* (Scolopendra) 10g to free the passage of semen and open the lower orifices.

➢ With loss of blood, add *hàn lián cǎo* (Herba Ecliptae) 10g and *nǚ zhēn zǐ* (Fructus Ligustri Lucidi) 10g to nourish yin and stanch bleeding.

➢ With non-liquefaction of semen, add *wū méi* (Fructus Mume) 10g, *hē zǐ* (Fructus Chebulae) 10g, and *gān cǎo* (Radix et Rhizoma Glycyrrhizae) 5g to transform yin with sour and sweet.

➢ With insomnia and profuse dreaming, add *zǎo rén* (Semen Ziziphi Spinosae) 10g, *yuǎn zhì* (Radix Polygalae) 10g, and *hé huān pí* (Cortex Albiziae) 10g to calm the spirit.

➢ With palpitations, add *bǎi zǐ rén* (Semen Platycladi) 10g, *dān shēn* (Radix et Rhizoma Salviae Miltiorrhizae Miltiorrhizae) 10g, and *fú líng*

(Poria) 15g to nourish the heart and calm the spirit.

(4) Spleen and Kidney Dual Deficiency

【Syndrome Characteristics】

Thin and clear semen, low sperm count, declined sexual desire, and impotence or premature ejaculation. Other symptoms and signs include weak legs with lumbar pain, aversion to cold, bright white complexion, fatigue, abdominal distention, loose stool, and poor appetite. The tongue appears pale with a thin white coating. Pulses are deep and thready.

【Treatment Principle】

Warm and tonify the spleen and kidney, tonify qi and engender sperm.

【Commonly Used Medicinals】

To tonify and regulate qi, fortify the spleen, and transform phlegm, select *fú líng* (Poria), *bái zhú* (Rhizoma Atractylodis Macrocephalae), *dǎng shēn* (Radix Codonopsis), *chén pí* (Pericarpium Citri Reticulatae), *gān cǎo* (Radix et Rhizoma Glycyrrhizae) and *fǎ bàn xià* (Rhizoma Pinelliae Praeparatum).

To tonify the kidney and engender sperm, select *tù sī zǐ* (Semen Cuscutae), *sāng shèn zǐ* (Fructus Mori), *gǒu qǐ zǐ* (Fructus Lycii), and *nǚ zhēn zǐ* (Fructus Ligustri Lucidi).

To warm the kidney and invigorate yang, select *bǔ gǔ zhī* (Fructus Psoraleae) and *shé chuáng zǐ* (Fructus Cnidii).

To tonify the kidney and secure essence, select *fù pén zǐ* (Fructus Rubi), *jīn yīng zǐ* (Fructus Rosae Laevigatae), and *wǔ wèi zǐ* (Fructus Schisandrae Chinensis).

Chē qián zǐ (Semen Plantaginis) may be selected to disinhibit dampness and free the passage of semen.

【Representative Formula】

Shǐ Zǐ Tāng (十子汤) modified with *Liù Jūn Zǐ Tāng* (六君子汤)

【Ingredients】

菟丝子	tù sī zǐ	15g	Semen Cuscutae
桑椹子	sāng shèn zǐ	15g	Fructus Mori
枸杞子	gǒu qǐ zǐ	15g	Fructus Lycii
女贞子	nǚ zhēn zǐ	15g	Fructus Ligustri Lucidi
补骨脂	bǔ gǔ zhī	15g	Fructus Psoraleae
蛇床子	shé chuáng zǐ	15g	Fructus Cnidii
覆盆子	fù pén zǐ	10g	Fructus Rubi
金樱子	jīn yīng zǐ	10g	Fructus Rosae Laevigatae
五味子	wǔ wèi zǐ	10g	Fructus Schisandrae Chinensis
茯苓	fú líng	10g	Poria
白术	bái zhú	10g	Rhizoma Atractylodis Macrocephalae
党参	dǎng shēn	10g	Radix Codonopsis
陈皮	chén pí	10g	Pericarpium Citri Reticulatae
法半夏	fǎ bàn xià	10g	Rhizoma Pinelliae Praeparatum
车前子	chē qián zǐ	20g	Semen Plantaginis
甘草	gān cǎo	3g	Radix et Rhizoma Glycyrrhizae

Decoct in 500 ml water until 100 ml remains. Take 50 ml warm, twice daily.

【Formula Analysis】

Tù sī zǐ (Semen Cuscutae), *sāng shèn zǐ* (Fructus Mori), *gǒu qǐ zǐ* (Fructus Lycii) and *nǚ zhēn zǐ* (Fructus Ligustri Lucidi) tonify the kidney and engender essence. *Bǔ gǔ zhī* (Fructus Psoraleae) and *shé chuáng zǐ* (Fructus Cnidii) warm the kidney and tonify yang. *Fù pén zǐ* (Fructus Rubi), *jīn yīng zǐ* (Fructus Rosae Laevigatae), and *wǔ wèi zǐ* (Fructus Schisandrae Chinensis) tonify the kidney and secure essence. *Fú líng* (Poria), *bái zhú* (Rhizoma Atractylodis Macrocephalae), *dǎng shēn* (Radix Codonopsis), *chén pí* (Pericarpium Citri Reticulatae), *gān cǎo* (Radix et Rhizoma Glycyrrhizae), and *fǎ bàn xià* (Rhizoma Pinelliae Praeparatum) act to tonify qi, fortify the spleen, regulate qi, and transform phlegm. *Chē qián zǐ* (Semen Plantaginis) disinhibits dampness to free the passage of semen.

Shǐ Zǐ Tāng (十子汤) is a modification of *Wǔ Zǐ Yǎn Zōng Wán* (五子衍宗丸). It can tonify both yin and yang, and is both moistening and drying. This formula is based on a principle from the *Yellow Emperor's Inner Classic* (黄帝内经 , *Huáng Dì Nèi Jīng*) which states, "Physical insufficiency should be warmed with qi" and, "Essence insufficiency should be tonified with flavors". When combined with *Liù Jūn Zǐ Tāng* (六君子汤), this formula acts to fortify the spleen, tonify the kidney, tonify qi, nourish blood, and replenish kidney essence.

【Modifications】

➢ With low sperm motility, add *shú fù zǐ* (Radix Aconiti Lateralis Praeparata) 10g and *ròu guì* (Cortex Cinnamomi) 3g to invigorate original yang and tonify life gate fire.

➢ With low sperm count, add *lù jiǎo jiāo* (Colla Cornus Cervi) 5g and *huáng jīng* (Rhizoma Polygonati) 15g to tonify the kidney and engender essence.

➢ With seminal emission, add *lián xū* (Stamen Nelumbinis) 10g and *qiàn shí* (Semen Euryales) 10g to astringe the essential qi.

➢ With lumbar pain, add *chuān duàn* (Radix Dipsaci) 15g and *sāng jì shēng* (Herba Taxilli) 15g to strengthen sinews and bones.

➢ With spleen and kidney yang deficiency, select *Wú Bǐ Shān Yào Wán* (无比山药丸).

The formula contains the following medicinals.

山药	*shān yào*	15g	Rhizoma Dioscoreae
熟地黄	*shú dì huáng*	15g	Radix Rehmanniae Praeparata
杜仲	*dù zhòng*	10g	Cortex Eucommiae
肉苁蓉	*ròu cōng róng*	10g	Herba Cistanches
茯苓	*fú líng*	15g	Poria
菟丝子	*tù sī zǐ*	15g	Semen Cuscutae
巴戟天	*bā jǐ tiān*	10g	Radix Morindae Officinalis
泽泻	*zé xiè*	10g	Rhizoma Alismatis

牛膝	*niú xī*	15g	Radix Achyranthis Bidentatae
五味子	*wǔ wèi zǐ*	10g	Fructus Schisandrae Chinensis
赤石脂	*chì shí zhī*	10g	Halloysitum Rubrum

(5) Damp-heat Pouring Downward

【Syndrome Characteristics】

Semen containing white blood cells and pus, low sperm count, low sperm survival rates, failure of semen liquefaction, and erection without ejaculation. Distention and discomfort of the testicles and pubic area appear following sexual intercourse. Others signs and symptoms include short voidings of reddish urine, burning and painful urination, genital itching and swelling, white turbid urine, thirst with desire for cold drinks, irritability, restlessness, and bound stool. Soreness and heaviness of the lumbus, legs, or head may also appear. The tongue appears red with yellow slimy coating. Pulses are wiry, slippery and rapid.

【Treatment Principle】

Clear and disinhibit damp-heat, disperse swelling, and relieve toxicity.

【Commonly Used Medicinals】

To clear damp-heat, select *lóng dǎn cǎo* (Gentianae Radix), *bì xiè* (Rhizoma Dioscoreae Hypoglaucae), *huáng bǎi* (Cortex Phellodendri Chinensis), *chē qián zǐ* (Semen Plantaginis), *huá shí* (Talcum), and *tōng cǎo* (Medulla Tetrapanacis).

To fortify the spleen and disinhibit dampness, select *yì yǐ rén* (Semen Coicis), *zé xiè* (Rhizoma Alismatis), and *fú líng* (Poria).

【Representative Formula】

Lóng Dǎn Xiè Gān Tāng (龙胆泻肝汤) modified with *Bì Xiè Shèn Shī Tāng* (萆薢渗湿汤).

【Ingredients】

| 龙胆草 | *lóng dǎn cǎo* | 10g | Gentianae Radix |
| 黄柏 | *huáng bǎi* | 10g | Cortex Phellodendri Chinensis |

通草	tōng cǎo	10g	Medulla Tetrapanacis
黄芩	huáng qín	10g	Radix Scutellariae
栀子	zhī zǐ	10g	Fructus Gardeniae
牡丹皮	mǔ dān pí	10g	Cortex Moutan
泽泻	zé xiè	10g	Rhizoma Alismatis
茯苓	fú líng	10g	Poria
当归	dāng guī	10g	Radix Angelicae Sinensis
萆薢	bì xiè	20g	Rhizoma Dioscoreae Hypoglaucae
车前子	chē qián zǐ	20g	Semen Plantaginis
薏苡仁	yì yǐ rén	20g	Semen Coicis
生地黄	shēng dì huáng	20g	Radix Rehmanniae Recens

Decoct in 500 ml water until 100 ml remains. Take 50 ml warm, twice daily.

【Formula Analysis】

Lóng dǎn cǎo (Gentianae Radix), *bì xiè* (Rhizoma Dioscoreae Hypoglaucae), *huáng bǎi* (Cortex Phellodendri Chinensis), *chē qián zǐ* (Semen Plantaginis), *huá shí* (Talcum), and *tōng cǎo* (Medulla Tetrapanacis) clear and disinhibit damp-heat. *Huáng qín* (Radix Scutellariae), *zhī zǐ* (Fructus Gardeniae) and *mǔ dān pí* (Cortex Moutan) discharge the liver and gallbladder, and clear heat in the blood aspect. *Yì yǐ rén* (Semen Coicis), *zé xiè* (Rhizoma Alismatis), and *fú líng* (Poria) fortify the spleen and disinhibit dampness. Exuberant fire easily injures yin-blood; therefore *shēng dì huáng* (Radix Rehmanniae Recens) and *dāng guī* (Radix Angelicae Sinensis) are included.

【Modifications】

➢ With pus in the semen, add *tǔ fú líng* (Rhizoma Smilacis Glabrae) 15g, *pú gōng yīng* (Herba Taraxaci) 15g, and *jīn yín huā* (Flos Lonicerae Japonicae) 10g to clear heat and relieve inflammation.

➢ With low sperm survival and motility rates, add *shān zhā* (Fructus Crataegi) 15g, *dān shēn* (Radix et Rhizoma Salviae Miltiorrhizae Miltiorrhizae) 10g, and *cāng zhú* (Rhizoma Atractylodis) 10g to disinhibit dampness and transform turbidity.

➢ With reduced lecithin levels, add *hé shǒu wū* (Radix Polygoni Multiflori) 10g and *gǒu qǐ zǐ* (Fructus Lycii) 10g to tonify the kidney and engender essence and marrow.

➢ With bloody semen, add *dà jì* (Herba Cirsii Japonici) 10g, *xiǎo jì* (Herba Cirsii) 10g, *hàn lián cǎo* (Herba Ecliptae) 10g, and *bái máo gēn* (Rhizoma Imperatae) 10g to clear heat, cool blood, and stanch bleeding.

➢ With kidney qi deficiency, add *tù sī zǐ* (Semen Cuscutae) 15g and *fù pén zǐ* (Fructus Rubi) 10g to tonify the kidney and secure essence.

➢ With bound stool, add *zhǐ qiào* (Fructus Aurantii) 10g and *dà huáng* (Radix et Rhizoma Rhei) 10g.

(6) Stagnation of Phlegm Turbidity

【Syndrome Characteristics】

Scant semen, low or absent sperm count, and ejaculation failure. Other symptoms and signs include swelling and pain of testicles, dizziness, blurred vision, chest oppression, nausea, palpitations, and obesity. The tongue appears fat with white slimy coating. Pulses are deep and slippery.

【Treatment Principle】

Transform phlegm, regulate qi, dissipate binding, and free the vessels.

【Commonly Used Medicinals】

To dry dampness, transform phlegm, regulate qi and regulate the middle, select *cāng zhú* (Rhizoma Atractylodis), *fú líng* (Poria), *bái zhú* (Rhizoma Atractylodis Macrocephalae), *chén pí* (Pericarpium Citri Reticulatae), *fǎ bàn xià* (Rhizoma Pinelliae Praeparatum), *dǎn nán xīng* (Arisaema cum Bile), *zhǐ shí* (Fructus Aurantii Immaturus), and *xiāng fù* (Rhizoma Cyperi).

To free the vessels, dissipate binding, and transform phlegm, select *lù lù tōng* (Fructus Liquidambaris) and *chuān shān jiǎ* (Squama Manis).

【Representative Formula】

Modified *Cāng Fù Dǎo Tán Tāng* (苍附导痰汤).

【Ingredients】

苍术	*cāng zhú*	10g	Rhizoma Atractylodis
陈皮	*chén pí*	10g	Pericarpium Citri Reticulatae
法半夏	*fǎ bàn xià*	10g	Rhizoma Pinelliae Praeparatum
胆南星	*dǎn nán xīng*	10g	Arisaema cum Bile
枳实	*zhǐ shí*	10g	Fructus Aurantii Immaturus
香附	*xiāng fù*	10g	Rhizoma Cyperi
茯苓	*fú líng*	10g	Poria
白术	*bái zhú*	10g	Rhizoma Atractylodis Macrocephalae
泽泻	*zé xiè*	10g	Rhizoma Alismatis
车前子	*chē qián zǐ*	15g	Semen Plantaginis
路路通	*lù lù tōng*	15g	Fructus Liquidambaris
穿山甲	*chuān shān jiǎ*	15g	Squama Manis

Decoct in 500 ml water until 100 ml remains. Take 50 ml warm, twice daily.

【Formula Analysis】

Cāng zhú (Rhizoma Atractylodis), *chén pí* (Pericarpium Citri Reticulatae), *fǎ bàn xià* (Rhizoma Pinelliae Praeparatum), *dǎn nán xīng* (Arisaema cum Bile), *zhǐ shí* (Fructus Aurantii Immaturus) and *xiāng fù* (Rhizoma Cyperi) dry dampness, transform phlegm, regulate qi, and harmonize the middle. *Fú líng* (Poria) and *bái zhú* (Rhizoma Atractylodis Macrocephalae) fortify the spleen and disinhibit dampness. *Zé xiè* (Rhizoma Alismatis) and *chē qián zǐ* (Semen Plantaginis) disinhibit dampness with bland percolation. *Lù lù tōng* (Fructus Liquidambaris) and *chuān shān jiǎ* (Squama Manis) transform phlegm, free the collaterals, and dissipate binding.

【Modifications】

➢ With non-liquefaction of semen, add *Chén Shì Huà Tán Shēng Yè*

Tāng (陈氏化痰生液汤) to eliminate phlegm turbidity and engender essential qi.

The formula contains the following medicinals.

浙贝母	*zhè bèi mǔ*	10g	Bulbus Fritillariae Thunbergii
玄参	*xuán shēn*	10g	Radix Scrophulariae
生牡砺	*shēng mǔ lì*	15g	Concha Ostreae Cruda
杏仁	*xìng rén*	10g	Semen Armeniacae Amarum
茯苓	*fú líng*	15g	Poria
路路通	*lù lù tōng*	15g	Fructus Liquidambaris

➤ With abnormal sperm, add *gǒu qǐ zǐ* (Fructus Lycii) 15g and *tù sī zǐ* (Semen Cuscutae) 15g to tonify the kidney and essence.

➤ With weak sperm activity, add *yì yǐ rén* (Semen Coicis) 15g and *shān zhā* (Fructus Crataegi) 15g to transform turbidity and open the orifices.

➤ With retrograde ejaculation, add *niú xī* (Radix Achyranthis Bidentatae) 15g and *wáng bù liú xíng* (Semen Vaccariae) 15g to disinhibit the lower orifice and direct downward movement.

➤ With obvious qi deficiency, add *huáng qí* (Radix Astragali) 15g and *dǎng shēn* (Radix Codonopsis) 15g to tonify qi.

➤ With bloody semen, add *hàn lián cǎo* (Herba Ecliptae) 10g and *ǒu jié* (Nodus Nelumbinis Rhizomatis) 10g to nourish yin and stanch bleeding.

➤ With constrained liver qi, add *yù jīn* (Radix Curcumae) 10g to regulate qi.

➤ With white turbidity, add *bì xiè* (Rhizoma Dioscoreae Hypoglaucae) 10g to separate clear from turbid.

➤ With lumbar pain, add *dù zhòng* (Cortex Eucommiae) 15g and *niú xī* (Radix Achyranthis Bidentatae) 15g to strengthen bones and sinews and relieve pain.

➤ With cold and dampness of the scrotum or spasmodic pain of the lower abdomen, add *wū yào* (Radix Linderae) 10g, *lì zhī hé* (Semen Litchi) 10g, and *yán hú suǒ* (Rhizoma Corydalis) 10g to warm the lower, invigorate qi, and relieve pain.

(7) Blood Stasis Obstruction

【Syndrome Characteristics】

Varicocele, stabbing pain with ejaculation, low sperm count or absent sperm, poor sperm motility, and red blood cells in the seminal fluid. Other symptoms and signs include dragging pain of the testes or fixed pain of the lower abdomen that becomes aggravated at night. The lips and tongue appear dark or purplish, with possible stasis spots.

Pulses are deep and rough, or thready and rough.

【Treatment Principle】

Invigorate blood, transform stasis, and free the seminal passage.

【Commonly Used Medicinals】

To invigorate blood and transform stasis, select *dān shēn* (Radix et Rhizoma Salviae Miltiorrhizae), *táo rén* (Semen Persicae), *hóng huā* (Flos Carthami), *chì sháo* (Radix Paeoniae Rubra), and *dāng guī* (Radix Angelicae Sinensis).

To transform stasis and free the seminal passage, select *wáng bù liú xíng* (Semen Vaccariae) and *lù lù tōng* (Fructus Liquidambaris).

【Representative Formula】

Modified *Xuè Fǔ Zhú Yū Tāng* (血府逐瘀汤).

【Ingredients】

柴胡	*chái hú*	10g	Radix Bupleuri
枳壳	*zhǐ qiào*	10g	Fructus Aurantii
牛膝	*niú xī*	10g	Radix Achyranthis Bidentatae
桃仁	*táo rén*	10g	Semen Persicae
红花	*hóng huā*	10g	Flos Carthami
赤芍	*chì sháo*	10g	Radix Paeoniae Rubra
当归	*dāng guī*	10g	Radix Angelicae Sinensis

穿山甲	*chuān shān jiǎ*	15g	Squama Manis
路路通	*lù lù tōng*	15g	Fructus Liquidambaris
丹参	*dān shēn*	20g	Radix et Rhizoma Salviae Miltiorrhizae
王不留行	*wáng bù liú xíng*	20g	Semen Vaccariae

Decoct in 500 ml water until 100 ml remains. Take 50 ml warm, twice daily.

【Formula Analysis】

In this formula, *dān shēn* (Radix et Rhizoma Salviae Miltiorrhizae Miltiorrhizae), *táo rén* (Semen Persicae), *hóng huā* (Flos Carthami), *chì sháo* (Radix Paeoniae Rubra), and *dāng guī* (Radix Angelicae Sinensis) act to invigorate blood and transform stasis. *Chuān shān jiǎ* (Squama Manis), *wáng bù liú xíng* (Semen Vaccariae) and *lù lù tōng* (Fructus Liquidambaris) transform stasis and free the seminal passage. *Chái hú* (Radix Bupleuri) and *zhǐ qiào* (Fructus Aurantii) regulate the qi dynamic. *Niú xī* (Radix Achyranthis Bidentatae) tonifies the kidney and invigorates blood, and also promotes the downward movement of medicinals.

To achieve best results, stasis-transforming medicinals should be combined with those that clear, warm, tonify, or break blood, depending on the presenting pattern and individual constitution.

【Modifications】

➢ With binding of phlegm and stasis, add *chén pí* (Pericarpium Citri Reticulatae) 10g, *fǎ bàn xià* (Rhizoma Pinelliae Praeparatum) 10g, *guā lóu* (Fructus Trichosanthis) 10g, and *yì yǐ rén* (Semen Coicis) 15g to eliminate phlegm and resolve stasis.

➢ With qi stagnation and blood stasis, add *qīng pí* (Pericarpium Citri Reticulatae Viride) 10g and *xiāng fù* (Rhizoma Cyperi) 10g to invigorate qi and blood.

➢ With blood stasis due to cold congealing, add *chuān liàn zǐ* (Fructus Toosendan) 3g, *wū yào* (Radix Linderae) 10g, and *xiǎo huí xiāng* (Fructus

Foeniculi) 10g to dissipate cold and invigorate blood.

➢ With heat brewing phlegm and blood, add *zhī zǐ* (Fructus Gardeniae) 10g, and *mǔ dān pí* (Cortex Moutan) 10g to clear heat and resolve stasis.

➢ With seminal stasis and low sperm count, add *huáng jīng* (Rhizoma Polygonati) 15g, *guī jiǎ* (Carapax et Plastrum Testudinis) 15g, and *wáng bù liú xíng* (Semen Vaccariae) 10g to resolve stasis and engender sperm.

➢ With kidney yang deficiency and blood stasis, add *bā jǐ tiān* (Radix Morindae Officinalis) 10g, and *shé chuáng zǐ* (Fructus Cnidi) 10g to warm the kidney and resolve stasis.

➢ With bloody semen, add powdered *sān qī* (Radix et Rhizoma Notoginseng) 3g, *hàn lián cǎo* (Herba Ecliptae) 10g, and *nǚ zhēn zǐ* (Fructus Ligustri Lucidi) 10g to nourish yin, clear heat, invigorate blood, and resolve stasis.

➢ With ejaculation failure, add *wú gōng* (Scolopendra) 10g and *fēng fáng* (Nidus Vespae) 10g to free the collaterals and open the orifices.

➢ With scant semen due to blood stasis and obstruction, apply *Chén Shì Huó Xuè Shēng Jīng Wán* (陈氏活血生精丸) to break blood and dispel stasis.

The formula contains the following medicinals.

三棱	*sān léng*	10g	Rhizoma Sparganii
莪术	*é zhú*	10g	Rhizoma Curcumae
红花	*hóng huā*	10g	Flos Carthami
当归尾	*dāng guī wěi*	10g	Radix Angelicae Sinensis
没药	*mò yào*	10g	Myrrha
丹参	*dān shēn*	10g	Radix et Rhizoma Salviae Miltiorrhizae

➢ With impotence, add *shé chuáng zǐ* (Fructus Cnidii) 10g, and *zǐ shí yīng* (Fluoritum) 10g to support yang.

➢ With stabbing pain of the seminal passage, add *hǔ pò* (Succinum) 10g, *pú huáng* (Pollen Typhae) 10g, and *xuán hú suǒ* (Rhizoma Corydalis)

10g to free the channels and relieve pain.

➤ With lower abdominal distention, add *wū yào* (Radix Linderae) 10g, and *xiǎo huí xiāng* (Fructus Foeniculi) 6g to invigorate qi, dissipate distention, and relieve pain.

➤ With welling-abscess caused by putrid blood stasis, add *Wǔ Wèi Xiāo Dú Yǐn* (五味消毒饮) to clear heat, relieve toxicity, invigorate blood, and resolve stasis.

The formula contains the following medicinals.

金银花	*jīn yín huā*	15g	Flos Lonicerae Japonicae
蒲公英	*pú gōng yīng*	15g	Herba Taraxaci
菊花	*jú huā*	10g	Flos Chrysanthemi
紫背天葵	*zǐ bèi tiān kuí*	10g	Semiaquilegia Adoxoides
紫花地丁	*zǐ huā dì dīng*	10g	Herba Violae

➤ With blood stasis and strangury with turbid urine, apply *Dāng Guī Tāng* (当归汤) to invigorate blood, resolve stasis, and separate clear from turbid.

The formula contains the following medicinals.

当归	*dāng guī*	10g	Radix Angelicae Sinensis
牛膝	*niú xī*	10g	Radix Achyranthis Bidentatae
滑石	*huá shí*	6g	Talcum
冬葵子	*dōng kuí zǐ*	10g	Fructus Malvae
瞿麦	*qú mài*	10g	Herba Dianthi

Additional Treatment Modalities

1. Chinese Patent Medicine

(1) *Liù Wèi Dì Huáng Wán* (六味地黄丸)

Take twice daily. Indicated for kidney yin insufficiency patterns.

(2) *Wǔ Zǐ Yǎn Zōng Wán* (五子衍宗丸)

Take twice daily. Indicated for kidney yin insufficiency patterns.

(3) *Jīn Guì Shèn Qì Wán* (金匮肾气丸)

Take twice daily. Indicated for kidney yang insufficiency patterns.

(4) *Guī Líng Jí* (龟龄集)

Take 1.5g, twice daily. Indicated for male infertility due to kidney yang deficiency and debilitation of life gate fire.

(5) *Rén Shēn Guī Pí Wán* (人参归脾丸)

Take twice daily. Indicated for qi and blood deficiency patterns.

(6) *Bǔ Shèn Yì Qì Wán* (补肾益气丸)

Take twice daily. Indicated for kidney qi deficiency patterns.

2. ACUPUNCTURE AND MOXIBUSTION

Current research indicates that treatment with acupuncture and moxibustion shows a definite therapeutic effect when applied in cases of male infertility. The following section includes the most effective and commonly applied clinical methods.

(1) Acupuncture for Male Immune Infertility

【Treatment Principle】

Tonify the liver and kidney, invigorate blood, and free the collaterals.

【Point Combination】

BL 18	*gān shù*	肝俞
BL 23	*shèn shù*	肾俞
LV 3	*tài chōng*	太冲
KI 3	*tài xī*	太溪

【Point Modification】

BL 15	*xīn shù*	心俞
BL 17	*gé shù*	膈俞
BL 22	*sān jiāo shù*	三焦俞
HT 7	*shén mén*	神门

| SJ 4 | *yáng chí* | 阳池 |
| SP 10 | *xuè hǎi* | 血海 |

Based on theories recorded in *Classic of Difficult Issues* (难 经 , *Nàn Jīng*), this point selection combines front-*mu* points with *yuan*-source points.

The pathomechanism here involves liver and kidney deficiency with blood stasis causing obstruction of the vessels. BL 18 (*gān shù*) combined with LV 3 (*tài chōng*), and BL 23 (*shèn shù*) combined with KI 3 (*tài xī*) act to tonify the liver and kidney, support the upright, and bank the origin. BL 15 (*xīn shù*) combined with HT 7 (*shén mén*) acts to tonify heart qi and invigorate qi and blood. BL 17 (*gé shù*) combined with SP 10 (*xuè hǎi*) invigorates blood and transforms stasis, and BL 22 (*sān jiāo shù*) combined with SJ 4 (*yáng chí*) acts to clear heat, relieve toxicity, eliminate pathogens, and clear and disinhibit the lower burner.

【Manipulation】

Treatment may be performed with the patient in a sitting position. Insert needles to a depth of 1.0-1.5 *cun*, and manipulate with rapid thrusting and rotation. Following the arrival of qi, apply flicking manipulations until the needling sensation begins to propogate. Follow with vigorous rotation for 2 minutes at 180-200 rotations per minute, according to the toleration of the patient. Repeat the manipulations after 10 minutes.

Next, puncture the secondary points and manipulate to obtain qi. Connect all points to a G6805 e-stim device set to dense-disperse wave at 14-26 pulses per second. Intensity may be adjusted to obtain a sensation of soreness, tingling, and distention, according to the toleration of the patient. Maintain stimulation for 30 minutes.

【Cautions】

Apply treatment once daily, with two months as one course. There is no need to restrain sexual life during treatment, but the use of condoms is strongly recommended.

(2) Acupuncture for Infertility due to Abnormal Semen

【Treatment Principle】

Tonify kidney and essence, regulate yin and yang.

【Point Combination】

RN 4	guān yuán	关元
KI 12	dà hè	大赫
SP 6	sān yīn jiāo	三阴交

RN 4 (*guān yuán*) is the intersection point of the conception vessel and the three yin channels of the foot. This point is known as the confluence of original yin and yang, also being the place where the original qi of the kidney is infused. Supplementation will invigorate the original qi of the kidney, strengthen the root of congenital constitution, and enrich reproductive essence.

SP 6 (*sān yīn jiāo*) is the intersection point of the three yin channels of the foot. It acts to fortify the spleen and enrich the source of engendering and transformation. It also tonifies kidney essence, regulates the qi of the three foot yin channels and also the penetrating and conception vessels. This point benefits the liver, spleen and kidney. SP 6 and RN 4 combined acts to regulate all of the yin channels, while also enhancing the functions of the conception vessel.

KI 12 (*dà hè*) is the intersection point of the kidney and the penetrating vessel. The penetrating vessel is known as the sea of blood because it stores the qi and blood of all twelve channels, five viscera, and six bowels. The penetrating vessel also serves as a root connection between the congenital and acquired constitutions. It meets the foot yang brightness channel at ST 30 (*qì chōng*), and then runs parallel with kidney channel.

This point combination acts to regulate yin and yang, tonify essence and kidney, promote the engendering of sperm, and increase seminal vitality. When the essence becomes effulgent, conception is possible.

Moxibustion using a medicinal cake is also quite effective as an adjunctive treatment. The main ingredients include *ròu guì* (Cortex Cinnamomi) and *fù zǐ* (Radix Aconiti Lateralis Praeparata). Both medicinals are acrid, sweet in flavor, and extremely hot. They enter the kidney channel to tonify both essence and kidney.

【Manipulation】

Treatment may be performed with the patient in a sitting position. Needle RN 4 and KI 12 bilaterally to a depth of 1.5-2 *cun*, according to the patient's physique. Following the arrival of qi, supplement with rotation until the needling sensation radiates to the glans penis and testes. Then needle SP 6 bilaterally, and supplement with rotation.

While retaining the needles, connect KI 12 bilaterally to an e-stim device set to dense-disperse wave at a frequency of 10Hz. Intensity may be adjusted according to the toleration of the patient.

Also apply a medicinal cake containing *ròu guì* (Cortex Cinnamomi) and *fù zǐ* (Radix Aconiti Lateralis Praeparata) to the triangular area formed by points RN 4 and KI 12. Place a 2g moxa cone on the cake and burn 3 cones, one after the other.

【Cautions】

Treatment may be applied once every other day, with three months as one course. There is no need to restrain sexual life during treatment, but the use of condoms is strongly recommended.

(3) Acupuncture for Infertility due to Low Sperm Count

【Treatment Principle】

Fortify the spleen, tonify the kidney, invigorate blood, and disinhibit dampness.

【Point Combination】

BL 23	shèn shù	肾俞
RN 4	guān yuán	关元
BL 20	pí shù	脾俞
ST 36	zú sān lǐ	足三里

【Point Modification】

➢ With kidney yang deficiency, add DU 4 to warm and tonify kidney yang.

➢ With kidney yin deficiency, add KI 3 to nourish kidney yin.

➢ With phlegm-damp brewing or damp-heat in the liver channel, add LV 3 and SP 9 to fortify the spleen, clear heat, and disinhibit dampness.

➢ With liver stagnation and blood stasis, add SP 10 and LV 14 to course the liver and invigorate blood.

【Manipulation】

Treatment may be performed with the patient in a sitting position. Needle the main points to a depth of 1.0-1.5 *cun*. Following the arrival of qi, manipulate with even supplementation and drainage for 2 minutes. Manipulate every 10 minutes, retaining the needles for 30 minutes.

【Cautions】

Treatment may be applied daily, with two months as one course. There is no need to restrain sexual life during treatment, but the use of condoms is strongly recommended.

(4) Pricking Therapy for Infertility due to Ejaculation Failure

【Point Combination】

The main stimulus points of the sacral plexus are located as follows.

➢ Point A is located at the midline of the body on the line between the highest points of the iliac crests. Point B is on the tip of the coccyx. The stimulus points are found 4 cm on either side of the midpoint of the line connecting point A and point B, at the outer edge of the sacroiliac joint.

➤ The other bilateral stimulus points are 1 to 2 cm below the posterior inferior iliac spine, between the extremities of the first and second lumbar vertebrae transverse processes.

Supplemental points include DU 20 (*bǎi huì*), and extra points *zhěn kǒng diǎn* (at the midpoint of a line connecting the midpoint of the posterior hairline and the occipital protruberance), *dà zhuī páng diǎn* (lateral to the spinous process of C-7), *dì shí xiōng zhuī páng diǎn*, (lateral to the spinous process of T-10) and *shēng zhí diǎn* (2 cm posterior to the temporal hairline on a line parallel to the frontal median line).

【Point Modification】

➤ With nervous exhaustion, add *zhěn kǒng diǎn*.

➤ With low sperm count, add *dì shí xiōng zhuī páng diǎn*.

➤ With reduced sexual function or impotence, add DU 20 (*bǎi huì*) or *shēng zhí diǎn*.

➤ With deficient constitution, add *dà zhuī páng diǎn*. Manipulate with mild intensity.

【Manipulation】

Apply local anesthesia and insert the pricking needle into the subcutaneous tissue and manipulate the needle with a drawing movement. The stimulation intensity will vary with each individual, according to their tolerance.

【Cautions】

Treatment may be applied once every 5-6 days, with two months as one course. There is no need to restrain sexual life during treatment, but the use of condoms is strongly recommended.

3. SIMPLE PRESCRIPTIONS AND EMPIRICAL FORMULAS

(1)

枸杞子	*gǒu qǐ zǐ*	15g	Fructus Lycii

To be consumed nightly for two months. Chew well before swallowing. Following routine semen testing, continue for another two months. Indicated for abnormal sperm due to kidney essence deficiency.

(2) *Nán Xìng Bú Yù Fāng* (男性不育方)

鱼鳔珠	yú biào zhū	10g	Piscis Vesica Aeris
紫河车	zǐ hé chē	10g	Placenta Hominis
炙狗肾	zhì gǒu shèn	15g	Testis et Penis Canis (fried with liquid)
何首乌	hé shǒu wū	10g	Radix Polygoni Multiflori
当归	dāng guī	10g	Radix Angelicae Sinensis
龟甲	guī jiǎ	15g	Carapax et Plastrum Testudinis
肉苁蓉	ròu cōng róng	15g	Herba Cistanches
杜仲	dù zhòng	10g	Cortex Eucommiae
菟丝子	tù sī zǐ	15g	Semen Cuscutae
沙苑子	shā yuàn zǐ	15g	Semen Astragali Complanati
淫羊藿	yín yáng huò	10g	Herba Epimedii
枸杞子	gǒu qǐ zǐ	10g	Fructus Lycii
茯苓	fú líng	15g	Poria
牛膝	niú xī	15g	Radix Achyranthis Bidentatae
补骨脂	bǔ gǔ zhī	10g	Fructus Psoraleae
熟附子	shú fù zǐ	10g	Radix Aconiti Lateralis Praeparata

Indicated for abnormal sperm due to kidney essence deficiency.

(3) *Jiā Wèi Jù Jīng Wán* (加味聚精丸)

丹参	dān shēn	10g	Radix et Rhizoma Salviae Miltiorrhizae
赤芍	chì sháo	10g	Radix Paeoniae Rubra
桂枝	guì zhī	5g	Ramulus Cinnamomi
桃仁	táo rén	5g	Semen Persicae
红花	hóng huā	5g	Flos Carthami
鹿角	lù jiǎo	10g	Cornu Cervi
橘核	jú hé	10g	Semen Citri Reticulatae
乌药	wū yào	10g	Radix Linderae
甘草	gān cǎo	5g	Radix et Rhizoma Glycyrrhizae

Indicated for abnormal semen due to kidney deficiency, or qi stagnation with blood stasis.

(4) *Yù Jīng Tāng* (育精汤)

何首乌	*hé shǒu wū*	10g	Radix Polygoni Multiflori
韭菜子	*jiǔ cài zǐ*	10g	Semen Allii Tuberosi
当归	*dāng guī*	5g	Radix Angelicae Sinensis
熟地黄	*shú dì huáng*	10g	Radix Rehmanniae Praeparata
覆盆子	*fù pén zǐ*	10g	Fructus Rubi
淫羊藿	*yín yáng huò*	10g	Herba Epimedii
牛膝	*niú xī*	15g	Radix Achyranthis Bidentatae
菟丝子	*tù sī zǐ*	15g	Semen Cuscutae

Indicated for abnormal sperm due to kidney essence deficiency.

(5) *Gōng Jī Zhí Jiǔ Hé Jì* (公鸡殖酒合剂)

鲜公鸡殖	*xiān gōng jī zhí*	10g	Fresh Cock Genitalia
淫羊藿	*yín yáng huò*	10g	Herba Epimedii
夜交藤	*yè jiāo tēng*	15g	Caulis Polygoni Multiflori
仙茅	*xiān máo*	15g	Rhizoma Curculiginis
路路通	*lù lù tōng*	10g	Fructus Liquidambaris
龙眼肉	*lóng yǎn ròu*	10g	Arillus Longan

Indicated for abnormal sperm due to kidney deficiency and blood stasis.

(6) *Shēng Jīng Tāng* (生精汤)

炒韭子	*chǎo jiǔ zǐ*	10g	Semen Allii Tuberosi (dry-fried)
菟丝子	*tù sī zǐ*	10g	Semen Cuscutae
补骨脂	*bǔ gǔ zhī*	10g	Fructus Psoraleae
肉苁蓉	*ròu cōng róng*	15g	Herba Cistanches
生地黄	*shēng dì huáng*	15g	Radix Rehmanniae Recens
熟地黄	*shú dì huáng*	15g	Radix Rehmanniae Praeparata
淫羊藿	*yín yáng huò*	10g	Herba Epimedii
枸杞子	*gǒu qǐ zǐ*	10g	Fructus Lycii

| 制首乌 | zhì shǒu wū | 10g | Radix Polygoni Multiflori Praeparata cum Succo Glycines Sotae |
| 紫河车 | zǐ hé chē | 10g | Placenta Hominis |

Indicated for abnormal sperm due to kidney essence deficiency.

(7) *Sì Yù Tāng* (嗣育汤)

党参	dǎng shēn	15g	Radix Codonopsis
白术	bái zhú	15g	Rhizoma Atractylodis Macrocephalae
茯苓	fú líng	10g	Poria
当归	dāng guī	10g	Radix Angelicae Sinensis
川芎	chuān sháo	10g	Radix Paeoniae Alba
白芍	bái sháo	10g	Radix Paeoniae Alba
生地黄	shēng dì huáng	10g	Radix Rehmanniae Recens
牡丹皮	mǔ dān pí	10g	Cortex Moutan
菟丝子	tù sī zǐ	10g	Semen Cuscutae
肉苁蓉	ròu cōng róng	10g	Herba Cistanches
淫羊藿	yín yáng huò	10g	Herba Epimedii
紫河车	zǐ hé chē	10g	Placenta Hominis
甘草	gān cǎo	6g	Radix et Rhizoma Glycyrrhizae

Indicated for low sperm survival rates due to spleen and kidney dual deficiency and blood stasis obstruction.

(8) *Yè Huà Xù Sì Tāng* (液化续嗣汤)

知母	zhī mǔ	15g	Rhizoma Anemarrhenae
黄柏	huáng bǎi	10g	Cortex Phellodendri Chinensis
生地黄	shēng dì huáng	15g	Radix Rehmanniae Recens
熟地黄	shú dì huáng	15g	Radix Rehmanniae Praeparata
仙茅	xiān máo	10g	Rhizoma Curculiginis
淫羊藿	yín yáng huò	10g	Herba Epimedii
牡丹皮	mǔ dān pí	10g	Cortex Moutan
丹参	dān shēn	15g	Radix et Rhizoma Salviae Miltiorrhizae
麦门冬	mài mén dōng	10g	Radix Ophiopogonis
天花粉	tiān huā fěn	10g	Radix Trichosanthis

玄参	*xuán shēn*	10g	Radix Scrophulariae
赤白芍	*chì bái sháo*	10g	Radix Paeoniae Alba
南瓜子	*nán guā zǐ*	10g	Semen Cucurbitae
枸杞子	*gǒu qǐ zǐ*	10g	Fructus Lycii
车前子	*chē qián zǐ*	10g	Semen Plantaginis

Indicated for non-liquefaction of semen due to kidney yin deficiency.

(9) Ingredients include one male frog, one bladder of a male pig, and 30 to 60g *gǒu qǐ zǐ* (Fructus Lycii). Place the frog and the *gǒu qǐ zǐ* (Fructus Lycii) into the bladder and tie off tightly. Place into an earthenware pot and add boiled water. Seal tightly and stew with low heat. After cooking, discard the dregs and internal organs. Consume the meat and broth in 2-3 portions. May be taken 2-3 times weekly for infertility due to abnormal sperm.

(10) Decoct *bā jǐ tiān* (Radix Morindae) 30g, *gǒu qǐ zǐ* (Fructus Lycii) 30g and *shú dì huáng* (Rehmanniae Radix Conquita) 30g until 250 ml remains. Decoct again and mix together to make 500 ml. Then add about 250g of fresh river eel to the decoction and cook for a while. Consume in 2 portions. Generally indicated for a variety of sexual disorders.

(11) *Shuǐ Zhì Yè Huà Tāng* (水蛭液化汤)

水蛭粉	*shuǐ zhì fěn*	2g	Hirudo
知母	*zhī mǔ*	30g	Rhizoma Anemarrhenae
黄柏	*huáng bǎi*	10g	Cortex Phellodendri Chinensis
天冬	*tiān dōng*	15g	Radix Asparagi
麦冬	*mài dōng*	15g	Radix Ophiopogonis
生地	*shēng dì*	30g	Radix Rehmanniae
玄参	*xuán shēn*	15g	Radix Scrophulariae
石斛	*shí hú*	5g	Caulis Dendrobii
木通	*mù tōng*	9g	Caulis Akebiae
甘草	*gān cǎo*	6g	Radix et Rhizoma Glycyrrhizae

Indicated for non-liquefaction of semen due to damp-heat pouring downward.

(12) *Yì Shèn Shū Gān Tāng* (益肾疏肝汤)

枸杞子	*gǒu qǐ zǐ*	20g	Fructus Lycii
菟丝子	*tù sī zǐ*	20g	Semen Cuscutae
桑椹子	*sāng shèn zǐ*	15g	Fructus Mori
山药	*shān yào*	15g	Rhizoma Dioscoreae
白芍	*bái sháo*	15g	Radix Paeoniae Alba
覆盆子	*fù pén zǐ*	15g	Fructus Rubi
仙灵脾	*xiān líng pí*	12g	Herba Epimedii
熟地	*shú dì*	12g	Radix Rehmanniae Praeparata
山茱萸	*shān zhū yú*	10g	Fructus Corni
紫河车粉（冲服）	*zǐ hé chē fěn*	15g	Placenta Hominis (infused)
全当归	*quán dāng guī*	9g	Radix Angelicae Sinensis
柴胡	*chái hú*	9g	Radix Bupleuri

Indicated for absent sperm due to kidney deficiency and liver constraint.

(13) *Bǔ Jīng Fāng* (补精方)

黄精	*huáng jīng*	20g	Rhizoma Polygonati
山药	*shān yào*	20g	Rhizoma Dioscoreae
党参	*dǎng shēn*	20g	Radix Codonopsis
炙黄芪	*zhì huáng qí*	20g	Radix Astragali
续断	*xù duàn*	20g	Radix Dipsaci
五味子	*wǔ wèi zǐ*	10g	Fructus Schisandrae Chinensis
覆盆子	*fù pén zǐ*	10g	Fructus Rubi
菟丝子	*tù sī zǐ*	10g	Semen Cuscutae
车前子（包）	*chē qián zǐ*	10g	Semen Plantaginis (wrapped)
当归	*dāng guī*	10g	Radix Angelicae Sinensis
茯苓	*fú líng*	10g	Poria

Indicated for low sperm count due to kidney essence deficiency with qi and blood dual deficiency.

(14) *Qiáng Jīng Jiān* (强精煎)

熟地黄	*shú dì huáng*	12g	Radix Rehmanniae Praeparata
淮山药	*shān yào*	12g	Rhizoma Dioscoreae
山萸肉	*shān zhū yú*	12g	Fructus Corni
全当归	*quán dāng guī*	12g	Radix Angelicae Sinensis
枸杞子	*gǒu qǐ zǐ*	12g	Fructus Lycii
紫河车	*zǐ hé chē*	15g	Placenta Hominis
炙僵蚕	*zhì jiāng cán*	15g	Bombyx Batryticatus (fried with liquid)
干地龙	*gān dì lóng*	15g	Pheretima (dried)
肉苁蓉	*ròu cōng róng*	10g	Herba Cistanches
鹿角片	*lù jiǎo piàn*	10g	Cornu Cervi (sliced)

Indicated for reduced sperm motility due to spleen and kidney dual deficiency with stagnation of the channels and collaterals.

(15) *Tù Sī Zǐ Tāng* (菟丝子汤)

菟丝子	*tù sī zǐ*	30g	Semen Cuscutae
肉苁蓉	*ròu cōng róng*	15g	Herba Cistanches
枸杞子	*gǒu qǐ zǐ*	15g	Fructus Lycii
五味子	*wǔ wèi zǐ*	15g	Fructus Schisandrae Chinensis
山茱萸	*shān zhū yú*	15g	Fructus Corni
何首乌	*hé shǒu wū*	20g	Radix Polygoni Multiflori
熟地	*shú dì*	20g	Radix Rehmanniae Praeparata
人参	*rén shēn*	5g	Radix et Rhizoma Ginseng
泽泻	*zé xiè*	10g	Rhizoma Alismatis

Indicated for abnormal sperm due to kidney essence deficiency.

(16) *Jiā Wèi Liù Wèi Wán* (加味六味丸)

熟地	*shú dì*	15g	Radix Rehmanniae Praeparata
山茱萸	*shān zhū yú*	15g	Fructus Corni
泽泻	*zé xiè*	15g	Rhizoma Alismatis
丹皮	*mǔ dān pí*	15g	Cortex Moutan
肉苁蓉	*ròu cōng róng*	15g	Herba Cistanches
山药	*shān yào*	30g	Rhizoma Dioscoreae

茯苓	fú líng	30g	Poria
丹参	dān shēn	30g	Radix et Rhizoma Salviae Miltiorrhizae
菟丝子	tù sī zǐ	10g	Semen Cuscutae
川草薢	chuān bì xiè	10g	Rhizoma Dioscoreae Hypoglaucae

Indicated for male immune infertility due to kidney deficiency and blood stasis.

PROGNOSIS

Male infertility should not be viewed as a single condition, but rather as the manifestation of a number of possible male reproductive system disorders. The prognosis for this condition is therefore generally associated with specific causative factors. The World Health Organization (WHO) has recognized the following sixteen categories of male infertility.

Dysfunction during sexual intercourse or ejaculatory impotence, immunological causes, abnormalities of sperm plasma, iatrogenic origin, systemic disease, congenital abnormality, acquired injury of the testes, varicocele, inflammation of male subsidiary gonad, endocrinal origin, idiopathic oligozoospermia, idiopathic asthenospermia, idiopathic teratozoospermia, obstructive azoospermia, idiopathic azoospermia, and causes of unknown origin.

It must be understood that these are sixteen separate disorders, each with distinctive differences in their etiology, pathogenesis and treatment. Their proper identification is therefore most important during clinical diagnosis, so as to provide optimum treatment and also a clear prognosis. The prognosis is relatively good in individuals with normal testes and the ability to generate sperm, and also in those where no structural disorder is present. Providing a cure proves more challenging in those presenting with infertility due to organic conditions. These include congenital hypoplasia of the testes, genuine azoospermia, and major structural deformities.

PREVENTIVE HEALTHCARE

Lifestyle Modification

Patients with infertility can take some control of their reproductive function by living healthy lifestyles. Smokers and drinkers display far lower sperm counts, since smoking and alcohol both deplete the body's supply of vitamin C. Experts also advise that a man should sleep at least 8 hours a day to maintain normal sexual function. Men might also be advised to avoid lounging in hot water bathtubs and steam baths, especially when they are planning a pregnancy. Spending more than 30 minutes in water at 40℃ or above can also lower sperm counts.

The traditionally recommended lifestyle practices were referred to as "sexual healthcare", and were further elaborated upon in a number of the Chinese medical classics.

The *Yellow Emperor's Inner Classic* (黄帝内经 , *Huáng Dì Nèi Jīng*) points out the benefits of a moderate sexual lifestyle. Engaging in sexual activity when one is intoxicated is considered to be especially improper, since this can "exhaust the essence".

The *Magic Pivot* (灵枢 · 邪气藏府病形篇 , *Líng Shū·Xié Qì Zàng Fǔ Bìng Xíng Piān*) states, "Engaging in sexual intercourse while intoxicated and sweating; followed by exposure to the wind; will damage the spleen." Also, "Over-indulgent sexual activities damage the kidney".

The *Thousand Gold Pieces Prescriptions* (千金要方 · 房中补益 , *Qiān Jīn Yào Fāng·Fáng Zhōng Bǔ Yì*) also points out, "Taking medicinals in order to benefit sexuality when under the age of forty will cause immediate disaster."

"Due to excessive greed, some people take a great number of tonifying medicinals so as to remain over-indulgent in sexual activities. Within a half-year, the essence and marrow become exhausted, and the date of death approaches."

The *Su Nǔ's Classic* (素女经 , *Sù Nǔ Jīng*) states, "Immediately after hair-washing or an exhausting trip, or with great joy or anger; it is improper to have intercourse of yin and yang."

The *Secrets of the Jade Bedroom* (玉房秘诀 , *Yù Fáng Mì Jué*) states, "Immediately after drinking and eating, the grain qi has not yet been transported. Having intercourse of yin and yang at this time will result in abdominal distention and white turbid urine. When pregnancy occurs under these circumstances, the resulting children will exhibit mania and withdrawl."

"When heavy burdens result in taxation fatigue, the mind and qi become unsettled. Having intercourse of yin and yang at this time will cause pain of the sinews and lumbus. When pregnancy occurs under these circumstances, the resulting children will be disabled or die at young age."

"Right after bathing, the hair and skin are not yet dry. Having intercourse of yin and yang at this time will cause a shortage of qi. When pregnancy occurs under these circumstances, the resulting children will be physically incomplete."

Though these traditional viewpoints are not fully accurate, they do reflect a relatively good understanding of the relationship between sexual activity and reproductive health. The ancient physicians certainly realized that improper sexual activity could produce negative effects on reproductive health, especially when a person is intoxicated, full, exhausted, nervous, or wet.

The *Sān Yuán Yán Shòu Cān Zàn Shū:Tiān Yuán Zhī Shòu:Yù Bù Kě Jué* (三元延寿参赞书 · 天元之寿 · 欲不可绝) describes the principles, methods, and contraindications which must be observed in order to maintain a healthy sexual lifestyle.

It states, "The sages do not prohibit sexual activities, but instead they advise people to maintain the true heavenly essence through restraint."

"A man at age sixty should constrain his essence instead of discharging it. However, if he is both healthy and capable, it is not recommended for him to restrain it for too long, as this may result in welling-abscesses." This statement points out that sexual activities are in fact necessary, and that overindulgence and excessive constraint can both lead to disease.

"It is recorded in *Discussions from Famous Physicians* (名医论 , *Míng Yī Lùn*) that when a person experiences endless but unfulfilled desire, his intention will physically manifest with a white slippery discharge. When this person overindulges in sexual activity, slackness of the ancestral sinew will appear."

The *Sān Yuán Yán Shòu Cān Zàn Shū:Tiān Yuán Zhī Shòu:Yù Bù Kě Qiáng Piān* (三元延寿参赞书 · 天元之寿 · 欲不可强篇) emphatically points out that one should never have sexual intercourse beyond one's capacity.

It states, "*Plain Questions* (素问 , *Sù Wèn*) points out that forcing [sexual activity] will damage the kidney qi and the hip bone. The commentary states that the forcing of sexual activity will cause essence depletion and kidney damage that results in marrow qi withering internally and a painful lumbus that cannot bend forward or upward."

"When one is impotent and so takes mineral medicinals to assist yang, kidney water will become exhausted, heart fire will scorch the five viscera, and dispersion-thirst will immediately occur."

"When insufficient water fails to extinguish exuberant fire, sores and welling-abscesses may appear."

"Sexual activities that follow a tiring journey will result in five taxations and deficiency detriment."

There is no benefit to having sexual intercourse beyond one's capacity. When the constitution is weak and sexual function is in decline, the taking of mineral-based medicinals to invigorate yang and warm the kidney will deplete the body even more.

The *Sān Yuán Yán Shòu Cān Zàn Shū:Tiān Yuán Zhī Shòu:YùYǒu Suǒ Jì Piān* (三元延寿参赞书 · 天元之寿 · 欲有所忌篇) states, "Taxation from sexual activity after overeating will cause the blood and qi to spill and percolate into the large intestine, which results in bloody stools with abdominal pain. This is called intestinal aggregation."

"Going into the bedroom when one is greatly intoxicated causes qi exhaustion and liver damage. For a man, this manifests with decreased semen and impotence." Also, "Having sexual relations when angry will lead to essence deficiency and qi exhaustion which results in welling-abscess and flat-abscess. Going in the bedroom in fear will lead to a deficiency of either yin or yang that can result in reversal, spontaneous sweating, and night sweating. The condition will accumulate and later manifest with taxation."

"Having intercourse before an incised wound has completely healed will disturb both blood and qi and cause the wound to putrefy."

"For those with red eyes, sexual activity should be prohibited in order to prevent internal obstruction."

"When seasonal diseases have not recovered, violating these prohibitions will cause the patient to die with his tongue protruding several *cun*."

Modern research also reveals a number of important facts related to lifestyle issues.

➢ A number of men are sensitive to nicotine and alcohol, with sperm-generating cells being especially affected. Smoking and drinking is associated with oligospermia, asthenospermia, and abnormal sperm morphology. Nicotine has been shown to decrease sexual hormone secretions and also increase the numbers of non-viable sperm, where alcoholism can result in a 50% reduction in seminal fluid volume. Although conception may be possible for drinkers and smokers, higher rates of complication are to be expected.

➢ The production of semen is closely related to proper nutrition. Zinc, copper, phosphorus, calcium, and vitamins E and A must be sufficiently present in the daily diet. When these essential substances are deficient, the production of semen can be seriously affected.

➢ The temperature range required for the production of semen is 35 to 36℃. The normal temperature of the scrotum is 1 to 8℃ lower than that of the abdominal cavity. Wearing tight trousers or taking hot baths will quickly raise the temperature of the scrotum and testicles, leading to oligospermia and reduced sperm survival rates. Blood circulation may become affected, which is also detrimental to seminal fluid production.

➢ Excessive sexual activity and interrupted intercourse can both lead to congestion of the urethra and prostate gland. Prostatitis affects liquefaction times, and also reduces sperm motility rates. Even though the testicles can produce as many as one hundred million sperm, excessive sexuality clearly decreases sperm counts and also rates of conception.

➢ Standing for long periods of time causes local congestion of the genital organs. This also affects prostate secretion, seminal vesicles, and sperm quality. When free movement of the scrotum becomes hindered, even during activity, seminal fluid production may be also significantly reduced.

➢ A man's predominant psychological state is also a factor in seminal fluid production. Men who suffer with depression or anxiety may also show reduced sperm counts. Optimistic attitudes have been shown to improve reproductive health in general and seminal fluid production in particular.

Dietary Recommendation

During the course of treatment, the daily diet should be generally light and nutritious. A daily broth prepared with *lián zǐ* (Semen

Nelumbinis), *yín ěr* (Tremella), *bǎi hé* (Bulbus Lilii) or *hóng zǎo* (Fructus Jujubae) can protect the spleen and stomach, benefit the kidney, and nourish essence. Tobacco, alcohol and acrid or spicy foods are to be generally avoided. Smoking and excessive alcohol drinking affects the production and maturation of semen, and also increases the number deformed sperm. The following section includes a variety of therapeutic medicinal recipes.

(1) *Guì Yuán Hóng Zǎo Tāng* (桂元红枣汤)

龙眼肉	*lóng yǎn ròu*	30g	Arillus Longan
红枣	*hóng zǎo*	30g	Fructus Jujubae
瘦肉	*shòu ròu*	30g	Pork Meat

Prepare as a broth and cook with steam. Indicated for patterns of qi and blood dual deficiency.

(2) *Chì Mǐ Zhōu* (赤米粥)

Take equal amounts of *chì xiǎo dòu* (Semen Phaseoli) and *yì yǐ rén* (Semen Coicis), and boil them to make porridge.

This nutritious recipe acts to fortify the spleen, disinhibit dampness, nourish blood, and benefit essence. Indicated for patterns of damp-heat in the lower burner.

(3) *Lù Jiǎo Zhōu* (鹿角粥)

鹿角粉	*lù jiǎo fěn*	5~10g	Cornu Cervi (powdered)
粳米	*jīng mǐ*	30~60g	Semen Oryzae

Make porridge with *jīng mǐ* (Semen Oryzae), then add *lù jiǎo fěn* (Cornu Cervi powder) and a little salt, and bring to a boil. Consume two servings each day.

This recipe supplements kidney yang, benefits essence and blood, and strengthens the sinews and bones. Indicated for impotence and premature ejaculation due to kidney yang insufficiency with essence and blood deficiency.

(4) *Lì Zhī Gān Bǎo Zhōu* (荔枝干煲粥)

Take about a dozen *lì zhī* (Fructus Litchi) fruits; discard the peels and seeds. Add rice, and boil together as porridge. Take daily for one month. Shān yào (Rhizoma Dioscoreae) and *lián zǐ* (Semen Nelumbinis) may also be added to enhance the therapeutic effect.

Lì zhī (Fructus Litchi) contains glucose, sucrose, fats, vitamins A, B, and G, folic acid, citric acid and malate. This recipe acts to engender fluids, benefit blood, and regulate qi.

(5) *Bǎi Yáng Shèn Gēng* (白羊肾羹)

肉苁蓉	*ròu cōng róng*	20g	Herba Cistanches
白羊肾	*bái yáng shèn*	2 pieces	White Lamb Kidney
羊脂	*yáng zhī*	50g	Lamb Fat
荜茇	*bì bá*	6g	Fructus Piperis Longi
草果	*cǎo guǒ*	3g	Fructus Tsaoko
橘皮	*jú pí*	3g	Citri Exocarpium
胡椒	*hú jiāo*	1g	Fructus Piperis

Also add salt, shēng jiāng (Rhizoma Zingiberis Recens) and spring onions. Stew over moderate heat.

This recipe acts to supplement kidney yang, benefit essence and blood, warm the middle, and dissipate cold. Indicated for impotence with aching lumbus and limp knees.

(6) *Bǔ Gǔ Zhǐ Hú Táo Gāo* (补骨脂胡桃膏)

补骨脂	*bǔ gǔ zhī*	300g	Fructus Psoraleae
胡桃肉	*hú táo ròu*	600g	Semen Juglandis
蜂蜜	*fēng mì*	300g	Honey

Steam *bǔ gǔ zhī* (Fructus Psoraleae) with wine; sun-dry and grind into powder. Dissolve *fēng mì* (Honey) in water and bring it to a boil. Then add mashed *hú táo* (Semen Juglandis) and the powdered *bǔ gǔ zhī*

(Fructus Psoraleae) and stir. Take 10g, twice daily.

This recipe acts to warm and tonify kidney yang. Indicated for kidney yang deficiency manifesting with impotence, seminal emission, frequent urination, and aching lumbus and knees. This preparation can stir fire and engender phlegm, so it is not recommended for patients with effulgent yin deficiency fire or kidney yang deficiency that manifests without seminal emission and an aching lumbus.

(7) *Hǎi mǎ* (Hippocampus), *lù ròu* (Cervi caro), *lù biān* (Cervi Testis et Penis), *yáng ròu* (Caprae seu Ovis Renes), *gǒu ròu* (Dog Meat), *niú ròu* (Bovis Caro), *má què* (Sparrow), *hé táo ròu* (Semen Juglandis) and *jiǔ cài* (Allii Tuberosi Folium) can be prepared and consumed to warm the kidney and invigorate yang. Indicated for infertility due to kidney yang deficiency and life gate fire debilitation manifesting with impotence, seminal efflux, premature ejaculation, seminal emission, and cold semen.

(8) *Zǐ hé chē* (Placenta Hominis), *dōng chóng xià cǎo* (Cordyceps), *hǎi shēn* (Stichopus Japonicus), *gé jiè* (Gecko) and *gē ròu* (Dove) can be prepared and consumed to tonify the kidney, replenish essence, and benefit marrow. Indicated for oligospermia, asthenospermia, seminal emission, and seminal efflux.

(9) *Niú nǎi* (Milk), *hēi mù ěr* (Black Agaric), *hóng zǎo* (Fructus Ziziphi), *lóng yǎn ròu* (Arillus Longan), *fēng mì* (Honey), *ē jiāo* (Colla Corii Asini), *sāng shèn* (Fructus Mori), *bō cài* (Spinach) and *pú táo* (Grape) may be prepared to tonify qi and blood. These foods can assist in the treatment of reduced sexual desire, impotence, and infertility.

(10) *Guī* (Tortoise), *biē* (Turtle), *sāng shèn* (Fructus Mori), *huáng huā yú* (Yellow Croaker), *niú suǐ* (Ox Marrow), *zhū suǐ* (Pig Marrow) and *mǔ lì* (Concha Ostreae) can enrich the kidney, replenish essence, and foster yin. Indicated for essence and blood deficiency with congenital deformity of

the genitals or penile agenesis.

(11) *Lián zǐ* (Semen Nelumbinis), *qiàn shí* (Semen Euryales), *bái guǒ* (Semen Ginkgo) and *lián xū* (Stamen Nelumbinis) act to secure the kidney and astringe essence. Indicated for seminal emission and seminal efflux.

(12) *Dōng guā* (Exocarpium Benincasae), *ní qiū* (Loach), *lián zǐ xīn* (Plumula Nelumbinis) and *sī guā* (Retinervus Luffae Fructus) act to clear and disinhibit damp-heat. Indicated for turbid semen and seminal heat.

Regulation of Emotional and Mental Health

A balanced emotional state is very beneficial to reproductive health. The conscious cultivatation of a positive mental attitude often proves beneficial to recovery. Patient education, discussions of personal and family history, and counseling specifically related to male infertility can be also helpful in many cases. Patients in counseling report feeling less upset about their infertility, less anxious and nervous, and also have fewer difficulties with sexual performance.

CLINICAL EXPERIENCE OF RENOWNED PHYSICIANS

Empirical Formulas

Due to intensive research into the treatment of male diseases with Chinese medicine, new protocols have been recently developed for the treatment of male infertility. Clinical practice records reveal a great number of highly effective empirical formulas for this particular condition.

1. *Shēng Jīng Tāng* (生精汤) (Wang Qi)

【Ingredients】

| 何首乌 | *hé shǒu wū* | 10g | Radix Polygoni Multiflori |
| 蜂房 | *fēng fáng* | 10g | Nidus Vespae |

鹿衔草	lù xián cǎo	10g	Herba Pyrolae
菟丝子	tù sī zǐ	15g	Semen Cuscutae
枸杞子	gǒu qǐ zǐ	15g	Fructus Lycii
蛇床子	shé chuáng zǐ	15g	Fructus Cnidii
淫羊藿	yín yáng huò	10g	Herba Epimedii
黄精	huáng jīng	15g	Rhizoma Polygonati
丹参	dān shēn	20g	Radix et Rhizoma Salviae Miltiorrhizae

【Indications】

Low sperm count due to kidney deficiency or blood stasis.

(*Wang Qi's Perspective on Male Diseases*. Zhengzhou: Henan Press of Science and Technology, 1997: 596.)

2. *Wēn Shèn Yì Jīng Wán* (温肾益精丸) (Luo Yuan-kai)

【Ingredients】

炮天雄	páo tiān xióng	180g	Aconiti Tuber Laterale Tianxiong (Stir-fried)
熟地	shú dì	180g	Radix Rehmanniae Praeparata
菟丝子	tù sī zǐ	480g	Semen Cuscutae
鹿角霜	lù jiǎo shuāng	120g	Cornu Cervi Degelatinatum
白术	bái zhú	480g	Rhizoma Atractylodis Macrocephalae
肉桂	ròu guì	30g	Cortex Cinnamomi

Make small honey-pills. Take 6g each time, twice daily.

【Indications】

Low sperm motility due to kidney yang deficiency and life gate fire debilitation.

(*Collected Discussions on Medicine with Luo Yuan-kai*. Beijing: People's Medical Publishing House, 1990: 43.)

3. *Shēng Jīng Zàn Yù Tāng* (生精赞育汤) (Hu Xi-ming)

【Ingredients】

| 淫羊藿 | yín yáng huò | 15g | Herba Epimedii |

肉苁蓉	*ròu cōng róng*	10g	Herba Cistanches
仙茅	*xiān máo*	15g	Rhizoma Curculiginis
枸杞子	*gǒu qǐ zǐ*	10g	Fructus Lycii

【Indications】

Azoospermia due to kidney essence deficiency.

(*Complete Collection of Secret Chinese Medicine Formulas*. The Middle Volume. Shanghai: Wenhui Publishing, 1989, 501.)

4. *QIÁNG JĪNG JIĀN* (强精煎) (HE QING-HU AND ZHOU SHEN)

【Ingredients】

紫丹参	*zǐ dān shēn*	15g	Radix et Rhizoma Salviae Miltiorrhizae
莪术	*é zhú*	15g	Rhizoma Curcumae
川牛膝	*chuān niú xī*	15g	Radix Cyathulae
柴胡	*chái hú*	10g	Radix Bupleuri
生牡蛎	*shēng mǔ lì*	30g	Concha Ostreae Cruda
生黄芪	*shēng huáng qí*	20g	Radix Astragali Cruda

【Indications】

Varicocele with infertility due to qi stagnation and blood stasis.

(*Outlines of Diagnosis and Treatment of Thousands of Diseases*. Beijing: World Scientific Publishing Company, 1997: 596.)

5. *YÈ HUÀ TĀNG* (液化汤) (HE QING-HU AND ZHOU SHEN)

【Ingredients】

知母	*zhī mǔ*	9g	Rhizoma Anemarrhenae
黄柏	*huáng bǎi*	9g	Cortex Phellodendri Chinensis
花粉	*huā fěn*	9g	Radix Trichosanthis
赤芍	*chì sháo*	9g	Radix Paeoniae Rubra
白芍	*bái sháo*	9g	Radix Paeoniae Alba
麦冬	*mài dōng*	9g	Radix Ophiopogonis
生地	*shēng dì*	12g	Radix Rehmanniae
熟地	*shú dì*	12g	Radix Rehmanniae Praeparata

玄参	xuán shēn	12g	Radix Scrophulariae
枸杞子	gǒu qǐ zǐ	12g	Fructus Lycii
淫羊藿	yín yáng huò	12g	Herba Epimedii
车前草	chē qián cǎo	12g	Herba Plantaginis
丹参	dān shēn	30g	Radix et Rhizoma Salviae Miltiorrhizae

【Indications】

Non-liquefaction of semen due to kidney yin deficiency and binding of damp and heat.

(*Outlines of Diagnosis and Treatment of Thousands of Diseases*. Beijing: World Scientific Publishing Company, 1997: 596.)

6. JIĀ WÈI BĂO ZHĒN WÁN (加味保真丸) (HE QING-HU, ZHOU SHEN)

【Ingredients】

党参	dǎng shēn	24~60g	Radix Codonopsis
生黄芪	shēng huáng qí	24~60g	Radix Astragali
桑寄生	sāng jì shēng	15g	Herba Taxilli
菟丝子	tù sī zǐ	15g	Semen Cuscutae
覆盆子	fù pén zǐ	24g	Fructus Rubi
仙灵脾	xiān líng pí	24g	Herba Epimedii
杜仲	dù zhòng	9g	Cortex Eucommiae

【Indications】

Infertility due to spleen and kidney dual deficiency.

(*Outlines of Diagnosis and Treatment of Thousands of Diseases*. Beijing: World Scientific Publishing Company, 1997: 594.)

7. SHĒNG JĪNG TĀNG (生精汤) (WANG YI-PING)

【Ingredients】

生地	shēng dì	15g	Radix Rehmanniae
首乌	shǒu wū	15g	Radix Polygoni Multiflori
川断	chuān duàn	15g	Radix Dipsaci

鸡血藤	jī xuè téng	15g	Caulis Spatholobi
枸杞子	gǒu qǐ zǐ	10g	Fructus Lycii
菟丝子	tù sī zǐ	10g	Semen Cuscutae
车前子	chē qián zǐ	10g	Semen Plantaginis
五味子	wǔ wèi zǐ	10g	Fructus Schisandrae Chinensis
覆盆子	fù pén zǐ	10g	Fructus Rubi
黄芪	huáng qí	20g	Radix Astragali
当归	dāng guī	12g	Radix Angelicae Sinensis
淫羊藿	yín yáng huò	15g	Herba Epimedii
红参	hóng shēn	9g	Radix et Rhizoma Ginseng Rubra

【Indications】

Abnormal sperm due to deficiency of the spleen and kidney.

(Experiences of Liu Jian-min in the Treatment of Male Infertility. *Journal of Traditional Chinese Medicine Literature*, 2000, (4): 20.)

8. *Dōng Gé Shēng Jīng Yǐn* (冬蛤生精饮) (Yang Zhu-xing, et al)

【Ingredients】

麦冬	mài dōng	15g	Radix Ophiopogonis
白芍	bái sháo	15g	Radix Paeoniae Alba
石菖蒲	shí chāng pú	15g	Rhizoma Acori Tatarinowii
合欢花	hé huān huā	15g	Flos Albiziae
茯苓	fú líng	15g	Poria
淫羊藿	yín yáng huò	15g	Herba Epimedii
枸杞	gǒu qǐ	20g	Fructus Lycii
知母	zhī mǔ	20g	Rhizoma Anemarrhenae
山药	shān yào	10g	Rhizoma Dioscoreae

Take two *gé jiè* (Gecko) and discard the heads, feet and skins. Bake to dry and grind to minute granules. Divide into four portions, and take with the decoction.

【Indications】

Infertility due to azoospermia.

(Miraculous Family Formulas from Famous Physicians of Chinese Medicine. Guangxi Nationalities Publishing House, 1992: 179.)

9. *Huà Yū Zàn Yù Tāng* (化瘀赞育汤) (Yang Zhu-xing)

【Ingredients】

柴胡	*chái hú*	9g	Radix Bupleuri
红花	*hóng huā*	9g	Flos Carthami
桃仁	*táo rén*	9g	Semen Persicae
赤芍	*chì sháo*	9g	Radix Paeoniae Rubra
川芎	*chuān xiōng*	9g	Rhizoma Chuanxiong
当归	*dāng guī*	9g	Radix Angelicae Sinensis
熟地	*shú dì*	30g	Radix Rehmanniae Praeparata
紫石英	*zǐ shí yīng*	30g	Fluoritum
枳壳	*zhǐ qiào*	5g	Fructus Aurantii
桔梗	*jié gěng*	5g	Radix Platycodonis
牛膝	*niú xī*	5g	Radix Achyranthis Bidentatae

【Indications】

Male infertility due to kidney deficiency, qi stagnation and blood stasis.

(Miraculous Family Formulas of Famous Senior Physicians of Chinese Medicine. Guangxi Nationalities Publishing House, 1992: 180.)

10. *Bǔ Shèn Yì Xuè Tián Jīng Tāng* (补肾益血填精汤) (Zhang Feng-qiang, Zheng Ying)

【Ingredients】

熟地	*shú dì*	12g	Radix Rehmanniae Praeparata
菟丝子	*tù sī zǐ*	12g	Semen Cuscutae
巴戟天	*bā jǐ tiān*	12g	Radix Morindae Officinalis
枸杞子	*gǒu qǐ zǐ*	12g	Fructus Lycii
山萸肉	*shān yú ròu*	12g	Fructus Corni
制首乌	*zhì hé shǒu wū*	12g	Radix Polygoni Multiflori Praeparata cum Succo Glycines Sotae
刺蒺藜	*cì jí lí*	12g	Fructus Tribuli

当归	*dāng guī*	10g	Radix Angelicae Sinensis
白茯苓	*bái fú líng*	10g	Poria
锁阳	*suǒ yáng*	10g	Herba Cynomorii
丹参	*dān shēn*	10g	Radix et Rhizoma Salviae Miltiorrhizae
鹿角胶	*lù jiǎo jiāo*	10g	Colla Cornus Cervi
龟甲	*guī jiǎ*	10g	Carapax et Plastrum Testudinis
蛇床子	*shé chuáng zǐ*	6g	Fructus Cnidii
砂仁	*shā rén*	6g	Fructus Amomi
小茴香	*xiǎo huí xiāng*	6g	Fructus Foeniculi

【Indications】

Male infertility due to kidney deficiency.

(*Secret Effective Formulas of the First Group of Famous Senior Physicians in Chinese Medicine*. International Culture Publishing House, 1996: 436.)

Selected Case Studies

1. MEDICAL RECORDS OF ZHAO XI-WU

Mr. Sun, age 29.

【Initial Visit】

No pregnancy after 4 years of marriage. Sperm count was 16×10^6/ml to 21×10^6/ml, with motility rates of 30% to 50%. Methyltestosterone had been applied previously without significant effect. Symptoms and signs included dizziness, fatigue, aching lumbus, aversion to cold, impotence, and premature ejaculation. The tongue coating appeared thin. Pulses were deep and thready; forceless at both *chi* positions.

【Pattern Differentiation】

Kidney yang insufficiency and insecurity of the essence gate.

【Treatment Principle】

Warm yang, replenish essence, and benefit qi.

【Prescription】

The prescribed formula contains the following medicinals.

天雄	tiān xióng	12g	Aconiti Tuber Laterale Tianxiong
白术	bái zhú	18g	Rhizoma Atractylodis Macrocephalae
肉桂	ròu guì	6g	Cortex Cinnamomi
生龙骨	shēng lóng gǔ	18g	Os Draconis Cruda
生牡蛎	shēng mǔ lì	18g	Concha Ostreae Cruda
韭菜子	jiǔ cài zǐ	15g	Semen Allii Tuberosi
当归	dāng guī	12g	Radix Angelicae Sinensis
肉苁蓉	ròu cōng róng	18g	Herba Cistanches
枸杞子	gǒu qǐ zǐ	9g	Fructus Lycii
巴戟天	bā jǐ tiān	12g	Radix Morindae Officinalis
党参	dǎng shēn	30g	Radix Codonopsis
淫羊藿	yín yáng huò	18g	Herba Epimedii
冬虫夏草	dōng chóng xià cǎo	6g	Cordyceps

【Second Visit】

Following 30 doses, impotence and premature ejaculation issues were resolved, aching of the lumbus and dizziness were relieved, and all other symptoms improved. Semen analysis showed a sperm count of 108.8×10^6/ml with motility rates of 80%. Soon afterward, the patient reported that his spouse had successfully conceived.

(Shan Shu-jian. *Clinical Experience of Ancient and Contemporary Experts: Male Diseases*. Beijing: China Press of Traditional Chinese Medicine, 1999: 166)

2. MEDICAL RECORDS OF LUO YUAN-KAI

Mr. Fang, age 30.

【Initial Visit】

January, 1986. The patient's spouse had become pregnant twice in the previous 3 years, but in both cases she suffered a miscarriage after 2 months. Gynecological examination however revealed no abnormality. Biphasic BBT, menstrual cycles, and bleeding volume all appeared normal. Examination of the patient revealed no obstruction or structural disorder present. Semen analysis revealed sperm count of 80×10^6/ml, motility rates of 40%, liquefaction time at 7.5 hours, and abnormal sperm numbers at 43%. Symptoms and signs included fatigue, occasional seminal emission, poor sleep quality, and a bitter taste in the mouth during the morning. His tongue appeared enlarged with a thin white coating. Pulses were thready and slightly wiry.

【Pattern Differentiation】

Original qi debilitation with kidney essence deficiency.

【Treatment Principle】

The treatment method here is to nourish the kidney and tonify qi.

【Prescription】

The prescribed formula contains the following medicinals.

熟地	*shú dì*	20g	Radix Rehmanniae Praeparata
淫羊藿	*yín yáng huò*	10g	Herba Epimedii
枸杞子	*gǒu qǐ zǐ*	15g	Fructus Lycii
肉苁蓉	*ròu cōng róng*	20g	Herba Cistanches
党参	*dǎng shēn*	25g	Radix Codonopsis
菟丝子	*tù sī zǐ*	20g	Semen Cuscutae
山萸肉	*shān yú ròu*	15g	Fructus Corni
白术	*bái zhú*	15g	Rhizoma Atractylodis Macrocephalae
炙甘草	*zhì gān cǎo*	6g	Radix et Rhizoma Glycyrrhizae Praeparata cum Melle

Zī Shèn Yù Tāi Wán (滋肾育胎丸) was also prescribed, 5g twice daily. Sexual activity should also be restrained.

A three month follow-up exam revealed sperm count reaching 75×10^6/ml, with motility rates still below 40%.

Stewed *rén shēn* (Radix et Rhizoma Ginseng) 6g was added to the daily prescription. 15 days constitutes one treatment course, with 10 days between courses.

【Second Visit】

One and a half months later, the patient's spirit was obviously improved. Sperm counts reached 9000×10⁴/ml, motility rates 50%, and abnormal sperm had decreased to 10%. At 6 weeks, sperm count reached 116×10⁶/ml, activity rates 65%, and abnormal sperm was at 10%.

Treatments continued until his spouse conceived in March, 1987. To protect the fetus, the spouse was prescribed with *Shòu Tāi Wán* (寿胎丸) modified with *Sì Jūn Zǐ Tāng* (四君子汤). Mild vaginal bleeding appeared during pregnancy, but the condition was promptly controlled. In January of 1988, she successfully gave birth to a healthy infant without complication.

(Shan Shu-jian. *Clinical Experience of Ancient and Contemporary Experts: Male Diseases*. Beijing: China Press of Traditional Chinese Medicine, 1999: 169, 170)

3. MEDICAL RECORDS OF CHEN WEN-BO

Mr. Zhang, age 30.

Infertility due to low sperm density for 5 years. 3 to 5 white blood cells were observed in each HP field of vision. Symptoms and signs included a moist scrotum, aching lumbus and limp legs, with occasional dizziness. His tongue appeared red with a white slimy coating, and pulses were slippery and rapid. The patient also reported a history of tuberculosis of the bilateral epididymides.

Xiān líng pí (Herba Epimedii), *lù róng* (Cornu Cervi Pantotrichum), *bā jǐ tiān* (Radix Morindae Officinalis), *tù sī zǐ* (Semen Cuscutae) and *gǒu qǐ zǐ* (Fructus Lycii) were prescribed.

At four weeks, semen analysis revealed the presence of white blood cells and pyocytes, with a sperm count of three to five per HP field of vision.

Jīn yín huā (Flos Lonicerae), *zǐ huā dì dīng* (Herba Violae), *zhī mǔ* (Rhizoma Anemarrhenae), *huáng bǎi* (Cortex Phellodendri Chinensis), *shēng dì* (Radix Rehmanniae Recens), *shǒu wū* (Radix Polygoni Multiflori), *gǒu qǐ zǐ* (Fructus Lycii), *chē qián cǎo* (Herba Plantaginis), and *pú gōng yīng* (Herba Taraxaci) were selected to clear heat, eliminate damp, nourish yin, and tonify the kidney. After a treatment course of three months, examination revealed normal sperm counts with no white blood cells or pyocytes present.

Dr. Chen Wen-bo believes that in addition to deficient patterns, the kidney may also be associated with conditions of pathological excess. The main patterns here include stasis obstructing the essence passage, damp-heat of the essence chamber, toxin disturbing the essence chamber, essence stagnation, and damp constraint of the essence chamber. Biomedical symptoms include varicocele, testicular tuberculosis, testitis, hydrocele, prostatitis, and gonorrhea. Without predominant symptoms of yin or yang deficiency, yang-invigorating medicinals are not recommended. Proper treatment should primarily nourish yin, while also also tonifying the kidney. For patterns of yang deficiency, the best approach is to apply the principle of "seeking yang within yin".

Ming dynasty physician Yue Pu-jia, author of *Miào Yī Zhāi Yī Xué Zhèng Yìn Biān* (妙一斋医学正印编) stated, "To assist yang with excessively warming medicinals is prohibited when treating men. In the long run, it is more appropriate to select moderate medicinals that act to restrain, and also those which secure true yin".

Qing dynasty physician Shi Shou-tang also discussed the selection of medicinals for male infertility in the text, *Yī Yuán* (医原). It states, "Medicinals should be selected that are warm and moist, or sweet and moist. Harsh, dry, metal and stone are most prohibited". He also said, "To treat fire within water, select medicinals that are warm and moist, rather than warm and dry. When yin humor becomes deficient, dry and harsh medicinals will deplete it even more. In mild cases, headache and toothache may appear. In severe cases, blurred vision, sores, flat-abscess, hemiplegia and crippling wilt will occur".

Dr. Chen's main treatment principle for male diseases is to nourish through tonification of the kidney to engender humor and replenish essence. He is strongly opposes the warming of yang with fierce tonification, especially without clear differentiation of deficiency and excess patterns.

(Shan Shu-jian. *Clinical Experience of Ancient and Contemporary Experts: Male Diseases*. Beijing: China Press of Traditional Chinese Medicine, 1999: 173, 174)

4. MEDICAL RECORDS OF LI WEN-GUANG

(1) Mr. He, age 35.

【Initial Visit】

The patient complained of being childless even though he had been married for six years. He reported low sexual desire, with activity only once every ten days. Other signs and symptoms included erectile dysfunction, forceless ejaculation, occasional impotence, aversion to cold, cold limbs, aching lumbus with limp legs, dizziness, tinnitus, and a bright white complexion. His tongue appeared pale with a white coating, and pulses thready and forceless. In three previous examinations, sperm survival rates remained at 10%. The biomedical diagnosis was male infertility secondary to necrospermia.

【Pattern Differentiation】

Kidney yang deficiency.

【Treatment Principle】

Warm the kidney and invigorate yang.

【Prescription】

Modified *Yáng Gāo Wán Tāng* (羊睾丸汤).

阳起石	yáng qǐ shí	30g	Actinolitum
淫羊藿	yín yáng huò	15g	Herba Epimedii
巴戟天	bā jǐ tiān	9g	Radix Morindae Officinalis

胡芦巴	*hú lú bā*	9g	Semen Trigonellae
仙茅	*xiān máo*	9g	Rhizoma Curculiginis
菟丝子	*tù sī zǐ*	9g	Semen Cuscutae
枸杞子	*gǒu qǐ zǐ*	9g	Fructus Lycii
鹿角霜	*lù jiǎo shuāng*	9g	Cornu Cervi Degelatinatum
续断	*xù duàn*	15g	Radix Dipsaci
黄芪	*huáng qí*	30g	Radix Astragali
当归	*dāng guī*	12g	Radix Angelicae Sinensis

Boiled goat testicles are used as a conductor; decoct the formula using the broth. The testes may also be consumed. To be taken once daily.

【Second Visit】

Following ten doses, sexual desire and ejaculation strength were much improved. He became free of all symptoms after thirty doses, with sperm survival rates reaching 65%. His spouse soon became pregnant and later gave birth to a healthy female infant.

(Leng Fang-nan. *Clinical Therapeutics of Male Diseases in Chinese Medicine*. Beijing: People's Medicinal Publishing House, 1991: 126)

(2) Mr. Liu, age 30.

【Initial Visit】

April, 1976. No pregnancy had occurred following three years of marriage. Routine examination showed 3 to 7 sperm in each HP field of view. The patient also reported pain of the testes for one year. Physical examination revealed nodes present in the right testicle, also painful upon palpation.

【Treatment Principle】

The treatment principle here is to clear heat, soften hardness, and relieve pain.

【Prescription】

The prescribed formula contains the following ingredients.

柴胡	*chái hú*	9g	Radix Bupleuri
橘核	*jú hé*	9g	Semen Citri Reticulatae

白芍	*bái sháo*	9g	Radix Paeoniae Alba
赤芍	*chì sháo*	9g	Radix Paeoniae Rubra
当归	*dāng guī*	12g	Radix Angelicae Sinensiss
桑椹子	*sāng shèn zǐ*	9g	Fructus Mori
金银花	*jīn yín huā*	24g	Flos Lonicerae Japonicae
野菊花	*yě jú huā*	12g	Flos Chrysanthemi Indici
瓜蒌仁	*guā lóu rén*	12g	Fructus Trichosanthis
生牡蛎	*shēng mǔ lì*	30g	Concha Ostreae Cruda
香附	*xiāng fù*	12g	Rhizoma Cyperi
丹参	*dān shēn*	15g	Radix et Rhizoma Salviae Miltiorrhizae
甘草	*gān cǎo*	6g	Radix et Rhizoma Glycyrrhizae

3 decocted doses were taken, with an interval of 1 or 2 days afterward.

【Second Visit】

April 16th: Patient reports testicular pain completely resolved.

Modified *Shēng Jīng Zhòng Yù Tāng* (生精种玉汤).

The prescribed formula contains the following medicinals.

淫羊藿	*yín yáng huò*	9g	Herba Epimedii
续断	*xù duàn*	12g	Radix Dipsaci
当归	*dāng guī*	9g	Radix Angelicae Sinensiss
枸杞子	*gǒu qǐ zǐ*	9g	Fructus Lycii
菟丝子	*tù sī zǐ*	9g	Semen Cuscutae
五味子	*wǔ wèi zǐ*	9g	Fructus Schisandrae Chinensis
覆盆子	*fù pén zǐ*	9g	Fructus Rubi
车前子	*chē qián zǐ*	9g	Semen Plantaginis
党参	*dǎng shēn*	15g	Radix Codonopsis
白术	*bái zhú*	9g	Rhizoma Atractylodis Macrocephalae
茯苓	*fú líng*	9g	Poria
陈皮	*chén pí*	9g	Pericarpium Citri Reticulatae
甘草	*gān cǎo*	9g	Radix et Rhizoma Glycyrrhizae

At a three month routine examination, sperm counts reached 0.5×10^6/ml. Continuing with the same formula, the patient was also advised to have sexual intercourse during his wife's next ovulatory period. His spouse successfully achieved pregnancy, later giving birth to a healthy female infant.

(Shan Shu-jian. *Clinical Experience of Ancient and Contemporary Experts: Male Diseases*. Beijing: China Press of Traditional Chinese Medicine, 1999: 178, 179)

(3) Mr. Li, age 36.

【**Initial Visit**】

June 9th, 1976. Childless after seven years of marriage, also with a history of prostatitis. More than ten examinations since 1971 had revealed non-liquefaction of semen within 24 hours. The patient had previously taken over 400 doses of kidney-warming and yang-invigorating medicinals, with no obvious effect. He also reported aching of the lumbus and profuse dreaming.

【**Treatment Principle**】

The treatment method here is to nourish yin and discharge fire.

【**Prescription**】

Modified *Yè Huà Tāng* (液化汤).

The prescribed formula contains the following medicinals.

知母	*zhī mǔ*	9g	Rhizoma Anemarrhenae
黄柏	*huáng bǎi*	9g	Cortex Phellodendri Chinensis
生地	*shēng dì*	12g	Radix Rehmanniae
熟地	*shú dì*	12g	Radix Rehmanniae Praeparata
白芍	*bái sháo*	9g	Radix Paeoniae Alba
赤芍	*chì sháo*	9g	Radix Paeoniae Rubra
丹参	*dān shēn*	30g	Radix et Rhizoma Salviae Miltiorrhizae
淫羊藿	*yín yáng huò*	15g	Herba Epimedii
丹皮	*dān pí*	9g	Cortex Moutan
车前子（包）	*chē qián zǐ*	9g	Semen Plantaginis (wrapped)
金银花	*jīn yín huā*	30g	Flos Lonicerae Japonicae
生甘草	*shēng gān cǎo*	6g	Radix et Rhizoma Glycyrrhizae (raw)

【Second Visit】

August 2nd. At dose 27, liquefaction time reached 30 minutes and sperm count 61×10^6/ml, with motility rates over 50%. Following 10 more doses, his spouse successfully conceived and gave birth to a male infant on July 22rd, 1977.

(Shan Shu-jian. *Clinical Experience of Ancient and Contemporary Experts: Male Diseases.* Beijing: China Press of Traditional Chinese Medicine, 1999: 180)

(4) Mr. Jia, age 35.

【Initial Visit】

July 26th, 1976. Childless after six years of marriage. The patient reported low sexual desire and intermittent aching of the lumbus. Routine examination revealed normal liquefaction time, with sperm count of 136×10^6/ml. The proportion of non-viable sperm was 2/3, with 34% appearing abnormal. The diagnosis here is male infertility due to deficiency of the kidney.

【Prescription】

The prescribed formula contains the following medicinals.

菟丝子	tù sī zǐ	9g	Semen Cuscutae
枸杞子	gǒu qǐ zǐ	9g	Fructus Lycii
五味子	wǔ wèi zǐ	6g	Fructus Schisandrae Chinensis
覆盆子	fù pén zǐ	9g	Fructus Rubi
车前子（包）	chē qián zǐ	9g	Semen Plantaginis (wrapped)
续断	xù duàn	15g	Radix Dipsaci
当归	dāng guī	15g	Radix Angelicae Sinensis
淫羊藿	yín yáng huò	15g	Herba Epimedii
鹿角霜	lù jiǎo shuāng	6g	Cornu Cervi Degelatinatum
肉桂	ròu guì	1.5g	Cortex Cinnamomi
熟地	shú dì	12g	Radix Rehmanniae Praeparata

【Second Visit】

After 15 doses, all previous symptoms had improved. October 8th examination showed normal liquefaction time, with a sperm count of 138×10^6/ml, a survival rate of 50%, and abnormal sperm at 34%. Following another 6 doses, his spouse conceived and later gave birth to a male infant on June 15th, 1977.

(Shan Shu-jian. *Clinical Experience of Ancient and Contemporary Experts: Male Diseases*. Beijing: China Press of Traditional Chinese Medicine, 1999: 181)

5. MEDICAL RECORDS OF WANG QI

(1) Mr. Zhang, age 32.

【Initial Visit】

October 10th, 1999.

Chief complaint: Childless after 3 years of marriage.

The reproductive health of his spouse appeared normal. Routine examination showed sperm survival rates of 42% with A-grade motility at 3%, and B-grade at 15%. PH value was 7.5, liquefaction time 30 minutes, sperm density 49×10^6/ml, and abnormal sperm at 15% with 2-3 white blood cells present. Blood serum hormone levels showed FSH, LH, PRL and testosterone all within normal ranges. Physical examination revealed normal gonadal development with no varicocele present. The patient appeared underweight, with symptoms and signs of fatigue, aversion to cold, and an occasionally aching lumbus. His tongue appeared pale with a thin white coating. Pulses were deep, thready and forceless.

【Biomedical Diagnosis】

Infertility secondary to asthenospermia.

【Pattern Differentiation】

Kidney yang deficiency.

【Treatment Principle】

Warm the kidney and assist yang.

【Prescription】

Modified *Yòu Guī Wán* (右归丸).

The modified formula contains the following medicinals.

菟丝子	tù sī zǐ	20g	Semen Cuscutae
熟地	shú dì	20g	Radix Rehmanniae Praeparata
黄芪	huáng qí	20g	Radix Astragali
枸杞子	gǒu qǐ zǐ	15g	Fructus Lycii
锁阳	suǒ yáng	15g	Herba Cynomorii
鹿角胶（另烊化冲服）	lù jiǎo jiāo	10g	Colla Cornus Cervi (infused)
仙茅	xiān máo	10g	Rhizoma Curculiginis
淫羊藿	yín yáng huò	12g	Herba Epimedii
当归	dāng guī	12g	Radix Angelicae Sinensis
制附子	zhì fù zǐ	6g	Radix Aconiti Lateralis Praeparata

One divided dose, twice daily. The patient was also advised to eat *hé táo rén* (Semen Juglandis) and eel. Following 20 doses, re-examination revealed sperm survival rates of 53% with A-grade sperm at 15% and B-grade at 20%. After 50 doses of the modified formula, his wife successfully conceived and later gave birth to a female infant.

(Sun Zi-xue, Chen Jian-she. Introduction to Dr. Wang Qi's Experience in the Treatment of Male Infertility. *Journal of Sichuan Traditional Chinese Medicine*, 2004, 22(1): 7-8)

(2) Mr. Liu, age 30.

【Initial Visit】

March 3rd, 2000.

Chief complaint: Childless after 2 and one-half years of marriage.

The reproductive health of his wife appeared normal. The patient had received a previous diagnosis of oligozoospermia. Physical examination revealed grade Ⅲ varicocele on the left side, but its effect on the size and texture of the left testicle was negligible. No other obvious abnormalities were found. Sperm density was $1.2×10^6$/ml, with FSH serum levels normal. Patient reported infrequent sensations of sinking and distention of the left testicle, which became aggravated following activity. His tongue appeared dark with static spots at the margin. Pulses were deep, thready and forceless.

【Biomedical Diagnosis】

Infertility secondary to oligozoospermia.

【Pattern Differentiation】

Kidney deficiency with stasis.

【Treatment Principle】

Tonify the kidney, replenish essence, invigorate blood, and free the collaterals.

【Prescription】

Wǔ Zǐ Yǎn Zōng Wán (五子衍宗丸) modified with *Táo Hóng Sì Wù Tāng* (桃红四物汤).

The modified formula contains the following medicinals.

菟丝子	*tù sī zǐ*	30g	Semen Cuscutae
黄芪	*huáng qí*	30g	Radix Astragali
枸杞子	*gǒu qǐ zǐ*	20g	Fructus Lycii
车前子（另包）	*chē qián zǐ*	20g	Semen Plantaginis (wrapped)
熟地黄	*shú dì huáng*	20g	Radix Rehmanniae Praeparata
覆盆子	*fù pén zǐ*	15g	Fructus Rubi
五味子	*wǔ wèi zǐ*	15g	Fructus Schisandrae Chinensis
当归	*dāng guī*	15g	Radix Angelicae Sinensis
赤芍	*chì sháo*	15g	Radix Paeoniae Rubra
桃仁	*táo rén*	15g	Semen Persicae
淫羊藿	*yín yáng huò*	15g	Herba Epimedii
鹿角胶（另烊化冲服）	*lù jiǎo jiāo*	10g	Colla Cornus Cervi (infused)
红花	*hóng huā*	12g	Flos Carthami
路路通	*lù lù tōng*	25g	Fructus Liquidambaris
水蛭（研末冲服）	*shuǐ zhì*	5g	Hirudo seu Whitmania (powdered and infused)

The patient was also advised to eat *hé táo rén* (Semen Juglandis) and *huā shēng rén* (Semen Arachidis), with acrid or spicy foods and celery being contraindicated. Some counseling was given to help establish confidence and a positive mental outlook. Following 90 doses, sperm density had reached $4.8×10^6$/ml. The prescription was changed to one dose every other day, or daily as needed. After 20 doses, his spouse successfully conceived and later gave birth to a healthy male infant in May, 2001.

(Sun Zi-xue, Chen Jian-she. Introduction to Dr. Wang Qi's Experience in the Treatment of Male infertility. *Journal of Sichuan Traditional Chinese Medicine*, 2004, 22(1): 7-8)

(3) Mr. Sun, age 29.

【Initial Visit】

June 25th, 1998. No pregnancy after three years of marriage. The reproductive health of his spouse appeared normal. Semen analysis from two hospitals showed non-liquefaction within one hour. The patient appeared overweight, and physical examination revealed no genital abnormality. He reported a preference towards alcohol, and also a feeling of moisture on his scrotum. His tongue appeared red with a thick yellow coating in the middle and rear. Pulses were slippery and rapid.

【Biomedical Diagnosis】

Infertility and non-liquefaction of semen.

【Pattern Differentiation】

Brewing and binding of damp-heat.

【Treatment Principle】

Clear heat, resolve toxin, and disinhibit damp.

【Prescription】

Modified *Chéng Shì Bì Xiè Fēn Qīng Yǐn* (程氏萆薢分清饮).

The prescribed formula contains the following ingredients.

草薢	*bì xiè*	15g	Rhizoma Dioscoreae Hypoglaucae
白蔻仁	*bái kòu rén*	15g	Fructus Amomi Cardamomi
黄柏	*huáng bǎi*	12g	Cortex Phellodendri Chinensis

知母	zhī mǔ	12g	Rhizoma Anemarrhenae
生苡仁	shēng yǐ rén	20g	Semen Coicis
车前子（另包）	chē qián zǐ	20g	Semen Plantaginis (wrapped)
败酱草	bài jiàng cǎo	20g	Herba Patriniae
土茯苓	tǔ fú líng	15g	Rhizoma Smilacis Glabrae
虎杖	hǔ zhàng	15g	Rhizoma et Radix Polygoni Cuspidati
赤芍	chì sháo	15g	Radix Paeoniae Rubra
菟丝子	tù sī zǐ	15g	Semen Cuscutae
淫羊藿	yín yáng huò	10g	Herba Epimedii

One decocted dose, twice daily. The patient was advised to avoid acrid and spicy foods, and to also restrain sexual activity.

After 10 doses, *zhī mǔ* (Rhizoma Anemarrhenae) and *huáng bǎi* (Cortex Phellodendri Chinensis) were removed to avoid the possibility of decreasing sperm activity. *Shēng mài yá* (raw Fructus Hordei Germinatus) 12g and *dì lóng* (Pheretima) 12g were added. Following another 30 doses, examination showed incomplete liquefaction at one hour. After 20 doses, examination revealed complete liquefaction at 50 minutes. His spouse conceived during September, and gave birth to a healthy male infant in June, 1999.

(Sun Zi-xue, Chen Jian-she. Introduction to Dr. Wang Qi's Experience in the Treatment of Male Infertility. *Journal of Sichuan Traditional Chinese Medicine*, 2004, 22(1):7-8)

6. Medical Records of Zhang Shu-cheng

Mr. Liu, age 33.

【Initial Visit】

Childless 6 years after marriage. His right testicle had been removed nine years previous due to seminoma, following 3 courses of radiotherapy. A number of hospitals had suggested azoospermatism. Physical examination found the residual testicle obviously enlarged with a volume of 6×5×3 cm. Sexual function was reported normal, with activity 1 to 3 times per week. Three separate examinations suggested azoospermatism, with a seminal fluid volume of 2.5 to 3.5 ml.

【Biomedical Diagnosis】

Male infertility secondary to azoospermatism due to radiotherapy.

【Treatment Principle】

Fortify the spleen, course the liver, invigorate blood, and nourish the kidney.

【Prescription】

Sperm-generating medicinals.

党参	dǎng shēn	15g	Radix Codonopsis
苍术	cāng zhú	10g	Rhizoma Atractylodis
白术	bái zhú	10g	Rhizoma Atractylodis Macrocephalae
白花蛇舌草	bái huā shé shé cǎo	10g	Herba Hedyotis Diffusae
菟丝子	tù sī zǐ	15g	Semen Cuscutae
女贞子	nǚ zhēn zǐ	15g	Fructus Ligustri Lucidi
五味子	wǔ wèi zǐ	10g	Fructus Schisandrae Chinensis
韭菜子	jiǔ cài zǐ	10g	Semen Allii Tuberosi
生地	shēng dì	15g	Radix Rehmanniae
首乌	shǒu wū	15g	Radix Polygoni Multiflori
蜈蚣	wú gōng	10g	Scolopendra
水蛭	shuǐ zhì	10g	Hirudo

【Second Visit】

After three months of treatment, high numbers of abnormal and immotile sperm were observed. By month four, the amount of motile sperm had increased, but with more than 90% appearing abnormal. At month six, the sperm count markedly increased to reach 0.25×10^6/ml, with motility rates of 40%. A-grade and B-grade sperm remained below 10%, with abnormal morphology present in 85%. Month seven showed sperm counts of 3×10^6/ml, abnormality rates of 70%, and motility reaching 55%-60%. The A-grade and B-grade counts reached 20% and 40%. His spouse achieved pregnancy during month eight, later giving birth to a healthy male infant. The child was found to be in good health at an 18 month follow-up exam.

(Zhang Shu-cheng, He Bin, Wang Hong-yi, et al. Exploring the Potential of Chinese Traditional Medicine on Spermatogonial Stem Cells. *Chinese Journal of Basic Medicine in Traditional Chinese Medicine*, 2001, 10(1):78)

7. MEDICAL RECORDS OF QI GUANG-CHONG

(1) Mr. Zhao, age 33.

【Initial Visit】

No pregnancy 3 years after marriage. Presenting signs and symptoms included deficient obesity, fatigue, poor appetite, and a bitter taste in the mouth. His tongue appeared pale red with teeth marks at the margins and a white slimy coating. Pulses were slippery.

CASA examination: seminal fluid appeared grayish white with a volume of 6.0 ml, liquefaction time at 60 minutes, a sperm count of 16×10^6/ml, and a grade IV motility rate of 18%. The biomedical diagnosis was male infertility secondary to asthenospermia and non-liquefaction of sperm.

【Pattern Differentiation】

Internal disturbance of phlegm turbidity.

【Treatment Principle】

Transform phlegm, eliminate turbidity, and benefit essence.

【Prescription】

Modified *Huà Jīng Jiān* (化精煎).

苍术	*cāng zhú*	10g	Rhizoma Atractylodis
姜半夏	*jiāng bàn xià*	10g	Rhizome Pinelliae Praeparata
厚朴	*hòu pò*	10g	Cortex Magnoliae Officinalis
胆南星	*dǎn nán xīng*	10g	Arisaema cum Bile
橘红	*jú hóng*	10g	Exocarpium Citri Rubrum

枳实	zhǐ shí	10g	Fructus Aurantii Immaturus
竹茹	zhú rú	10g	Caulis Bambusae in Taenia
石菖蒲	shí chāng pú	10g	Rhizoma Acori Tatarinowii
茯苓	fú líng	10g	Poria
生姜	shēng jiāng	10g	Rhizoma Zingiberis Recens
甘草	gān cǎo	3g	Radix et Rhizoma Glycyrrhizae

【Second Visit】

June 18th.The liquefaction period reached 40 minutes. The previous prescription was continued.

【Third Visit】

July 20th. Examination revealed a seminal volume of 4 ml with a liquefaction period of 20 minutes. The sperm count reached $73×10^6$/ml, motility rates 55%, and grade IV sperm 29%.

(Ma Chuan-fang. Experiences of Qi Guang-chong in the Diagnosis and Treatment of Male Infertility due to Non-liquefaction of Semen. *Jiangxi Journal of Traditional Chinese Medicine*, 2001, 32 (10): 18)

(2) Mr. Liu, age 31.

【Initial Visit】

December 8th, 1999. CASA examination: seminal fluid volume of 1.5 ml with a liquefaction period of 60 minutes. The sperm count reached $54×10^6$/ml, motility rates 37%, and grade I motility 19%. Grade I varicocele was also present on the left side. His tongue appeared red with a white slimy coating. Pulses were slippery and rapid.

【Prescription】

Modified *Qīng Jīng Jiān* (清精煎).

白花蛇舌草	bái huā shé shé cǎo	15g	Herba Hedyotis Diffusae
红藤	hóng téng	15g	Caulis Sargentodoxae
萆薢	bì xiè	10g	Rhizoma Dioscoreae Hypoglaucae
柴胡	chái hú	10g	Radix Bupleuri
黄柏	huáng bǎi	10g	Cortex Phellodendri Chinensis

知母	zhī mǔ	10g	Rhizoma Anemarrhenae
制大黄	zhì dà huáng	10g	Radix et Rhizoma Rhei Praeparata
丹皮	dān pí	10g	Cortex Moutan
王不留行（包煎）	wáng bù liú xíng	10g	Semen Vaccariae (wrapped)
车前子（包煎）	chē qián zǐ	15g	Semen Plantaginis (wrapped)
丹参	dān shēn	15g	Radix et Rhizoma Salviae Miltiorrhizae
碧玉散（包煎）	Bì Yù Sǎn	15g	Green Jade Powder (wrapped)

【Second Visit】

The prescription was continued for four weeks until the following visit on January 3rd, 2000.

CASA examination results: seminal fluid volume of 2.5 ml with a liquefaction period of 20 minutes. Sperm counts reached $62×10^6$/ml, motility rates 27%, and grade Ⅰ motility rates 19%. The previous formula was continued for another 2 months. The patient later reported that his spouse had become pregnant near the end of February.

(Ma Chuan-fang. Experiences of Qi Guang-chong in the Diagnosis and Treatment of Male Infertility due to Non-liquefaction of Semen. *Jiangxi Journal of Traditional Chinese Medicine*, 2001, 32 (5): 18, 19)

(3) Mr. He, age 45.

【Initial Visit】

March 24th, 1999. CASA examination results: seminal fluid appeared slightly yellow, with a volume of 2.0 ml. Liquefaction time was over 60 minutes, with sperm counts of $40×10^6$/ml and grade Ⅰ motility rates at 19%. His tongue appeared dark red with teeth marks at the margins and a thin white coating. Pulses were thready and wiry. This presentation indicates a pattern of static blood obstructing the lower.

【Treatment Principle】

Invigorate blood, transform stasis, and free the essence.

【Prescription】

Modified *Tōng Jīng Jiān* (通精煎).

丹参	dān shēn	15g	Radix et Rhizoma Salviae Miltiorrhizae
桃仁	táo rén	10g	Semen Persicae
莪术	é zhú	15g	Rhizoma Curcumae
川牛膝	chuān niú xī	15g	Radix Cyathulae
当归	dāng guī	10g	Radix Angelicae Sinensis
柴胡	chái hú	10g	Radix Bupleuri
黄芪	huáng qí	20g	Radix Astragali
生牡蛎（先煎）	shēng mǔ lì	30g	Concha Ostreae Cruda (decoct first)

【Second Visit】

May 19th. Re-examination showed a liquefaction period of 50 minutes. The formula was continued, with the addition of sān qī fěn (Radix et Rhizoma Notoginseng powder) 4g (taken twice daily by mouth), and zhì shǒu wū (Radix Polygoni Multiflori Praeparata cum Succo Glycines Sotae) 15g.

【Third Visit】

June 16th. His tongue appeared slightly dark with a thin white coating, and pulses were thready. Seminal fluid volume reached 3 ml, with a liquefaction period of 15 minutes. Sperm counts reached $92×10^6$/ml with grade I motility rates at 36%, and an overall motility rate of 80%. The former prescription was continued with the addition of Bǔ Zhōng Yì Qì Wán (补中益气丸) 8g, to be taken 2 or 3 times daily.

(Ma Chuan-fang. Experiences of Qi Guang-chong in the Diagnosis and Treatment of Male Infertility due to Non-liquefaction of Semen. *Jiangxi Journal of Traditional Chinese Medicine*, 2001, 32 (5): 18, 19)

(4) Mr. Hu, age 33.

【Initial Visit】

January 8th, 1999.

Chief complaint: No pregnancy three years after marriage.

The patient had been diagnosed with non-liquefaction of semen. Previous treatment with both Chinese medicinals and biomedicine had been unremarkable. His sexual desire was quite low, with activity only once each month, and with some degree of erectile dysfunction. He also reported aching of the lumbus with limp knees. The tongue appeared pale with a thin white coating, and pulses were thready.

CASA examination revealed a seminal volume of 1.5 ml, liquefaction period of 60 minutes, sperm count of 44×10^6/ml, motility rate of 80%, and grade I motility at 27%.

The presenting pattern here is kidney essence insufficiency. The treatment method is to warm yang and tonify the kidney to invigorate essence.

【Prescription】

Modified *Qiáng Jīng Jiān* (强精煎).

炒带子蜂房	chǎo dài zǐ fēng fáng	15g	Vespae Nidus (with spawn, stir-fried)
淫羊藿	yín yáng huò	15g	Herba Epimedii
鹿角片（先煎）	lù jiǎo piàn	10g	Cornu Cervi (sliced, decocted first)
肉苁蓉	ròu cōng róng	10g	Herba Cistanches
锁阳	suǒ yáng	10g	Herba Cynomorii
沙苑子	shā yuàn zǐ	10g	Semen Astragali Complanati
当归	dāng guī	10g	Radix Angelicae Sinensis
熟地	shú dì	15g	Radix Rehmanniae Praeparata
黄精	huáng jīng	15g	Rhizoma Polygonati
何首乌	hé shǒu wū	15g	Radix Polygoni Multiflori
川断	chuān duàn	10g	Radix Dipsaci
大枣	dà zǎo	20g	Fructus Jujubae

【Second Visit】

May 28th. After more than 2 months, the CASA examination revealed a seminal fluid volume reaching 4.5 ml, sperm count of 40×10^6/ml, a liquefaction period at 20 minutes, and motility rates of 60% with grade I motility at 40%. He also reported that his wife had successfully achieved pregnancy since his last visit.

(Ma Chuan-fang. Experiences of Qi Guang-chong in the Diagnosis and Treatment of Male Infertility due to Non-liquefaction of Semen. *Jiangxi Journal of Traditional Chinese Medicine*, 2001, 32 (5): 18, 19)

(5) Mr. Chen, age 31.

【**Initial Visit**】

April 20th, 1997. No pregnancy after 5 years of marriage, with the condition of his spouse appearing normal. Several past semen analyses all revealed non-liquefaction of semen. The results of previous biomedical and Chinese medicinal treatments were all unremarkable.

Symptoms and signs included tinnitus, dry mouth with the desire to drink, and night sweating, especially after sexual activity. His tongue appeared red with little coating.

CASA examination revealed a seminal fluid volume of 1.5 ml, liquefaction time over 60 minutes, a sperm count of 61×10^6/ml, and a motility rate of 42% with grade I motility at 19%.

【**Pattern Differentiation**】

Effulgent yin deficiency fire scorching the essence chamber with brewing turbidity.

【**Treatment Principle**】

Nourish yin and downbear fire to engender essence.

【**Prescription**】

Modified *Zī Jīng Jiān* (滋精煎) .

天冬	*tiān dōng*	10g	Radix Asparagi
麦冬	*mài dōng*	10g	Radix Ophiopogonis
生地	*shēng dì*	15g	Radix Rehmanniae
熟地	*shú dì*	15g	Radix Rehmanniae Praeparata
山茱萸	*shān zhū yú*	10g	Fructus Corni
山药	*shān yào*	10g	Rhizoma Dioscoreae
知母	*zhī mǔ*	10g	Rhizoma Anemarrhenae
丹皮	*dān pí*	10g	Cortex Moutan
炙龟板 (先煎)	*zhì guī bǎn*	10g	Carapax et Plastrum Testudinis Praeparata cum Melle (decoct first)

炙鳖甲（先煎）	zhì biē jiǎ	10g	Carapax Trionycis Praeparata cum Melle (decoct first)
赤芍	chì sháo	10g	Radix Paeoniae Rubra
白芍	bái sháo	10g	Radix Paeoniae Alba
甘草	gān cǎo	3g	Radix et Rhizoma Glycyrrhizae

【Second Visit】

May 18th. CASA revealed a seminal volume of 2.5 ml, liquefaction time of 30 minutes, sperm count of $65×10^6$/ml, and motility rates of 62% with grade I motility at 19%. The symptoms of effulgent yin deficiency fire had been relieved to some degree, so the previous formula was continued.

After one month, CASA examination showed a liquefaction period of 20 minutes, with sperm counts and motility rates also improved. *Dà Bǔ Yīn Wán* (大补阴丸) and *Jīn Guì Shèn Qì Wán* (金匮肾气丸) were then prescribed at 6g each, three times daily.

Three months later his spouse conceived and later gave birth to a healthy male infant.

(Ma Chuan-fang. Experiences of Qi Guang-chong in the Diagnosis and Treatment of Male Infertility due to Non-liquefaction of Semen. *Jiangxi Journal of Traditional Chinese Medicine*, 2001, 32 (5): 18, 19)

8. MEDICAL RECORDS OF XU FU-SONG

(1) Mr. Liu, age 34.

【Initial Visit】

No pregnancy 6 years after marriage even though the reproduction health of his wife appeared normal. The semen analyses were as follows: seminal fluid volume 3 ml, pH value 7.4, liquefaction period 40 minutes, sperm density $177.08×10^6$/ml, survival rate 25.3%, and a+b+c+d was 4.85%+ 13.40%+7.38%+74.87%.

【Biomedical Diagnosis】

Male infertility secondary to oligospermia and non-liquefaction of sperm.

【Pattern Differentiation】

Kidney essence insufficiency.

【Treatment Principle】

Tonify kidney and nourish essence.

【Prescription】

Jù Jīng Tāng (聚精汤).

地黄	*dì huáng*	15g	Radix Rehmanniae Recens
何首乌	*hé shǒu wū*	15g	Radix Polygoni Multiflori
沙苑子	*shā yuàn zǐ*	10g	Semen Astragali Complanati
枸杞子	*gǒu qǐ zǐ*	15g	Fructus Lycii
茯苓	*fú líng*	15g	Poria
薏苡仁	*yì yǐ rén*	15g	Semen Coicis
巴戟天	*bā jǐ tiān*	10g	Radix Morindae Officinalis

【Second Visit】

The results of semen analysis were as follows: seminal fluid volume 3.8 ml, pH value 7.4, liquefaction period 30 minutes, sperm density 170.14×10^6/ml, sperm survival rate 52.94%, and a+b+c+d was 34.80%+13.73%+4.41%+47.06%.

(Zheng Hui-nan, Yang Wen-tao, Xu Fu-song. Clinical observation of *Ju Jing Tang* in the Treatment of 50 Cases of Male Infertility. *Research of Traditional Chinese Medicine*, 2002, 18 (4): 3)

(2) Mr. Yan, age 28.

【Initial Visit】

April 6th, 1988. No pregnancy after 4 years of marriage. The patient reported normal sexual activity, and gynecological examination of his spouse suggested no abnormality. Routine seminal analysis was also within normal range. However, antisperm antibody (AsAb) in the blood serum tested positive (1:16).

Signs and symptoms included thirst with a desire to drink, night sweating, aching and limp lumbus, dizziness, tinnitus, dripping urination, and bound stool. His tongue appeared red with little coating. Pulses were wiry, thready and slightly rapid. The patient also appeared slightly underweight.

【Pattern Differentiation】

Yin deficiency and damp-heat of the liver and kidney.

【Treatment Principle】

Nourish yin, downbear fire, and disinhibit and clear damp-heat.

【Prescription】

Modified *Zhī Bǎi Dì Huáng Tāng* (知柏地黄汤).

【Second Visit】

After 3 months, serum AsAb tested negative, and semen analysis results were normal. The previous methods were continued for two more months in order to strengthen the therapeutic effect. At this point his spouse became pregnant and later gave birth to a healthy male infant.

(Shan Shu-jian. *Clinical Experience of Ancient and Contemporary Experts: Male Diseases*. Beijing: China Press of Traditional Chinese Medicine, 1999: 208, 209)

(3) Mr. Zhang, age 36.

【Initial Visit】

June 14th, 1988.

No pregnancy after 5 years of marriage. The patient reported normal sexual activity, and semen analysis revealed normal sperm. Gynecological examination of his spouse also suggested no abnormality. He had been treated at several hospitals with both biomedicines and Chinese medicinals for more than 3 years, but without result.

Serum AsAb levels had been examined in both parties, and results showed the spouse negative with the patient testing positive (1:16). After 6 months and two treatment courses with prednisone with Chinese medicinals, there had been little result.

Signs and symptoms included loose stool, yellow urine, aching weakness of the lumbus, dull pain of the left lower abdomen, a bland taste, reduced food intake, and a lusterless facial complexion. His tongue appeared red with a thin white and slightly yellow coating. Pulses were thready and weak. The patient reported often catching colds, and he also appeared overweight.

【Pattern Differentiation】

Lung and spleen dual deficiency with internal brewing of damp-heat.

【Treatment Principle】

Tonify the lung, fortify the spleen, clear the intestines, and purge heat.

【Prescription】

Shēn Líng Bái zhú Wán (参苓白术丸) and *Xiāng Lián Wán* (香连丸). To be decocted once daily.

【Second Visit】

After 3 months, the patient reported normal stools and other symptomatic improvement, with no occurrence of influenza. Serum AsAb had tested negative, and semen analysis results were also within normal ranges. The previous formula was continued in order to strengthen the therapeutic effect. At a follow-up visit in December 1989, the patient reported that his spouse had successfully given birth to a healthy daughter.

(Shan Shu-jian. *Clinical Experience of Ancient and Contemporary Experts: Male Diseases*. Beijing: China Press of Traditional Chinese Medicine, 1999: 209)

(4) Mr. Zhang, age 35.

【Initial Visit】

Chief complaint: No pregnancy 5 years after marriage.

The patient reported normal sexual activity, and semen analysis results were within normal ranges. Serum AsAb testing was positive. The main symptoms included fatigue, occasional tinnitus, dry mouth, and an aching lumbus with limp legs. His tongue appeared red with little coating. Pulses were thready and rapid.

【Biomedical Diagnosis】

Male immune infertility.

【Pattern Differentiation】

Liver and kidney yin deficiency.

【Treatment Principle】

Nourish and tonify the kidney and liver.

【Prescription】

Liù Wèi Dì Huáng Wán (六味地黄丸) modified with *Dà Bǔ Yīn Wán* (大补阴丸).

生地黄	*shēng dì huáng*	10g	Radix Rehmanniae Recens
熟地黄	*shú dì huáng*	10g	Radix Rehmanniae Praeparata
泽泻	*zé xiè*	10g	Rhizoma Alismatis
牡丹皮	*mǔ dān pí*	10g	Cortex Moutan
山茱萸	*shān zhū yú*	10g	Fructus Corni
枸杞子	*gǒu qǐ zǐ*	10g	Fructus Lycii
黄精	*huáng jīng*	10g	Rhizoma Polygonati
山药	*shān yào*	10g	Rhizoma Dioscoreae
知母	*zhī mǔ*	10g	Rhizoma Anemarrhenae
鳖甲	*biē jiǎ*	30g	Carapax Trionycis
牡砺	*mǔ lì*	30g	Concha Ostreae
瘪桃干	*biē táo gān*	15g	Prunus persica (L.) Batsch
碧玉散	*Bì Yù Sǎn*	15g	Green Jade Powder

【Second Visit】

After 4 months, semen analysis and serum AsAb tested normal. Treatment was continued for 2 months, at which time his spouse achieved a successful pregnancy.

(Xu Yong-jian, Wang Jiu-kuan. Experiences of Dr. Xu Fu-song in the Treatment of Male infertility According to Syndrome Differentiation. *New*

Journal of Traditional Chinese Medicine, 1997, (5): 7

9. Medical Records of Xie Hai-zhou

Mr. Yang, age 34.

【Initial Visit】

No pregnancy 10 years after marriage. Signs and symptoms included impotence, premature ejaculation, aching lumbus, lassitude of the spirit and general fatigue. His tongue appeared enlarged and tender with teeth marks. Pulses were weak, particularly at both *chi* positions. Semen analysis showed sperm survival rates of only 10%-20%.

【Pattern Differentiation】

Kidney yang debilitation with yin essence depletion.

【Treatment Principle】

Warm the kidney, invigorate yang, benefit yin, and replenish essence.

【Prescription】

Jiǔ Zǐ Wán (韭子丸) modified with *Wǔ Zǐ Yǎn Zōng Wán* (五子衍宗丸).
The prescribed formula contains the following medicinals.

海狗肾	*hǎi gǒu shèn*	1 pair	Callorhini Testes et Penis
韭菜子	*jiǔ cài zǐ*	15g	Semen Allii Tuberosi
蛇床子	*shé chuáng zǐ*	10g	Fructus Cnidii
五味子	*wǔ wèi zǐ*	10g	Fructus Schisandrae Chinensis
菟丝子	*tù sī zǐ*	30g	Semen Cuscutae
补骨脂	*bǔ gǔ zhī*	12g	Fructus Psoraleae
桑螵蛸	*sāng piāo xiāo*	30g	Oötheca Mantidis
覆盆子	*fù pén zǐ*	15g	Fructus Rubi
生山药	*shēng shān yào*	15g	Rhizoma Dioscoreae
车前子	*chē qián zǐ*	9g	Semen Plantaginis
盐炒知母	*yán chǎo zhī mǔ*	9g	Rhizoma Anemarrhenae (Stir-fried with salt)
盐炒黄柏	*yán chǎo huáng bǎi*	9g	Cortex Phellodendri Chinensis (Stir-fried with salt)
全当归	*quán dāng guī*	12g	Radix Angelicae Sinensis

【Second Visit】

The patient was advised to restrain sexual activity, and to also lead a more regular lifestyle. Following 60 doses, impotence and premature ejaculation resolved, the spirit improved, pulses became more powerful, and the survival rate of sperm increased to 70%.

Shú dì (Radix Rehmanniae Praeparata), *bái sháo* (Radix Paeoniae Alba) and *shān yú ròu* (Fructus Corni) were added to further nourish yin and benefit essence. 30 doses were prescribed.

【Third Visit】

For the next course of treatment, *zhī mǔ* (Cortex Phellodendri Chinensis) and *huáng bǎi* (Cortex Phellodendri Chinensis) were removed, and *qiāng huó* (Rhizoma et Radix Notopterygii), *yì mǔ cǎo* (Herba Leonuri), *dān pí* (Cortex Moutan) and *chuān xiōng* (Rhizoma Chuanxiong) were added. 20 doses were prescribed.

Following a total of 110 doses, all symptoms had resolved and the sperm survival rate reached 80%-90%. The patient eventually reported that his spouse had successfully conceived.

(Shan Shu-jian. *Clinical Experience of Ancient and Contemporary Experts: Male Diseases*. Beijing: China Press of Traditional Chinese Medicine, 1999: 176)

10. MEDICAL RECORDS OF XUE MENG

(1) Congenital Disease with Exhaustion of Kidney Water (Absent Emission)

Mr. Li, age 41.

【Initial Visit】

No pregnancy after more than 10 years of marriage. The patient had been underdeveloped when he was younger, and now appeared underweight. Seminal emission was absent during sexual activity. He was able to achieve erection in the early mornings, but he was unable to maintain it for very long. Biomedical treatments, Chinese medicinals, acupuncture, moxibustion, and qigong had all been ineffective. Prostate massage was unable to produce seminal fluid, so a semen examination had not been performed.

Symptoms and signs included yellow complexion, lassitude, aching lumbus, and reduced food intake. His tongue appeared crimson with a thin coating. Pulses were wiry and thin, deep and weak at the left *chi* position.

【Pattern Differentiation】

This presentation indicates a pattern of congenital kidney yin deficiency failing to restrain ministerial fire. As the fire continues to stir, true yin becomes more depleted. Reproduction is not possible without a sufficient source of water.

【Prescription】

During the first stage of treatment, *Zhù Yìng Zī Shēng Tāng* (助应资生 汤) was prescribed with added *shí chāng pú* (Rhizoma Acori Tatarinowii) 9g, *zhì yuǎn zhì* (Radix Polygalae Praeparata cum Melle) 9g, *lù lù tōng* (Fructus Liquidambaris) 9g, *chǎo zhī mǔ* (stir-fried Rhizoma Anemarrhenae) 10g, *zhì biē jiǎ* (Carapax Trionycis Praeparata cum Melle) 18g, and *zhì guī bǎn* (Carapax et Plastrum Testudinis Praeparata cum Melle) 18g.

【Second Visit】

Appetite was greatly improved after 10 doses, and his complexion appeared moist with a healthy red color. He was also able to maintain an erection, and seminal emission appeared.

Qiáng Jīng Yì Shèn Jiāo Náng (强 精 益 肾 胶 囊) was then prescribed along with with *Guī Líng Jí* (龟龄集). His spouse conceived after 2 months, and later gave birth to a healthy male infant.

(Shan Shu-jian. *Clinical Experience of Ancient and Contemporary Experts: Male Diseases*. Beijing: China Press of Traditional Chinese Medicine, 1999: 184)

(2) Excessive Seminal Leakage Leading to Kidney Origin Impairment (Spermatorrhea)

Mr. Ji, age 27.

Childless after four years after marriage. Examination of his spouse revealed no abnormality. The patient reported a history of excessive masturbation in the past. He complained of long-term seminal emission at a frequency of 7 to 8 times per month, sometimes with sexual dreams. He also reported some sexual dysfunction and an indifferent attitude toward sexuality.

Examination: Seminal fluid appeared thin with a sperm count of 360×10^4/ml, sperm survival rates of 20%, and a motility rate of 35%.

Symptoms and signs included aching lumbus with limp knees, dizziness, blurred vision, physical cold, and general fatigue. His tongue appeared pale. Pulses were deep, thready and rapid.

This syndrome is associated with long-term spermatorrhea. The kidney fails to store essence, leading to a condition of deficiency taxation. *Zhù Yìng Zī Shēng Tāng* (助应资生汤) was selected to tonify the kidney, support yang, and secure the root.

Sāng piāo xiāo (Oötheca Mantidis) 9g, *cì wèi pí* (Erinacei Pellis) 9g, *duàn lóng gǔ* (calcined Os Draconis) 18g, and *duàn mǔ lì* (calcined Concha Ostreae) 18g were added to astringe the lower origin. *Qiáng Jīng Yì Shèn Wán* (强精益肾丸) was also selected to replenish essence.

Soon after, the symptom of seminal emission resolved completely. After 3 months, his spouse became pregnant and later gave birth to a gave birth healthy female infant.

(Chan Shu-jian. *Clinical Experience of Ancient and Contemporary Experts: Male Diseases*. Beijing: China Press of Traditional Chinese Medicine, 1999: 185)

(3) Forceless Erection Due to Kidney Yang Insufficiency (Impotence)

Mr. Zhang, age 32.

No pregnancy after five years of marriage. Patient reports a history of powerless erections during sexual intercourse. The erections were originally strong at the beginning, but could not be maintained over time. His condition gradually led to functional impotence, with only partial and temporary erection.

Examination: Reduced sperm counts with very low motility, poor liquefaction time.

Urination, defecation, and diet were all reported normal. Complexion appeared darkish, and his voice quality was low and deep. His tongue appeared pale with a thin coating. Pulses were thready and slow.

Chorionic gonadotropin, *Lù Róng Jīng* (鹿茸精) injections and *Nán Bǎo* (男宝) had been administered without obvious effect.

This presentation indicates a pattern of kidney qi deficiency cold leading to slackness of the ancestral sinew.

The prescribed formula contained the following medicinals.

Zhù Yìng Zī Shēng Tāng (助应资生汤) with added *dǎng shēn* (Radix Codonopsis) 30g, *lù jiǎo jiāo* (Colla Cornus Cervi) (infused) 9g, *xiǎo huí xiāng* (Fructus Foeniculi) 9g, *shú dì* (Radix Rehmanniae Praeparata) 18g, *bǔ gǔ zhī* (Fructus Psoraleae) 12g, and *dà wú gōng* (Scolopendra), 3 pieces.

After 6 weeks, treatment continued with the formula *Qiáng Jīng Yì Shèn Wán* (强精益肾丸). The patient later reported that he no longer suffered from impotence, and that his spouse had recently become pregnant.

(Shan Shu-jian. *Clinical Experience of Ancient and Contemporary Experts: Male Diseases*. Beijing: China Press of Traditional Chinese Medicine, 1999: 185)

(4) Damp-Heat Pouring Downward Leading to True Essence Turbidity (Prostatitis)

Mr. Zhou, age 36.

No pregnancy after 6 years of marriage. Symptoms and signs included aching lumbus, abdominal distention, frequent incontinence in very small amounts, and urinary urgency. He reported an occasional pulling sensation and spasm of the testicles, and a moist scrotum. A white secretion obstructing the urinary meatus often appeared with a stabbing pain in the penis. He had been previously diagnosed with chronic prostatitis.

The TCM pattern indicates taxation strangury.

Examination: Seminal fluid appeared white and cream-colored, with a volume of 2 ml. The sperm survival rate was 30% with grade III motility, and a sperm liquefaction period of 31 minutes. Prostate examination also revealed lower than normal lecithin levels. The tongue coating appeared greasy at the root. Pulses were soggy and thready.

This case seemed to confirm a statement from the *Yellow Emperor's Inner Classic:* "Excessive sexual desire leads to excessive sexual activity. Slackness of the ancestral sinew and wilting will then occur, accompanied by a white discharge."

This presentation indicates a pattern of lower burner damp-heat attacking the essence and kidney. The primary treatment method here is to tonify, but only with the proper application of discharging medicinals. First eliminate excess, and then tonify deficiency. Tonification without discharging will "strengthen excess" in this case, which is always contraindicated.

Zhù Yìng Zī Shēng Tāng (助应资生汤) and *Zhī Bǎi Dì Huáng Wán* (知柏地黄丸) were selected.

The prescribed formula contains the following medicinals.

生黄芪	shēng huáng qí	30g	Radix Astragali (raw)
白茅根	bái máo gēn	30g	Rhizoma Imperatae
生地	shēng dì	18g	Radix Rehmanniae
熟地	shú dì	18g	Radix Rehmanniae Praeparata
山萸肉	shān yú ròu	15g	Fructus Corni
扁蓄	biǎn xù	15g	Herba Polygoni Avicularis
瞿麦	qú mài	15g	Herba Dianthi

薜荔果	*xuē lì guǒ*	15g	Ficus Pumila L
白花蛇舌草	*bái huā shé shé cǎo*	15g	Herba Hedyotis Diffusae
莪术	*é zhú*	12g	Rhizoma Curcumae
菟丝子	*tù sī zǐ*	12g	Semen Cuscutae
桑寄生	*sāng jì shēng*	12g	Herba Taxilli
炒知母	*chǎo zhī mǔ*	12g	Rhizoma Anemarrhenae
黄柏	*huáng bǎi*	12g	Cortex Phellodendri Chinensis

Following 40 doses, aching of the lumbus and abdominal distention were resolved, and urinination returned to normal. At a one year follow-up visit, he reported that his previous complaints had not returned, and also that his spouse had recently given birth.

【Attachment】

A. *Zhù Yìng Zī Shēng Tāng* (助应资生汤) contains the following ingredients.

潼蒺藜	*tóng jí lí*	20g	Semen Astragali Complanati
枸杞子	*gǒu qǐ zǐ*	20g	Fructus Lycii
仙茅	*xiān máo*	20g	Rhizoma Curculiginis
菟丝子	*tù sī zǐ*	20g	Semen Cuscutae
薏米	*yì mǐ*	20g	Semen Coicis
清炙黄芪	*qīng zhì huáng qí*	30g	Radix Astragali Praeparata cum Melle
淫羊藿	*yín yáng huò*	30g	Herba Epimedii
当归	*dāng guī*	15g	Radix Angelicae Sinensis
胡芦巴	*hú lú bā*	15g	Semen Foeni-Graeci
巴戟肉	*bā jǐ ròu*	15g	Radix Morindae Officinalis
韭菜子	*jiǔ cài zǐ*	15g	Semen Allii Tuberosi
北沙参	*běi shā shēn*	15g	Radix Glehniae
大蜈蚣（不去头足，忌经炉火烘焙）	*dà wú gōng (head and feet unbaked)*	3 pieces	Scolopendra

B. *Qiáng Jīng Yì Shèn Wán* (强精益肾丸)

| 潼蒺藜 | *tóng jí lí* | 60g | Semen Astragali Complanati |
| 枸杞子 | *gǒu qǐ zǐ* | 60g | Fructus Lycii |

仙茅	xiān máo	60g	Rhizoma Curculiginis
菟丝子	tù sī zǐ	60g	Semen Cuscutae
薏苡仁	yì yǐ rén	60g	Semen Coicis
清炙黄芪	qīng zhì huáng qí	90g	Radix Astragali Praeparata cum Melle
淫羊藿	yín yáng huò	90g	Herba Epimedii
北沙参	běi shā shēn	45g	Radix Glehniae
熟地	shú dì	60g	Radix Rehmanniae Praeparata
肉苁蓉	ròu cōng róng	45g	Herba Cistanches
阳起石	yáng qǐ shí	45g	Actinolitum
鱼鳔胶	yú biào jiāo	500g	Piscis Vesica Aeris
羊睾丸	yáng gāo wán	2 pairs	sheep testicle
猪脊髓	zhū jǐ suǐ	5 pieces	pig marrow
羊脊髓	yáng jǐ suǐ	5 pieces	sheep marrow
大蜈蚣	dà wú gōng	9 pieces	Scolopendra

Grind the medicinals and make honeyed pills, 15g twice daily. The powder may also be encapsulated, 15 capsules twice daily. Smoking and drinking are prohibited, and sexual activity should be restrained. Acrid or spicy foods are also contraindicated.

(Shan Shu-jian. *Clinical Experience of Ancient and Contemporary Experts: Male Diseases*. Beijing: China Press of Traditional Chinese Medicine, 1999: 186)

11. Medical Records of Yang Zong-meng

Mr. Huang complained of being childless after seven years of marriage.

Examination in the urology department revealed a sperm count of 800×10^4 per ml, with 10 to 15 WBC and few RBC present. *Jīn Guì Shèn Qì Wán* (金匮肾气丸) and *Nán Bǎo* (男宝) had been taken along with chorionic gonadotropin injections for a long period of time. Sperm count fluctuated, but never reaching 60×10^6/ml.

His tongue appeared dark red with a thin yellow coating. Pulses were deep, wiry, thready and rapid. Patient also reported morning diarrhea persisting for several years.

This presentation indicates a pattern of liver constraint transforming into heat disturbing the essence chamber, manifesting with premature ejaculation. The essence contained in the associated viscera had also become damaged, resulting in low sperm counts and infertility.

Dān Zhī Xiāo Yáo Sǎn (丹栀逍遥散) was first selected. Modifications included the addition of *zhú yè* (Folium bambusae), *zhī mǔ* (Rhizoma Anemarrhenae), *fáng fēng* (Radix Saposhnikoviae), and *chǎo yīn chén* (stir-fried Herba Artemisiae Scopariae). *Bái zhú* (Rhizoma Atractylodis Macrocephalae) was removed, and *bái fú líng* (Poria) was replaced with *tǔ fú líng* (Rhizoma Smilacis Glabrae).

After 7 doses, the signs of heat affecting the heart and spleen had become resolved. Sperm count also had increased slightly, reaching 20×10^6/ml.

At this point, the formula was changed to *Zhī Bǎi Dì Huáng Tāng* (知柏地黄汤) modified with *dān pí* (Cortex Moutan), *chì fú líng* (Poria Rubra) and *qīng yán* (Halitum) added, and *tǔ fú líng* (Rhizoma Smilacis Glabrae) removed. At dose 20, all symptoms were relieved. Sperm count also remained between 60×10^6 and 1000×10^6/ml. Soon after, the patient reported that his spouse had successfully conceived.

(Shan Shu-jian. *Clinical Experience of Ancient and Contemporary Experts: Male Diseases*. Beijing: China Press of Traditional Chinese Medicine, 1999: 187)

12. MEDICAL RECORDS OF LI PEI-SHENG

(1) Mr. Li, age 20.

The patient reported a lack of sexual desire for many years. His medical history revealed that he had suffered from chronic fright wind during childhood, which contributed to a condition of physical deficiency and underdevelopment. Presenting signs and symptoms included intellectual torpor, pale complexion, coldness of the limbs, and a preference for warmth with an aversion to cold. Pulses were thready and weak.

This presentation indicates a pattern of kidney yang deficiency manifesting with male infertility. The treatment principle involves warming and tonification of kidney yang to benefit essence, replenish marrow, and promote sexual function.

Fù Zǐ Tāng (附子汤) was modified with the following medicinals: *yín yáng huò* (Herba Epimedii), *xiān máo* (Rhizoma Curculiginis), *lù jiǎo jiāo* (Colla Cornus Cervi), *guī jiǎ jiāo* (Colla Carapax et Plastrum Testudinis), *chǎo dù zhòng* (Cortex Eucommiae), *sāng shèn zǐ* (Fructus Mori), *tù sī zǐ* (Semen Cuscutae), *wǔ wèi zǐ* (Fructus Schisandrae Chinensis), *gǒu qǐ zǐ* (Fructus Lycii), *bǔ gǔ zhī* (Fructus Psoraleae), *hú táo ròu* (Juglandis Semen), *sāng piāo xiāo* (Oötheca Mantidis), *ròu cōng róng* (Herba Cistanches) and *shú dì* (Radix Rehmanniae Praeparata).

After two years of treatment, the patient displayed greater vitality and his sexual function also returned. His spouse eventually conceived and later gave birth.

(Shan Shu-jian. Clinical Experience of Ancient and Contemporary Experts: Male Diseases. Beijing: China Press of Traditional Chinese Medicine, 1999: 190)

(2) Mr. Zhou, age 30.

The patient complained of being childless after many years of marriage. Signs and symptoms included tidal reddening of the face, vexing heat in the five hearts, irritability, thirst, and disturbed sleep. His tongue appeared crimson with a yellow coating. Pulses were thready and rapid.

This presentation clearly indicates interior heat due to yin deficiency.

Medical history revealed that the patient had masturbated excessively during adolescence, also experiencing frequent nocturnal emission. Sexual activity remained excessive after marriage, eventually leading to poor erection and thin semen.

The treatment principle here is to primarily foster yin and replenish the middle, while secondarily downbearing fire with bitter and cold medicinals. By doing so, yang will not become hyperactive, and yin will remain stored.

Prescription: *Zhī Bǎi Dì Huáng Tāng* (知柏地黄汤) modified with *bái wéi* (Radix et Rhizoma Cynanchi Atrati), *zhì guī bǎn* (Carapax et Plastrum), *tiān dōng* (Radix Asparagi), *bái sháo* (Radix Paeoniae Alba), and *chǎo tù sī zǐ* (stir-fried Semen Cuscutae).

The patient was advised to remain abstinent, and also counseled to cultivate a positive attitude. He returned to the clinic after having taken 20 doses over a period of one month. The symptoms of yin deficiency and internal heat had become alleviated.

Jí Líng Gāo Fāng (集灵膏方) was then prescribed. The basic formula contains *xī yáng shēn* (Radix Panacis Quinquefolii), *tiān dōng* (Radix Asparagi), *mài dōng* (Radix Ophiopogonis), *shēng dì* (Radix Rehmanniae Recens), *shú dì* (Radix Rehmanniae Praeparata), and *yín yáng huò* (Herba Epimedii).

Dù zhòng (Cortex Eucommiae), *sāng shèn zǐ* (Fructus Mori), *tù sī zǐ* (Semen Cuscutae), *wǔ wèi zǐ* (Fructus Schisandrae Chinensis), *jīn yīng zǐ* (Fructus Rosae Laevigatae), *gǒu qǐ zǐ* (Fructus Lycii), *shān yào* (Rhizoma Dioscoreae), *shān yú ròu* (Fructus Corni), *guī jiǎ jiāo* (Colla Carapax et Plastrum Testudinis), and *guǎng yú biào jiāo* (Gelatinum Aeris Piscis Vesica) were also added.

The patient displayed greater vitality over a period of time, and sexual activity returned to normal. The following year, he happily reported that his spouse had given birth.

(Shan Shu-jian. *Clinical Experience of Ancient and Contemporary Experts: Male Diseases*. Beijing: China Press of Traditional Chinese Medicine, 1999: 191)

(3) Mr. Ding, age 35.

The patient was married but childless due to male frigidity. He also displayed depressive personality traits. Other signs and symptoms included rib-side distention, glomus in the chest, belching, insomnia, aching lumbus, and premature ejaculation. His pulses were wiry and fine.

This presentation indicates a pattern of kidney yin deficiency with liver constraint. The treatment principle here is to enrich kidney water and regulate liver qi. Care must be taken to avoid stagnation affecting the qi dynamic of the liver and stomach.

Zī Shèn Shēng Gān Sǎn (滋肾生肝散) was selected.

The medicinals include *dì huáng* (Radix Rehmanniae), *shān yào* (Rhizoma Dioscoreae), *shān yú ròu* (Fructus Corni), *fú líng* (Poria), *dān pí* (Cortex Moutan), *zé xiè* (Rhizoma Alismatis), *chái hú* (Radix Bupleuri), *dāng guī* (Radix Angelicae Sinensis), *bái zhú* (Rhizoma Atractylodis Macrocephalae), *wǔ wèi zǐ* (Fructus Schisandrae Chinensis), and *zhì gān cǎo* (Radix et Rhizoma Glycyrrhizae Praeparata cum Melle).

Dān shēn (Radix et Rhizoma Salviae Miltiorrhizae Miltiorrhizae), *bái sháo* (Radix Paeoniae Alba) and *méi guī huā* (Flos Rosae Rugosae) were added to emolliate the liver and harmonize the nutrient aspect.

Yù jīn (Radix Curcumae), *hé huān huā* (Flos Albiziae) and *zhǐ qiào* (Fructus Aurantii) were also added to soothe constraint and regulate qi. The symptoms of liver-stomach disharmony were completely relieved after 20 doses.

At the second visit, *Zī Shèn Shēng Gān Sǎn* (滋肾生肝散) was continued with the addition of *gǒu qǐ zǐ* (Fructus Lycii), *tù sī zǐ* (Semen Cuscutae), *sāng shèn* (Fructus Mori), *yín yáng huò* (Herba Epimedii), *dù zhòng* (Cortex Eucommiae) and *shā rén* (Fructus Amomi).

The primary treatment principle here is to tonify kidney yin. The patient was also advised to remain abstinent, and also counseled to maintain a positive attitude with an open mind. After continuing treatment through the winter, his vitality had obviously increased and premature ejaculation was no longer an issue. His spouse successfully conceived later in the year.

(Shan Shu-jian. *Clinical Experience of Ancient and Contemporary Experts: Male Diseases*. Beijing: China Press of Traditional Chinese Medicine, 1999: 192)

(4) Mr. Li, age 30.

The patient reported often becoming ill due to an irregular diet, especially after consuming even slightly cold-natured foods. Other symptoms and signs included poor appetite and loose stools, a white tongue coating, and generally weak pulses.

This presentation indicates deficiency cold of the spleen and stomach. The treatment principle here is to fortify the spleen and warm the middle.

Modifications of *Xiāng Shā Liù Jūn Zǐ Tāng* (香砂六君子汤) and *Lǐ Zhōng Tāng* (理中汤) are generally indicated for this pattern.

➢ With stomach cold, add *gāo liáng jiāng* (Rhizoma Alpiniae Officinarum) and *xiāng fù* (Rhizoma Cyperi).

➢ With belching, add *dài zhě shí* (Haematitum) and *xuán fù huā* (Flos Inulae).

➢ With abdominal distention, add *hòu pò* (Cortex Magnoliae Officinalis) and *dà fù pí* (Pericarpium Arecae).

➢ With food stagnation, add *jiāo mài yá* (scorch-fried Fructus Hordei Germinatus), *jiāo shān zhā* (scorch-fried Fructus Crataegi), *jiāo shén qǔ* (scorch-fried Massa Medicata Fermentata), and *jī nèi jīn* (Endothelium

Corneum Gigeriae Galli).

➤ With cold-heat complex, tenesmus, and red and white stool, add *mù xiāng* (Radix Aucklandiae) and *chǎo chuān lián* (Rhizoma Coptidis).

The above treatments had been applied for several years, effectively managing his condition. He later complained that his spouse was not able to become pregnant.

Xiāng Shā Lǐ Zhōng Wán (香砂理中丸), and *Shēn Líng Bái Zhú Sǎn* (参苓白术散) were combined with the addition of *qiàn shí* (Semen Euryales) and *jīn yīng zǐ* (Fructus Rosae Laevigatae). The formula was made into pills and taken daily. After several months, his appetite markedly improved. Soon after the condition of his spleen and stomach returned to normal, his spouse was able to conceive.

(Shan Shu-jian. *Clinical Experience of Ancient and Contemporary Experts: Male Diseases*. Beijing: China Press of Traditional Chinese Medicine, 1999: 193)

13. Case Studies of Gu Heng-fang

(1) Mr. Chen, age 30. Initial visit: Apr.16th, 1983.

No pregnancy 5 years after marriage. The patient reported that he could not maintain a full erection or ejaculate on his wedding night. Since that time, the situation was repeated whenever he attempted to have sexual relations. Before marriage, he had suffered from dream-disturbed sleep and occasional nocturnal emission, but with no other complaints.

Signs and symptoms included irritability, profuse dreaming, frequent nocturnal emission, dizziness, lassitude, and sexual frigidity. Examination revealed no genital abnormality.

The patient was prescribed *Gōng Jī Zhí Jiǔ Hé Jì* (公鸡殖酒合剂). Psychological counseling was also conducted, as he had recently become separated from his spouse. After 20 days they were reunited, and advised to attempt intercourse. At a 2 month follow-up visit, they reported that their sexual activity had become normal. Urine testing at that time revealed that his wife had become pregnant.

(Shan Shu-jian. *Clinical Experience of Ancient and Contemporary Experts: Male Diseases*. Beijing: China Press of Traditional Chinese Medicine, 1999: 196)

(2) Mr. He, age 38.

Childless after 13 years of marriage. Examination of his spouse revealed no abnormality, and sexual activity was reported normal. Semen analysis showed a sperm count of 6-20 million/ml with survival rates of 35%. The patient reported no other complaints. After a period of treatment with *Gōng Jī Zhí Jiǔ Hé Jì* (公鸡殖酒合剂), sperm counts reached 100 million/ml. At dose 120, his spouse was found to have become pregnant.

(Shan Shu-jian. *Clinical Experience of Ancient and Contemporary Experts: Male Diseases*. Beijing: China Press of Traditional Chinese Medicine, 1999: 196)

(3) Mr. Chen, age 31.

The patient complained of sexual impotence. During six years of marriage, he had never been able to complete the act of sexual intercourse. The patient reported having had good health and no unhealthy habits prior to the marriage. The dysfunction first appeared on his wedding night. After achieving and maintaining a healthy erection, he suddenly felt sensations of coldness in the lower abdomen. At this point, his penis became not only flaccid but also extremely contracted, causing a great deal of anxiety. Tiger balm was applied around the umbilicus and genitals, and the sensations of cold immediately subsided. However, the same situation was repeated at each future attempt. Later conflicts between his mother and wife had also caused the patient great anxiety and serious marital difficulties.

Symptoms and signs included dizziness, blurred vision, insomnia, nocturnal emission, lassitude, and sexual frigidity. Semen analysis revealed slightly reduced sperm counts, but with no other abnormalities present.

Following 2 courses of *Gōng Jī Zhí Jiǔ Hé Jì* (公鸡殖酒合剂), the patient reported that sexual activity had returned to normal, and also that his wife had become pregnant.

【Note】

Gōng Jī Zhí Jiǔ Hé Jì (公鸡殖酒合剂) is known as an ancient family prescription. It is very effective in the treatment of male infertility associated with impotence, premature ejaculation, and abnormal semen.

The formula contains the following medicinals.

鲜公鸡殖	*xiān gōng jī zhí*	200g	Fresh Cock Genitalia
淫羊藿	*yín yáng huò*	100g	Herba Epimedii
夜交藤	*yè jiāo téng*	100g	Polygoni Multiflosi Caulis
仙茅	*xiān máo*	100g	Rhizoma Curculiginis
路路通	*lù lù tōng*	100g	Fructus Liquidambaris
桂圆肉	*guì yuán ròu*	100g	Longanae Arillus
50度米酒	*mǐ jiǔ*	2500g	Oryzae Vinum (50%)

Preparation methods, usage and precautions:

A. After removing the the cock genitalia by castration, the parts should be immediately weighed and then soaked in wine. Do not wash with water or leave exposed to the air for any period of time.

B. Combine with all medicinals put into a tightly sealed container, store for 30 days.

C. Take 20 ml of the liquid each morning and every afternoon before meals and 40 ml before bedtime. 60 days is regarded as one course of treatment. If one course is not effective, treatment may be continued for a second course. Some patients may appear flushed for a short time after taking.

D. During treatment, avoid cold-natured foods such as radish and cabbage.

E. Sexual intercourse should be avoided during the first treatment course. According to tradition, the couple should also live apart during this period of time.

(Shan Shu-jian. *Clinical Experience of Ancient and Contemporary Experts: Male Diseases*. Beijing: China Press of Traditional Chinese Medicine, 1999: 196)

14. CASE STUDIES OF BAN XIU-WEN

Mr. Zheng, age 32.

【Initial Visit】

May 22ⁿᵈ, 1988. No pregnancy after 4 years of marriage. Examination of his spouse revealed no abnormality. Symptoms and signs included occasional dizziness, blurred vision, aching lumbus with limp knees, difficult falling asleep, profuse dreaming, and bound stool once every other day. The patient reported normal appetite, urination, and sexual desire. The tongue appeared with little coating and a red tip. Pulses were thready and rapid, at 90 bpm.

Semen analysis: Seminal fluid appeared grey-white, with a volume of 3 ml. Sperm count reached 40×10^6/ml with motility rates at 10%. Liquefaction time was poor, and non-viable sperm numbers reached 90%.

【Pattern Differentiation】

This presentation indicates a pattern of true yin insufficiency with deficiency fire further depleting yin essence.

【Treatment Principle】

Invigorate water to restrain fire.

【Prescription】

The prescribed formula contains the following medicinals.

熟地	*shú dì*	15g	Radix Rehmanniae Praeparata
山萸肉	*shān yú ròu*	10g	Fructus Corni
山药	*shān yào*	15g	Rhizoma Dioscoreae
牡丹皮	*mǔ dān pí*	10g	Cortex Moutan
茯苓	*fú líng*	10g	Poria
泽泻	*zé xiè*	6g	Rhizoma Alismatis
麦冬	*mài dōng*	10g	Radix Ophiopogonis
当归	*dāng guī*	10g	Radix Angelicae Sinensis
白芍	*bái sháo*	6g	Radix Paeoniae Alba
女贞子	*nǔ zhēn zǐ*	10g	Fructus Ligustri Lucidi
素馨花	*sù xīn huā*	6g	Flos Jasmini Officinalis
红花	*hóng huā*	2g	Flos Carthami

One decocted daily dose.

Semen analysis at dose 20 revealed motility rates of 30%, non-viable sperm at 50%, and a normal liquefaction period. The treatment had shown good therapeutic effect, so the previous prescription was continued.

Tài zǐ shēn (Radix Pseudostellariae) 15g, *xiǎo mài* (Fructus Tritici Levis) 20g, *jiāo téng* (Caulis Polygoni Multiflori) 20g, and *hàn lián cǎo* (Herba Ecliptae) 15g were also added.

After 12 doses, examination showed motility rates of 50%, non-viable sperm at 10%, and sperm counts approaching normal.

Modified *Wǔ Zǐ Yǎn Zōng Wán* (五子衍宗丸).

The prescribed formula contains the following medicinals.

菟丝子	*tù sī zǐ*	15g	Semen Cuscutae
女贞子	*nǔ zhēn zǐ*	10g	Fructus Ligustri Lucidi
枸杞子	*gǒu qǐ zǐ*	10g	Fructus Lycii
五味子	*wǔ wèi zǐ*	6g	Fructus Schisandrae Chinensis
车前子	*chē qián zǐ*	6g	Semen Plantaginis
覆盆子	*fù pén zǐ*	10g	Fructus Rubi
太子参	*tài zǐ shēn*	15g	Radix Pseudostellariae

当归身	dāng guī shēn	10g	Radix Angelicae Sinensis
白芍	bái sháo	6g	Radix Paeoniae Alba
玉兰花	yù lán huā	6g	Magnolia
红枣	hóng zǎo	10g	Fructus Ziziphi

The patient recovered after 30 doses, and his spouse concieved the following month.

(Shan Shu-jian. *Clinical Experience of Ancient and Contemporary Experts: Male Diseases*. Beijing: China Press of Traditional Chinese Medicine, 1999: 198, 199)

15. Case Studies of Liu Ming-han

Mr. Fan, age 30.

【Initial Visit】

Sept. 24th, 1979. No pregnancy after 4 years of marriage. Examination of his spouse revealed no abnormality, and sexual activity was reported to be normal. Semen examination revealed a complete absence of viable sperm and extremely low sperm counts. No other clinical symptoms were found present.

The patient was prescribed *Yì Jīng Líng* (益 精 灵) on Oct. 13th. By December 16[th,] sperm counts had reached 16 million/ml with motility rates of 35%. Routine semen analysis on January 21st revealed a sperm count of 92×10^6/ml and motility rates of 60%. On March 20th, the patient reported that his spouse had not menstruated for 50 days. She then tested positive for pregnancy and later gave birth in November of that year.

【Note】

Yì Jīng Líng (益精灵) is a compound preparation generally applied to improve sperm quality.

According to the *Materia Medica of Ri Hua-zi* (日 华 子 诸 家 本 草 , *Rì Huá Zǐ Zhū Jiā Běn Cǎo*), the sovereign medicinal *yín yáng huò* (Herba

Epimedii) is generally indicated for male infertility due to yang deficiency.

It is assisted by medicinals that benefit the kidney and invigorate yang such as *suǒ yáng* (Herba Cynomorii), *bā jǐ tiān* (Radix Morindae Officinalis), *fù piàn* (Aconiti Tuber Laterale), *ròu guì* (Cortex Cinnamomi), *ròu cōng róng* (Herba Cistanches), *jiǔ cài zǐ* (Semen Allii Tuberosi), *tù sī zǐ* (Semen Cuscutae), and *chōng wèi zǐ* (Fructus Leonuri). *Guī jiāo* (Testudinis Plastri Gelatinum), *lù jiǎo jiāo* (Colla Cornus Cervi), *shú dì huáng* (Radix Rehmanniae Praeparata), *gǒu qǐ zǐ* (Fructus Lycii), *sāng shèn* (Fructus Mori), and *shān yú ròu* (Fructus Corni) are also selected to nourish yin and replenish essence. *Huáng qí* (Radix Astragali) and *dāng guī* (Radix Angelicae Sinensis) tonify both qi and blood. *Gān cǎo* (Radix et Rhizoma Glycyrrhizae) harmonizes the middle and fortifies the spleen. *Chē qián zǐ* (Semen Plantaginis) regulates and disinhibits the water passages to promote proper emission.

This formula was composed in light of the statement, "Yin can not be generated without yang, and yang will not grow without yin". It acts to effectively nourish yin and invigorate yang while also tonifying both qi and blood. Furthermore, it acts to promote conception by nourishing essence and also coursing its passage.

(Shan Shu-jian. *Clinical Experience of Ancient and Contemporary Experts: Male Diseases*. Beijing: China Press of Traditional Chinese Medicine, 1999: 202)

16. Case Studies of Liang Hua-cai

(1) Yang Hyperactivity with Yin Debilitation

Mr. Shang, age 28.

【Initial Visit】

May 20th, 1986. No pregnancy after 4 years of marriage. Physical examination of both parties revealed no abnormality. Previous semen analyses had shown a seminal fluid volume of 2-4 ml, sperm count of 400-600×10⁶/ml, motility rates of 70%-80%, PH levels of 7.0-7.5, and normal liquefaction. The patient reported normal healthy erections. His penis typically became erect soon after falling asleep each night, but with an unbearable sore and distending sensation. Other symptoms and signs included dizziness, distending sensation of the head, thirst with a desire to drink, dry stool, and reddish urine. His tongue appeared red with a thin yellow coating. Pulses were rapid.

【Pattern Differentiation】

Yang hyperactivity with yin debilitation, water and fire failing to aid each other.

【Treatment Principle】

Repress yang, support yin, and invigorate water to restrain fire.

【Prescription】

Èr Zhì Wán (二至丸) modified with *Dà Bǔ Yīn Wán* (大补阴丸).

The prescribed formula contains the following medicinals.

女贞子	*nǔ zhēn zǐ*	20g	Fructus Ligustri Lucidi
炙龟板	*zhì guī bǎn*	20g	Carapax et Plastrum Testudinis Praeparata cum Melle
生地	*shēng dì*	20g	Radix Rehmanniae
熟地	*shú dì*	20g	Radix Rehmanniae Praeparata
旱莲草	*hàn lián cǎo*	15g	Herba Ecliptae
知母	*zhī mǔ*	15g	Rhizoma Anemarrhenae
地骨皮	*dì gǔ pí*	15g	Cortex Lycii
黄柏	*huáng bǎi*	15g	Cortex Phellodendri Chinensis
丹皮	*dān pí*	10g	Cortex Moutan

One divided daily dose, decocted three times. Mix the first and second decoctions together and divide into 3 equal portions, to be taken after meals. Pour the third into a bath basin and add cold water until the solution approaches body temperature. Soak the hips for 10 minutes each time. Also avoid smoking, drinking, acrid and spicy foods, and any fish without scales.

After 3 weeks of treatment, the erectile symptoms began to gradually resolve. Semen analysis revealed a seminal fluid volume of 5 ml, sperm counts of 180×10^6/ml, motility rates of 80%, pH levels of 7.0, and with normal liquefaction. To secure the therapeutic effect, 3 doses of the former formula were made into honey pills, 10g taken 2 to 3 times daily. His spouse conceived and gave birth to a healthy male infant on July 30th, 1987.

(Shan Shu-jian. *Clinical Experience of Ancient and Contemporary Experts: Male Diseases*. Beijing: China Press of Traditional Chinese Medicine, 1999: 203)

(2) Yin and Yang Repelling Each Other

Mr. Hao, age 30.

【Initial Visit】

Dec. 12th, 1985. No pregnancy 5 years after marriage. Sexual activity was reported normal, and physical examination of both parties revealed no abnormality. Previous semen analysis had revealed the following: seminal fluid volume 24 ml, sperm count >450 million/ml, and motility rates of 70%-80%. Signs and symptoms included a bitter taste in the mouth, hot sensations of the palms and soles, yellow and reddish urine, bound stool, lower abdominal distention, and coldness of the limbs, joints, and calves. His tongue appeared red with a yellow greasy coating. Pulses were wiry and rapid.

【Pattern Differentiation】

This presentation indicates a pattern of yin and yang repelling each other. Internal heat constraint forces yin outwards, causing yin and yang to become non-interdependant.

【Treatment Principle】

The treatment principle here is to clear heat, nourish yin, invigorate blood, and free the essence. The primary objective is to restore the normal and harmonious balance of yin and yang.

【Prescription】

The prescribed formula contains the following medicinals.

黄连	huáng lián	10g	Rhizoma Coptidis
焦山栀	jiāo shān zhī	10g	Fructus Gardeniae Praeparatus
阿胶珠	ē jiāo zhū	10g	Colla Corii Asini
旱莲草	hàn lián cǎo	10g	Herba Ecliptae
水牛角	shuǐ niú jiǎo	15g	Cornu Bubali
女贞子	nǚ zhēn zǐ	15g	Fructus Ligustri Lucidi
杜仲炭	dù zhòng tàn	15g	Cortex Eucommiae Carbonisatus
鸡血藤	jī xuè téng	15g	Caulis Spatholobi
益母草	yì mǔ cāo	15g	Herba Leonuri
生地	shēng dì	15g	Radix Rehmanniae
熟地	shú dì	15g	Radix Rehmanniae Praeparata
制首乌	zhì shǒu wū	20g	Radix Polygoni Multiflori Praeparata
鳖甲	biē jiǎ	20g	Carapax Trionycis

The administration methods and contraindications are the same as in the previous case.

【Second Visit】

On the second visit, after 7 days, all clinical manifestations had resolved. Semen analysis revealed the following: seminal fluid volume of 4 ml, sperm counts of 198×10^6/ml, motility rates of 80%, and with normal liquefaction. Another 7 dosages of the formula were prescribed.

Semen analysis on Feb. 5th showed a seminal volume 4.5 ml, sperm counts of 150 million/ml, and motility rates of 80%. His spouse soon became pregnant later and gave birth to a healthy male infant on March 15th.

(Shan Shu-jian. *Clinical Experience of Ancient and Contemporary Experts: Male Diseases*. Beijing: China Press of Traditional Chinese Medicine, 1999: 205)

(3) Stasis Obstructing the Essence Chamber

Mr. Han, age 31.

【Initial Visit】

Mar. 18th, 1986. No pregnancy after 4 years of marriage. Examination of his spouse revealed no abnormality. Repeated semen analyses showed no liquefaction within 24 hours, and sperm counts could not be evaluated. The patient had received a variety of treatments from many doctors in the past, with no significant effect. He also reported a history of frequent and excessive masturbation before marriage.

Symptoms and signs included dizziness and a distending sensation of the head, and stabbing pain of the lumbus and heels. He also occasionally experienced stabbing pains when having sexual intercourse, with some discomfort during ejaculation. The seminal fluid appeared thick and clotted. His tongue appeared dark purple with stasis maculae. Pulses were deep, wiry and rough.

【Pattern Differentiation】

Stasis obstructing the essence orifice.

【Treatment Principle】

Invigorate blood and free the essence.

【Prescription】

The prescribed formula contains the following medicinals.

当归	dāng guī	10g	Radix Angelicae Sinensis
生蒲黄	shēng pú huáng	10g	Pollen Typhae Cruda
王不留行	wáng bù liú xíng	10g	Semen Vaccariae
制首乌	zhì shǒu wū	20g	Radix Polygoni Multiflori Praeparata
龟板	guī bǎn	20g	Testudinis Plastrum
鸡血藤	jī xuè téng	15g	Caulis Spatholobi
益母草	yì mǔ cǎo	15g	Herba Leonuri
怀牛膝	huái niú xī	15g	Radix Achyranthis Bidentatae
女贞子	nǚ zhēn zǐ	15g	Fructus Ligustri Lucidi

熟地	shú dì	15g	Radix Rehmanniae Praeparata
灵脂	líng zhī	15g	Faeces Togopteri
血竭	xuè jié	5g	Sanguis Draconis

The administration methods and contraindications are the same as in the previous case.

50 ml yellow rice wine was selected as a conductor. Divide into two parts, and add to the water of the first two decoctions.

After 35 doses, the semen analysis revealed a seminal volume of 3 ml, sperm count of 350×10^6/ml, motility rates of 70%, and a liquefaction time of 25 minutes.

Shēng pú huáng (Pollen Typhae Cruda), *wǔ líng zhī* (Faeces Togopteri), *xuè jié* (Sanguis Draconis), *wáng bù liú xíng* (Semen Vaccariae) and the yellow rice wine were removed from the formula, and *huáng bǎi* (Cortex Phellodendri Chinensis) 10g and *zhī mǔ* (Rhizoma Anemarrhenae) 10g were added.

After 20 days, semen analysis revealed a seminal volume of 5 ml, sperm count of 150 million/ml, motility rates of 80%, and a liquefaction time of 20 minutes. To consolidate the therapeutic effect, 3 doses were made into honey-pills. 10g, 2 to 3 times daily. A follow-up visit in July, 1987 revealed that his spouse had been pregnant for more than 7 months.

(Shan Shu-jian. *Clinical Experience of Ancient and Contemporary Experts: Male Diseases*. Beijing: China Press of Traditional Chinese Medicine, 1999: 206)

17. CASE STUDIES OF YAN DE-XIN

Mr. Li, age 40.

【Initial Visit】

The patient reported no ejaculation for 11 years. He had received previous treatment from a number of doctors, but without significant effect. The semen appeared normal, with normal sperm counts. Even though he displayed a young and vital appearance, he reported very low sexual desire, and also seemed reluctant to speak. His tongue appeared purple with a thin coating. Pulses were deep and rough.

【Pattern Differentiation】

Liver constraint often leads to irritability or reticence, and also dysfunction of the qi dynamic. Qi stagnation leads to blood stasis which can obstruct the essence orifice, thus affecting sexual function and ejaculation.

【Treatment Principle】

Course qi and regulate blood.

【Prescription】

Xuè Fǔ Zhú Yū Tāng (血府逐瘀汤) was prescribed with the addition of yang-invigorating *zǐ shí yīng* (Fluoritum), *shé chuáng zǐ* (Fructus Cnidii) and *jiǔ cài zǐ* (Semen Allii Tuberosi).

Significant results were obtained after 7 doses, and the patient recovered after 30 doses. His wife gave birth to a healthy son the following year.

(Shan Shu-jian. *Clinical Experience of Ancient and Contemporary Experts: Male Diseases*. Beijing: China Press of Traditional Chinese Medicine, 1999: 218)

18. CASE STUDIES OF YANG QIAN-QIAN

(1) Mr. Liang, age 39.

【Initial Visit】

Apr 28th, 1984. No pregnancy after 4 years of marriage. Ejaculation was absent except for an occasional seminal emission. He had previously been diagnosed with "functional non-ejaculation" and then prescribed with *zǐ hé chē* (Placenta Hominis), *lù lù tōng* (Fructus Liquidambaris), *shān yú ròu* (Fructus Corni) and *lù xián cǎo* (Herba Pyrolae). 10 months of treatment had shown no significant effect.

Signs and symptoms included pain of the penis during sexual intercourse and a reddish complexion. His tongue appeared red with a yellow coating. Pulses were wiry and forceful.

【Pattern Differentiation】

Qi and yin dual deficiency, and damp-heat obstruction due to long-term astringing and tonification.

【Treatment Principle】

Tonify qi, engender essence, clear and disinhibit damp-heat, free the orifices, and relieve pain.

【Prescription】

Huáng Qí Huá Shí Tāng (黄芪滑石汤) was modified with the following medicinals.

蒲公英	*pú gōng yīng*	9g	Herba Taraxaci
川萆薢	*chuān bì xiè*	12g	Rhizoma Dioscoreae Hypoglaucae
黄皮核	*huáng pí hé*	9g	Semen Clausenae Lansii

Following treatment with 7 doses, ejaculation occurred during sexual intercourse. His spouse was found pregnant within one month.

(2) Mr. Zou, age 37.

【Initial Visit】

No ejaculation had occurred in 12 years of marriage, even with masturbation. However, profuse seminal emission appeared once every 2 months. He had been treated in several local hospitals without significant result. Physical examination revealed varicocele: right Ⅰ°, left Ⅱ°. Other signs included yellowish urine, a yellow tongue coating, and wiry pulses.

【Pattern Differentiation】

Damp-heat obstructing the orifices.

【Prescription】

Huáng Qí Huá Shí Tāng (黄芪滑石汤) was modified with the following medicinals.

| 川贝 | chuān bèi | 10g | Bulbus Fritillariae Cirrhosae |
| 射干 | shè gān | 9g | Rhizoma Belamcandae |

Ejaculation occured following dose 10. The patient also reported powerful feelings of physical and mental well-being.

(Shan Shu-jian. *Clinical Experience of Ancient and Contemporary Experts: Male Diseases*. Beijing: China Press of Traditional Chinese Medicine, 1999: 221-222)

【Attachment】

Huáng Qí Huá Shí Tāng (黄芪滑石汤)

黄芪	huáng qí	17g	Radix Astragali
滑石	huá shí	15g	Talcum
甘草	gān cǎo	5g	Radix et Rhizoma Glycyrrhizae
楮实子	chǔ shí zǐ	9g	Fructus Broussonetiae
茯苓	fú líng	15g	Poria
车前子	chē qián zǐ	27g	Semen Plantaginis
菟丝子	tù sī zǐ	15g	Semen Cuscutae
肉苁蓉	ròu cōng róng	10g	Herba Cistanches
南豆花	nán dòu huā	9g	Flos Dolichoris Album
穿山甲	chuān shān jiǎ	9g	Squama Manis
王不留行	wáng bù liú xíng	9g	Semen Vaccariae

19. CASE STUDIES OF LIU YUN-PENG

(1) Mr. Ai, age 35.

【Initial Visit】

July 1996. No pregnancy after 2 years of marriage. Examination of his spouse revealed normal reproductive function. Sperm count was 4.5×10^6/ml with a 50% motility rate.

Symptoms and signs included frequent profuse dreaming with emission, feverish sensations of the palms and soles, weak erection during intercourse, and aching lumbus with limp knees. The patient also reported a preference for alcohol and cigarettes.

After examination of the tongue and pulse, *Zhī Bǎi Dì Huáng Tāng* (知柏地黄汤) was modified with *Wǔ Zǐ Wán* (五子丸) to nourish kidney yin and purge ministerial fire. 2 doses were prescribed every 3 days. After 5 months of treatment, his spouse achieved a healthy pregnancy.

【Prescription】

The prescribed formula contains the following medicinals.

知母	*zhī mǔ*	9g	Rhizoma Anemarrhenae
黄柏	*huáng bǎi*	9g	Cortex Phellodendri Chinensis
山药	*shān yào*	9g	Rhizoma Dioscoreae
山茱萸	*shān zhū yú*	9g	Fructus Corni
茯苓	*fú líng*	9g	Poria
泽泻	*zé xiè*	9g	Rhizoma Alismatis
熟地	*shú dì*	9g	Radix Rehmanniae Praeparata
丹皮	*dān pí*	9g	Cortex Moutan
车前子	*chē qián zǐ*	9g	Semen Plantaginis
五味子	*wǔ wèi zǐ*	9g	Fructus Schisandrae Chinensis
覆盆子	*fù pén zǐ*	9g	Fructus Rubi
枸杞子	*gǒu qǐ zǐ*	20g	Fructus Lycii
菟丝子	*tù sī zǐ*	20g	Semen Cuscutae
芡实	*qiàn shí*	9g	Semen Euryales
莲须	*lián xū*	9g	Stamen Nelumbinis
金樱子	*jīn yīng zǐ*	9g	Fructus Rosae Laevigatae
龙骨	*lóng gǔ*	30g	Os Draconis
牡蛎	*mǔ lì*	30g	Concha Ostreae

(2) Mr. Wang, age 32.

【Initial Visit】

October, 1997. No pregnancy after 6 years of marriage. Medical history showed chronic prostatitis, with typical discomfort of the perineum and epididymis. The sperm count was 72×10^6/ml, motility rates 80%, abnormal sperm 20%, and liquefaction was poor. The patient also reported somewhat frequent urination and urinary urgency which became aggravated after drinking or consuming acrid or spicy foods. His tongue appeared red with a yellow coating. Pulses were deep, wiry and forceless.

Qián Liè Xiàn Yán Fāng (前列腺炎方) was prescribed at 2 doses every 3 days. After 3 months of treatment, his spouse achieved a healthy pregnancy.

【Prescription】

Qián Liè Xiàn Yán Fāng (前列腺炎方).

蒲公英	*pú gōng yīng*	30g	Herba Taraxaci
败酱草	*bài jiàng cǎo*	30g	Herba Patriniae
丹参	*dān shēn*	15g	Radix et Rhizoma Salviae Miltiorrhizae
枸杞子	*gǒu qǐ zǐ*	30g	Fructus Lycii
王不留行	*wáng bù liú xíng*	15g	Semen Vaccariae
赤芍	*chì sháo*	15g	Radix Paeoniae Rubra
白芍	*bái sháo*	15g	Radix Paeoniae Alba
炮甲	*páo jiǎ*	9g	Squama Manis (stir-fried)
石韦	*shí wéi*	9g	Folium Pyrrosiae
乳香	*rǔ xiāng*	9g	Olibanum
没药	*mò yào*	9g	Myrrha
桃仁	*táo rén*	9g	Semen Persicae
红花	*hóng huā*	9g	Flos Carthami

(3) Mr. Chen, age 24.

【Initial Visit】

Jul 12th, 1997.

Chief complaint: No pregnancy 2 years after marriage.

The patient reported distending fullness of the chest and rib-side, lassitude, and poor appetite. His tongue appeared red with a thin yellow coating. Pulses were wiry and forceless. The sperm count was 54×10^6/ml with a motility rate of 40%.

【Pattern Differentiation】

Essence obstruction due to liver constraint with blood stasis.

【Treatment Principle】

Course the liver, resolve stasis, free and disinhibit the sperm orifices, and supplement essence.

【Prescription】

Xuè Fǔ Zhú Yū Tāng (血府逐瘀汤) was modified with the addition of *tù sī zǐ* (Semen Cuscutae) 15g and *gǒu qǐ zǐ* (Fructus Lycii) 15g to tonify kidney essence. After 15 doses, examination showed that sperm quality had returned to normal. His spouse eventually achieved a healthy pregnancy.

(Huang Ying. Experiences of Liu Yun-peng in the Treatment of Male Infertility. *Hubei Journal of Traditional Chinese Medicine*, 1998, 20 (6): 8, 9)

Discussions

1. YUE FU-JIA: CONSIDERATIONS OF THE HEART AND SPLEEN

Dr. Yue's approach to the treatment of male infertility certainly incorporates the following the statements of fact: "Fertility is the duty of the kidney", and "The key to reproduction is security of the essence". Infertility formulas generally consist of medicinals that primarily tonify the kidney and benefit essence. However, Dr. Yue also takes the condition of the heart and spleen into consideration during treatment. The engendering and transformation of kidney essence relies on the nourishment provided by the acquired essence. "Spirit, essence, qi, and blood are all engendered and transformed by spleen-earth." To benefit the kidney, one may therefore apply medicinals that primarily fortify the spleen. Once the spleen and stomach become fortified, "The origin of reproduction will be obtained, and the engendering of essence will occur swiftly." The majority of his formula choices for male fertility reflect this principle. Representative formulas include *Zhōng Hé Zhòng Zǐ Wán* (中和种子丸) and *Bǔ Shèn Jiàn Pí Yì Qì Zhòng Zǐ Jiān Fāng* (补肾健脾益气种子

煎方).

Furthermore, "Although infertility is related to the kidney, it is also rooted in the heart." It is also said, "To promote fertility, sufficient kidney water is essential, and heart fire must be especially calm." "The heart stores blood and the kidney stores essence. When essence and blood are both sufficient, reproduction is then made possible."

Dr. Yue often applies medicinals that benefit the heart, such as *Xīn Shèn Zhòng Zǐ Wán* (心肾种子丸) and *Bǔ Xīn Zī Shèn Wán* (补心滋肾丸). Although the kidney is the primary focus, it is quite clear that one must also consider the condition of the heart and spleen in the treatment of male infertility.

(Qin Guo-zheng. *Theory and Clinical Aspects of Male Diseases*. Beijing: China Medical Science and Technology Press, 1st edition, 1997: 167)

2. WANG QI: CLINICAL EXPERIENCE WITH MALE INFERTILITY

(1) Etiology and Pathomechanism

A. Pathomechanism: Kidney deficiency with damp-heat, stasis, and internal toxins.

The traditional point of view regarding infertility always tends to focus on patterns of kidney deficiency. Due to changes in society and the natural environment perhaps, Dr. Wang finds that this approach is not always effective in the modern clinic. He first stated in 1998 that the pathomechanism most common in modern cases of male infertility is kidney deficiency with damp-heat, stasis, and internal toxins. He considers kidney deficiency as the root pattern, and the patterns of damp-heat, stasis, and internal toxins as branch manifestations.

Dr. Wang views oligospermia and asthenospermia resulting from decreased male hormone levels or over-indulgence in sexual activities as belonging to the category of kidney deficiency. The category of damp-heat patterns include those conditions associated with inflammation or prostatitis which may include asthenospermia, necrozoospermia, or non-liquefaction of semen. These conditions often result from the excessive consumption of alcohol, tobacco, or acrid and spicy foods. Chronic inflammation of the reproductive system, varicocele, and seminal duct obstruction should be viewed as patterns of stagnation. Sexually transmitted diseases, effects of radiation, and acute inflammation of the seminal duct are considered as manifestations of internal toxins. Any one of these four possibilities may lead to infertility, or they may also appear in combination.

B. Nature of the Disease: Patterns of excess are predominant

Emotional irregularities, contraction of external pathogens, excessive sexual activity, alcohol abuse, and preferences for greasy, sweet, acrid and spicy foods are the main etiologies of male infertility. These factors lead to damp-heat, stasis, and internal toxins, all of which belong to the category of excess. Clinical presentations that indicate patterns of congenital deficiency and kidney qi deficiency cold are actually quite rare.

C. Associated Viscera: Liver, spleen and kidney

Dr. Wang states that healthy male fertility depends on the proper and coordinated functioning of the viscera, bowels, qi, blood, channels and collaterals. The liver, spleen and kidney are the viscera most involved with conditions of male fertility. The kidney stores essence and governs reproduction. The spleen is the source of qi and blood, governor of transportation and transformation, and it also acts to nourish the congenital essence. The liver stores blood and governs free-coursing. Essence and blood engender one another, and are also closely related to the transportation of qi and blood. When the viscera are not functioning properly, male infertility may appear as a result of damp-heat, phlegm turbidity, and static blood.

(2) Clinical Treatment

A. Combining Disease and Pattern Differentiation

Male infertility patients often present with no obvious clinical symptoms or physical signs. Dr. Wang therefore emphasizes the importance of proper disease differentiation. He suggests first using biomedical technology to clarify the diagnosis and etiologies, and to then select the treatment principles accordingly. For pattern differentiation, he emphasizes observation of the semen. White, thin and profuse semen indicates patterns of cold or deficiency. Yellow thick semen indicates the presence of heat or excess patterns. This approach essentially unites disease diagnosis and pattern differentiation by combining semen analysis with CM pattern differentiation.

The biomedical diagnosis of reproductive system inflammation is usually considered in pattern differentiation as lower burner damp-heat, and low male hormone levels are generally related to kidney deficiency. In treatment, low hormone levels usually require tonifying medicinals, especially those with hormone-like effects. These include *shé chuáng zǐ* (Fructus Cnidii), *xiān líng pí* (Herba Epimedii), *lù fēng fáng* (Nidus Vespae) and *xiān máo* (Rhizoma Curculiginis). The treatment principles for reproductive system inflammation are to clear heat, disinhibit dampness, resolve toxin, invigorate blood, and transform stasis.

Low levels of Zn and Mn in the semen may be treated with medicinals rich in such elements, such as *huáng jīng* (Rhizoma Polygonati), *gǒu qǐ* (Fructus Lycii), and *xiān líng pí* (Herba Epimedii).

Semen that fails to liquidize often involves a lack of protease, and may be treated with medicinals rich in enzymes, such as *jī nèi jīn* (Endothelium Corneum Gigeriae Galli), *gǔ yá* (Fructus Setariae Germinatus), *mài yá* (Fructus Hordei Germinatus), *shān zhā* (Fructus Crataegi), and *wū méi* (Fructus Mume).

B. Common Treatment Methods

Male infertility often involves abnormalities of the seminal fluid and sperm. In clinic, Dr. Wang's treatments generally focus on the condition of the liver, spleen and kidney. The main syndromes are kidney deficiency, damp-heat and static toxins. Quite often, several methods and several formulas are applied together. The most commonly applied clinical methods are as follows.

Tonification:

This approach includes nourishing kidney essence, warming the kidney to assist yang, and tonification of qi and blood. This approach is indicated for conditions of oligospermia, asthenospermia, azoospermia and necrozoospermia.

Commonly selected formulas include *Wǔ Zǐ Yǎn Zōng Wán* (五子衍宗丸), *Yòu Guī Wán* (右归丸), *Liù Wèi Dì Huáng Wán* (六味地黄丸), *Sì Jūn Zǐ Tāng* (四君子汤), and *Sì Wù Tāng* (四物汤).

Commonly applied medicinals include *guī bǎn jiāo* (Colla Carapax et Plastrum Testudinis), *lù jiǎo jiāo* (Colla Cornus Cervi), *shǒu wū* (Radix Polygoni Multiflori), *huáng jīng* (Rhizoma Polygonati), *gǒu qǐ zǐ* (Fructus Lycii), *nǚ zhēn zǐ* (Fructus Ligustri Lucidi) and *shān yú ròu* (Fructus Corni).

Tù sī zǐ (Semen Cuscutae), *zǐ hé chē* (Placenta Hominis), *bǔ gǔ zhī* (Fructus Psoraleae), *xiān líng pí* (Herba Epimedii), *xiān máo* (Rhizoma Curculiginis), and *shā yuàn zǐ* (Semen Astragali Complanati) may be selected to tonify the kidney and assist yang.

Huáng qí (Radix Astragali), *hóng shēn* (Radix et Rhizoma Ginseng Rubra), *dǎng shēn* (Radix Codonopsis), *dāng guī* (Radix Angelicae Sinensis) and *bái sháo* (Radix Paeoniae Alba) act to tonify qi and blood and engender essence.

Invigorating blood and freeing the collaterals:

This approach is indicated for conditions of seminal duct obstruction, prostatitis, and non-liquefaction of semen.

Commonly selected formulas include *Shào fŭ Zhú Yū Tāng* (少腹逐瘀汤) and *Táo Hóng Sì Wù Tāng* (桃红四物汤).

Commonly applied medicinals include *dān shēn* (Radix et Rhizoma Salviae Miltiorrhizae), *yì mŭ căo* (Herba Leonuri), *shuĭ zhì* (Hirudo), *dāng guī* (Radix Angelicae Sinensis), *wáng bù liú xíng* (Semen Vaccariae), *lù lù tōng* (Fructus Liquidambaris), *hóng huā* (Flos Carthami), *chuān xiōng* (Rhizoma Chuanxiong), *chì sháo* (Radix Paeoniae Rubra), *dān pí* (Cortex Moutan), *zé lán* (Herba Lycopi), and *chăo shān jiă* (stir-fried Squama Manis).

Clearing damp-heat and resolving toxins:

This approach is indicated for abnormal semen associated with infectious factors.

Commonly selected formulas include *Chéng Shì Bì Xiè Fēn Qīng Yĭn* (程氏萆薢分清饮), *Sān Rén Tāng* (三仁汤), and *Wŭ Wèi Xiāo Dú Yĭn* (五味消毒饮).

Commonly applied medicinals include *bì xiè* (Rhizoma Dioscoreae Hypoglaucae), *bài jiàng căo* (Herba Patriniae), *lóng dăn căo* (Gentianae Radix), *zhī mŭ* (Rhizoma Anemarrhenae), *zhī zĭ* (Fructus Gardeniae), *yì yĭ rén* (Semen Coicis), *chē qián zĭ* (Semen Plantaginis), *jīn yín huā* (Flos Lonicerae Japonicae), *lián qiáo* (Fructus Forsythiae), *zé lán* (Herba Lycopi), *huáng băi* (Cortex Phellodendri Chinensis), *tŭ fú líng* (Rhizoma Smilacis Glabrae), and *hŭ zhàng* (Rhizoma et Radix Polygoni Cuspidati).

Dr. Wang emphasizes that bitter and cold herbs such as *lóng dăn căo* (Gentianae Radix), *huáng băi* (Cortex Phellodendri Chinensis) and *zhī zĭ* (Fructus Gardeniae) must be applied in small dosages and for only a short duration. Long-term use may produce a negative effect on sperm motility. In general, medicinals that clear and disinhibit may damage yin essence and should therefore be applied with caution.

C. Psychological and Nutritional Counseling

Most male infertility patients experience high levels of stress due to an often long disease history and the increasing desire to have children. In Dr. Wang's experience, psychological counseling can improve patient compliance while also helping patients cultivate a confident and optimistic attitude. He also recommends a diet rich in amino acids, zinc, and vitamins. Some of these foods include sesame, peanuts, walnuts, millet, spinach, carrots, tomatoes, and eel. Highly nutritious foods can increase sperm quality and also benefit glandular function. Greasy or spicy foods and alcoholic beverages should be avoided, and smoking is prohibited.

(Sun Zi-xue, Chen Jian-she. Introduction to the Experience of Male Infertility Treatment by Professor Wang Qi. *Journal of Sichuan Traditional Chinese Medicine*, 2004, 22 (1): 7, 8)

3. LI GUANG-WEN: EXPERIENCES IN MALE INFERTILITY

(1) Pattern Differentiation, Semen Analysis, and Counseling

Male infertility cases come with their own set of particular characteristics. The four examinations may not completely reveal the root of the disease, since many patients will not display any obvious physical symptoms. In these cases, semen analysis results should be combined with pattern differentiation.

The presence of abnormal semen and sperm is clearly associated with the condition of the kidney. Low sperm counts, low seminal volume or the absence of sperm indicates deficiencies of qi and blood and kidney essence insufficiency. Low sperm motility or low numbers of viable sperm indicate kidney qi deficiency.

In terms of biomedicine, high numbers of non-viable sperm indicate a dysfunction of sperm production, deficiencies of vitamins A and E, or inflammation. In Chinese medicine, reproductive dysfunction is generally viewed as kidney qi deficiency, where reproductive system inflammation matches the syndrome of effulgent yin deficiency fire. The most effective clinical approach is to consider the presenting symptoms and signs along with the results of semen analysis.

Non-liquefaction of semen is usually associated with chronic prostatitis, and these patients may also present with symptoms of urinary tract infection. This presentation indicates a pattern of effulgent kidney fire, yin deficiency, and damp-heat. Semen that appears red or with red blood cells observed under a microscope usually indicates liver channel damp-heat scorching the blood collaterals. Pus cells present in the semen points to damp-heat in the lower burner. In this way, laboratory analysis becomes a further expansion of the four examinations. Combining pattern differentiation with semen analysis creates a more accurate diagnosis, which naturally leads to a clear and effective treatment plan.

Psychological guidance and counseling should be provided along with medical treatment. Patients should be advised to engage in a healthy lifestyle that involves less sexual activity, physical taxation, and anger. The excessive consumption of alcoholic beverages and rich flavors are also to be avoided. Patients should attempt to control sexual desire, since reduced sexual activity results in more active sperm and higher rates of conception. Excessive sexual intercourse over-consumes essence and blood, injures the liver and kidney, and ultimately damages reproductive health.

For male infertility cases, and especially those with sexual dysfunction, the predominant mental-emotional state becomes a very important factor. The typical stress and anxiety regarding reproductive issues can negatively effect sperm production and sexual function. Impotence and disorders of ejaculation are very often a direct result of mental-emotional factors. Therefore, psychological counseling leads to better treatment results by helping to reduce stress and foster optimistic attitudes with issues related to sexuality.

(Liu Jing-jun. Clinical Experience on Male infertility Treatment by Dr. Li Guang-wen. *New Journal of Traditional Chinese Medicine*, 1999, (2): 10)

(2) Treating Oligospermia with *Shēng Jīng Zhòng Yù Tāng* (生精种玉汤)

Sperm counts lower than 60,000,000/ml result in a reduced chance of achieving pregnancy. Oligospermia is often associated with patterns of kidney qi deficiency with qi and blood dual deficiency. Symptoms and signs include fatigue, dizziness, tinnitus, forgetfulness, and aching of the lumbus. Other symptoms may include impotence, premature ejaculation, and seminal emission. Some patients present no obvious clinical symptoms, nor any apparent changes in the pulse or tongue.

The primarily treatment principle here is to benefit kidney essence while also tonifying qi and blood.

Shēng Jīng Zhòng Yù Tāng (生精种玉汤) is based on traditional formulas such as *Qī Zǐ Sǎn* (七子散), *Qìng Yún Sǎn* (庆云散), and *Wǔ Zǐ Yǎn Zōng Wán* (五子衍宗丸).

The basic formula contains the following medicinals.

黄芪	huáng qí	30g	Radix Astragali
淫羊藿	yín yáng huò	15g	Herba Epimedii
川断	chuān duàn	15g	Radix Dipsaci
首乌	shǒu wū	12g	Radix Polygoni Multiflori
当归	dāng guī	12g	Radix Angelicae Sinensis
桑椹子	sāng shèn zǐ	9g	Fructus Mori
枸杞子	gǒu qǐ zǐ	9g	Fructus Lycii
菟丝子	tù sī zǐ	9g	Semen Cuscutae
五味子	wǔ wèi zǐ	9g	Fructus Schisandrae Chinensis
覆盆子	fù pén zǐ	9g	Fructus Rubi
车前子	chē qián zǐ	9g	Semen Plantaginis

【Modifications】

➢ With abdominal distention and poor appetite, add *mù xiāng* (Radix Aucklandiae) 9g and *chén pí* (Pericarpium Citri Reticulatae) 9g.

➢ With reduced libido or forceless ejaculation, add *yáng qǐ shí* (Actinolitum) 30g and *bā jǐ tiān* (Radix Morindae Officinalis) 9g.

➢ With qi deficiency, add *dǎng shēn* (Radix Codonopsis) 30g.

➢ With insomnia and profuse dreaming, add *chǎo zǎo rén* (Semen Ziziphi Spinosae) 15g and *hé huān huā* (Flos Albiziae) 9g.

In the formula *Shēng Jīng Zhòng Yù Tāng* (生精种玉汤), *xiān líng pí* (Herba Epimedii), *chuān duàn* (Radix Dipsaci), and *tù sī zǐ* (Semen Cuscutae) act to warm the kidney, invigorate kidney qi and yang, and promote sperm production. *Shǒu wū* (Radix Polygoni Multiflori), *gǒu qǐ zǐ* (Fructus Lycii) and *sāng shèn zǐ* (Fructus Mori) tonify the liver and kidney and replenish essence. *Fù pén zǐ* (Fructus Rubi) and *wǔ wèi zǐ* (Fructus Schisandrae Chinensis) secure the kidney and astringe essence. *Chē qián zǐ* (Semen Plantaginis) purges deficiency fire of the kidney. Its mobile and disinhibiting nature also acts to prevent congestion. *Huáng qí* (Radix Astragali) tonifies qi, and *dāng guī* (Radix Angelicae Sinensis) nourishes blood.

Because essence and blood are mutually engendering, kidney essence will become sufficient only when qi and blood are effulgent. Moreover, new sperm takes about 74 days to mature, so 3 months of treatment may be required to achieve an observable effect. The peak effect on sperm production lasts for about one year, after which the therapeutic effect will begin to decline.

(Shan Shu-jian. *Clinical Experience of Ancient and Contemporary Experts: Male Diseases*. Beijing: China Press of Traditional Chinese Medicine, 1999: 177-182)

(3) *Yè Huà Tāng*(液化汤) for Non-liquefaction of Semen

In normal conditions, semen will liquidize within 30 minutes of ejaculation. Non-liquefaction refers to cases where semen will not liquidize within one hour. In some cases, this process may take up to 24 hours. This condition is often accompanied by chronic prostatitis, with patients often reporting a history of intemperate sexual activity. The most acute clinical cases may display an overactive libido, where in chronic cases the libido is often reduced.

This presentation often indicates patterns of effulgent kidney fire scorching body fluids, which then manifests with non-liquefaction of semen. The treatment principle here is to tonify kidney yin and purge fire.

Yè Huà Tāng (液化汤) is a modified version *of Zhī Bǎi Dì Huáng Tāng* (知柏地黄汤).

The basic formula contains the following medicinals.

知母	*zhī mǔ*	9g	Rhizoma Anemarrhenae
黄柏	*huáng bǎi*	9g	Cortex Phellodendri Chinensis
生地	*shēng dì*	9g	Radix Rehmanniae
熟地	*shú dì*	9g	Radix Rehmanniae Praeparata
赤芍	*chì sháo*	9g	Radix Paeoniae Rubra
白芍	*bái sháo*	9g	Radix Paeoniae Alba
丹皮	*dān pí*	9g	Cortex Moutan
天冬	*tiān dōng*	9g	Radix Asparagi
花粉	*huā fěn*	9g	Radix Trichosanthis
茯苓	*fú líng*	9g	Poria
车前子	*chē qián zǐ*	9g	Semen Plantaginis
连翘	*lián qiáo*	12g	Fructus Forsythiae
丹参	*dān shēn*	30g	Radix et Rhizoma Salviae Miltiorrhizae
淫羊藿	*yín yáng huò*	15g	Herba Epimedii
生甘草	*shēng gān cǎo*	6g	Radix et Rhizoma Glycyrrhizae

In this formula, *zhī mǔ* (Rhizoma Anemarrhenae), *huáng bǎi* (Cortex Phellodendri Chinensis), *shēng dì huáng* (Radix Rehmanniae Recens), *shú dì huáng* (Radix Rehmanniae Praeparata), and *lián qiáo* (Fructus Forsythiae) act to nourish yin, clear heat, and resolve toxins.

Fú líng (Poria) and *chē qián zǐ* (Semen Plantaginis) disinhibit dampness with bland percolation.

Dān shēn (Radix et Rhizoma Salviae Miltiorrhizae), *dān pí* (Cortex Moutan), and *chì sháo* (Radix Paeoniae Rubra) invigorate blood and eliminate stasis.

Tiān dōng (Radix Asparagi), *huā fěn* (Radix Trichosanthis), and *bái sháo* (Radix Paeoniae Alba) increase humor and engender fluids.

Xiān líng pí (Herba Epimedii) warms the kidney, assists yang, and restrains the cold properties of *zhī mǔ* (Rhizoma Anemarrhenae) and *huáng bǎi* (Cortex Phellodendri Chinensis).

Shēng gān cǎo (raw Radix et Rhizoma Glycyrrhizae) resolves toxins and also acts to harmonize the formula.

These medicinals act in combination to nourish yin, downbear fire, dispel stasis, and disinhibit dampness.

Among all of the medicinals listed here, only *zhī mǔ* (Rhizoma Anemarrhenae) and *huáng bǎi* (Cortex Phellodendri Chinensis) possess the ability to reduce nerve sensitivity and thus reduce an overactive libido. However, *xiān líng pí* (Herba Epimedii) acts to prevent possible over-inhibition that may result from the use of *zhī mǔ* (Rhizoma Anemarrhenae) and *huáng bǎi* (Cortex Phellodendri Chinensis) by increasing the libido and seminal fluid. For patients with an extremely low libido, the dosage of *xiān líng pí* (Herba Epimedii) can be increased to 15-30g. The elegant construction of this formula maintains a delicate balance, which is also the key to its proper application.

(Shan Shu-jian. *Clinical Experience of Ancient and Contemporary Experts: Male Diseases*. Beijing: China Press of Traditional Chinese Medicine, 1999: 177, 182)

(4) *Shēng Jīng Zhòng Yù Tāng* (生精种玉汤) and *Yè Huà Tāng* (液化汤) for High Sperm Mortality

Healthy semen will reveal high sperm counts with normal morphology and sperm survival rates. When mortality rates are higher than 40%; this is referred to as necrozoospermia. Its pathogenesis is associated with two main patterns. Effulgent kidney fire often manifests with inflammation of the reproduction system. Kidney qi deficiency also leads to reduced reproductive function and a poor general health condition.

Prostatitis and spermatocystitis are the most commonly seen inflammatory conditions of the reproductive system. Cases of prostatitis usually present with frequent and painful urination and urinary urgency. The libido may increase prior to or at the onset of the inflammation, and then become reduced as the inflammatory condition continues to progress. Prostatic fluid will show increased numbers of white blood cells (more than 10 per HP field of view), and also decreased lecithin levels.

Spermatocystitis often coexists with prostatitis. The symptoms are similar, often with discomfort of the perineum following ejaculation. The featured symptom of spermatocystitis is the presence of bloody semen.

The treatment principle for necrozoospermia due to prostatitis or spermatocystitis is to nourish yin, clear heat, invigorate blood, and transform stasis.

The recommended formula contains the following medicinals.

金银花	jīn yín huā	30g	Flos Lonicerae Japonicae
丹皮	dān pí	30g	Cortex Moutan
蒲公英	pú gōng yīng	15g	Herba Taraxaci
生地	shēng dì	15g	Radix Rehmanniae
续断	xù duàn	15g	Radix Dipsaci
当归	dāng guī	12g	Radix Angelicae Sinensis
知母	zhī mǔ	9g	Rhizoma Anemarrhenae
黄柏	huáng bǎi	9g	Cortex Phellodendri Chinensis
赤芍	chì sháo	9g	Radix Paeoniae Rubra
白芍	bái sháo	9g	Radix Paeoniae Alba
生甘草	shēng gān cǎo	9g	Radix et Rhizoma Glycyrrhizae (raw)

Zhī mǔ (Rhizoma Anemarrhenae), *huáng bǎi* (Cortex Phellodendri Chinensis) and *bái sháo* (Radix Paeoniae Alba) nourish yin and purge fire.

Dān pí (Cortex Moutan), *chì sháo* (Radix Paeoniae Rubra) and *dāng guī* (Radix Angelicae Sinensis) invigorate blood and transform stasis. *Jīn yín huā* (Flos Lonicerae Japonicae), *pú gōng yīng* (Herba Taraxaci) and *shēng gān cǎo* (raw Radix et Rhizoma Glycyrrhizae) act to clear heat and resolve toxins. *Xù duàn* (Radix Dipsaci) acts to replenish kidney essence. These medicinals combined can effectively reduce inflammation of the prostate gland and seminal vesicles, and also benefit sperm survival and motility rates.

With necrozoospermia and non-liquefaction of semen, select *Yè Huà Tāng* (液化汤) with added *xù duàn* (Radix Dipsaci) 15g and *dāng guī* (Radix Angelicae Sinensis) 12g.

For prostatitis or spermatocystitis patients with low libido and a poor general physical condition, apply *Shēng Jīng Zhòng Yù Tāng* (生精种玉汤) with an increased dosage of *dāng guī* (Radix Angelicae Sinensis) and *xù duàn* (Radix Dipsaci).

In the treatment of male infertility due to abnormal semen, the following aspects should be emphasized so as to increase the chance of conception.

A. The spouse should take 6 doses of *Yù Lín Zhū* (毓麟珠) starting on the 7th day following the onset of menstruation. One daily dose; with one day off after dose 3. Sexual activity is also prohibited during this time, because optimum hormone levels are required in order to conceive. *Yù Lín Zhū* (毓麟珠) not only promotes ovulation, but also improves the function of the corpus luteum. This can also promote conception because the capacity of sperm becomes improved.

B. Accurately calculate the date of ovulation and plan for sexual intercourse at the proper time. Normally, the ovulation period begins 14 days before menstruation, plus or minus 2 days. The date of ovulation can be accurately predicted through measurement of the basal body temperature.

C. Physician Yuan Liao-yun was quoted in *The Compendium of Benefiting Females* (济阴纲目 , *Jì Yīn Gāng Mù*) which states, "The methods of gathering essence include: lessening desire, reducing taxation, quieting anger, abstaining from alcohol, and being cautious with flavors."

The *Jade Ruler of Gynecology* (妇科玉尺 , *Fù Kē Yù Chǐ*) also states, "When men seek reproduction, it is essential to clear the mind and reduce desire." Reducing the frequency of sexual activity, emotional regulation, and proper diet are all essential in the treatment of male infertility.

(Shan Shu-jian. *Clinical Experience of Ancient and Contemporary Experts: Male Diseases*. Beijing: China Press of Traditional Chinese Medicine, 1999: 177-182)

4. HUA LIANG-CAI: EXPERIENCES IN MALE INFERTILITY

(1) The Theory of Essence Stagnation

Congenital essence is one of the fundamental substances of human life. It is normally a mobile substance just like qi, blood, and seminal fluid. Essence stasis refers to a pathological stagnation in which a number of abnormal conditions may result.

The production and transportation of semen are affected by a variety of factors, and many of these can lead to essence stagnation and stasis. The main causes may be associated with any of the following factors.

A. Masturbation

Excessive masturbation is considered to be an unnatural physiological and psychological behavior. Furthermore, the masturbatory release of semen is a fundamentally different process than in that of sexual intercourse. The incomplete release of seminal fluid can lead to patterns of semen stagnating in the essence chamber.

B. Obstruction of the seminal duct

Sperm generation and emission may become dysfunctional due to inflammation, tumors, adhesions, surgery, or trauma. These factors may also result in the stagnation of essence.

C. Urinary and reproductive disorders

Prostatitis or prostate gland enlargement, testitis, epididymitis, spermophlebectasia, spermatocystitis, and hydrocele of the tunica vaginalis directly effect the generation and emission of sperm, also contributing to patterns of stagnation and stasis.

D. Abuse of tonifying medicinals or hormonal drugs

Tonifying medicinals are only effective when their prescription is based on accurate pattern differentiation. When improper tonification is applied, normal semen production may become interrupted. Particular caution must be exercised with yang-invigorating medicinals, as their improper application may lead to an imbalance of yin and yang, scorching of the semen, and stagnation of essence. Modern hormonal biomedicines also directly effect semen production, and their overuse may also contribute to patterns of essence stagnation.

E. Poor genital blood flow

Due to professional needs, some people must wear overly restricting clothing. This can affect the circulation of qi and blood in the pudendum, restricting the supply of blood and oxygen to the testicles. This can result in an accumulation of dampness and toxins, and also essence stagnation.

F. Emotional factors

Long-term depression and other emotional disturbances can cause qi and blood stagnation, which may lead to disorders of semen production and emission.

G. Bleeding or blood stasis

Local bleeding due to trauma, high fever due to febrile disease, and excessive consumption of warm and yang-invigorating medicinals can all cause blood congestion in the reproductive system. Blood stasis then leads to an oxygen deficiency with tissue degeneration or even atrophy of the reproductive system. This clearly affects the generation of semen and its emission.

H. Phlegm-damp obstruction

Disorders in the mechanism of bodyfluids may result from spleen and stomach dysfunction, and also the excessive consumption of greasy and sweet foods. Dampness then accumulates and becomes transformed into phlegm. Phlegm moves along with qi and stagnates in the essence chamber, interfering with the production and release of semen. Changes in the components of seminal fluid occur when when phlegm and semen bind with one another, also leading to essence stagnation.

Clinical manifestations of essence stagnation

➢ Stabbing pain in the kidney region, heels, soles of the feet, testicles, penis, and lower abdomen. Testicular sensations of heaviness and distending pain may also appear, usually becoming aggravated following sleep or inactivity, and improved with movement.

➢ Sexual dysfunction: Most typical are impotence, premature ejaculation, weak erection during intercourse, and incomplete or painful ejaculation. Occasionally, spontaneous or persistent erection may also occur.

➢ No ejaculation during intercourse, but with seminal emission at other times. Retrograde ejaculation, which refers to semen being released into the bladder during intercourse.

➢ Sensations of heaviness and pain of the perineum with inhibited or dripping urination.

➢ Premature graying or hair loss accompanied by numbness, itching or sharp pain in the area of the eyebrows, beard and pubic hair.

➢ Tinnitus and hearing loss, with tinnitus typically appearing low in pitch like tidal water.

➢ Poor mental concentration, dizziness, forgetfulness, and insomnia.

➢ Thick clotted semen with poor liquifaction, low semen volume, normal or even elevated sperm counts, excessive numbers of abnormal sperm, or absent sperm.

➢ Rough pulses with the tongue body appearing dark or with purplish patches.

➢ Little response to kidney-tonifying and essence-replenishing medicinals, or with symptoms that become worse after long-term or excessive application.

2 to 3 of the above symptoms are sufficient to make an accurate diagnosis.

Treatment: The key approach is to invigorate blood and free the essence, because essence and blood are mutually engendering. Essence stasis also suggests blood stasis, so when blood becomes invigorated, the essence also becomes freed.

The representative formula is *Huó Xuè Tōng Jīng Tāng* (活血通精汤).

当归	*dāng guī*	10g	Radix Angelicae Sinensis
制首乌	*zhì shǒu wū*	20g	Radix Polygoni Multiflori Praeparata
鸡血藤	*jī xuè téng*	15g	Caulis Spatholobi
怀牛膝	*huái niú xī*	15g	Radix Achyranthis Bidentatae
益母草	*yì mǔ cǎo*	20g	Herba Leonuri
血竭	*xuè jié*	5g	Sanguis Draconis
金毛狗脊	*jīn máo gǒu jǐ*	15g	Rhizoma Cibotii

Huáng Jiǔ (yellow rice wine) is added to the decoction as a conductor.

This formula contains a number of blood-invigorating medicinals which enter the kidney channel. Its main actions are to invigorate and nourish blood while engendering and freeing the essence. It also displays adaptogenic effects in disorders of azoospermia, oligospermia, abnormal sperm morphology, necrozoospermia, high sperm count, and retrograde ejaculation.

Gǔ suì bǔ (Rhizoma Drynariae), *chuān xù duàn* (Radix Dipsaci), *pú huáng* (Pollen Typhae), *wǔ líng zhī* (Faeces Togopteri), *táo rén* (Semen Persicae), *hóng huā* (Flos Carthami), *tǔ biē chóng* (Eupolyphaga seu Steleophaga), *chuān shān jiǎ* (Squama Manis), and *wáng bù liú xíng* (Semen Vaccariae) may also be added to the formula according to pattern differentiation.

For patients with azoospermia or asthenospermia, better treatment results may be achieved with the addition of medicinals that tonify the kidney, invigorate yang, and replenish essence. In these cases, the principle approach is to first free the essence, and then follow with tonification.

(Qin Guo-zheng. *Clinical Theory of Male Medicine*. Beijing: China Medical Science and Technology Press, 1997: 269)

(2) Restraining Yang and Supporting Yin in the Treatment of Male Infertility due to High Sperm Density

Abnormally high sperm counts reaching 200,000,000/ml can also result in male infertility, although the relationship between high sperm density and male infertility is still unclear at present. One possibility is that high sperm density may reduce sperm motility, which also reduces the opportunity for fertilization of the ovum. High sperm density may be associated with patterns of exuberant yang and yin debilitation. The corresponding treatment principle here is to inhibit yang while nourishing yin. Inhibiting yang means to inhibit the mechanism of sperm production, whereas nourishing yin means to promote sperm growth capability. In this way the unit volume sperm count may be reduced, and yet the individual sperm will develop with greater vigor and higher motility rates.

(Shan Shu-jian. *Clinical Experience of Ancient and Contemporary Experts: Male Diseases*. Beijing: China Press of Traditional Chinese Medicine, 1999: 203)

5. Qi Guang-chong: Disease Differentiation, Etiology, and Syndrome Differentiation in Male Infertility

(1) Obesity and Phlegm-damp

Patients in whom the semen analysis is unremarkable will typically not receive biomedical treatment. Many of these individuals will then choose to receive long-term Chinese medicinal treatments that focus on tonification of kidney essence, but without result. Dr. Qi notes that many of these cases are associated with obesity. In addition to affecting the general health of an individual, obesity also may also hinder sexual functioning and reproductive health. Obese male infertility patients most often present with patterns of spleen yang deficiency. This pattern may appear as a result of devitalized spleen yang, or splenic transportation failure and phlegm-damp retention due to the excessive consumption of raw, cold, rich and sweet foods. When the spleen fails to properly transport and transform, dampness and phlegm will accumulate, and this may manifest with obesity. Even though the kidney is the root of the congenital foundation, it is also closely related with the spleen, which is the root of the acquired foundation. The spleen in turn provides qi and blood to nourish the kidney and the congenital foundation. When the spleen fails to transport and transform, both phlegm and damp-heat may accumulate. In cases of male infertility associated with obesity, the proper treatment principle is to invigorate the spleen, transform phlegm, percolate dampness, and clear heat.

(2) Sinew Tumors and Blood Stagnation

Dr. Qi considers varicocele as belonging to the Chinese medicine category of sinew tumors. When seminal analysis is inconclusive, the possible presence of sinew tumors should be considered. Blood stasis often leads to qi stagnation, and qi stagnation will further aggravate the blood stasis condition. Qi and blood stagnation can lead to malnourishment of the testes, (known as the external kidney), and also impair the kidney function of storing essence and governing reproduction. For patients of this type, further laboratory analysis may reveal reduced sperm motility and sperm survival rates, which also may indicate the presence of varicocele. Patterns of blood stasis should be addressed with medicinals that invigorate blood and free the essence.

(3) Mental Depression and Liver Stagnation

Many patients present chronic infertility with no clearly identifiable cause. Dr. Qi has observed that these individuals often exhibit increasing mental depression due to the stressful and long-term expenditure of time, energy and money. The liver and kidney share the same origin, and essence and blood are mutually engendering. Prolonged depression therefore may result in failure of the liver to store blood and govern free coursing, which also influences the ability of the kidney to store essence and govern reproduction. Patterns of liver qi stagnation should be considered as a primary cause in these types of male infertility cases. The proper treatment principle here is to course the liver and resolve stagnation.

(4) Asymptomatic Patients and Kidney Deficiency

Some male infertility patients present with an absence of physical symptoms, and laboratory analysis results are also unremarkable. In these cases, Dr. Qi explains that the primary focus of treatment should address the condition of the kidney, which is considered as the root of reproduction.

First, the kidney is the congenital foundation which also determines the quality of the acquired foundation. Normal visceral function is closely related to kidney qi, as well as the sufficiency of qi and blood. If the congenital foundation is weak and the kidney essence is deficient, the kidney will fail to govern reproductive function.

Second, exterior pathogenic factors and environmental factors may also damage the kidney. This damage leads to the consumption of kidney essence, which also results in the kidney failing to govern reproduction.

Third, kidney essence rarely becomes exuberant, but often becomes debilitated. In other words, kidney essence tends to conditions of deficiency rather than of excess. Kidney deficiency is usually responsible for cases of male infertility that present with no apparent cause. Treatment in these cases should mainly focus on nourishing the kidney essence. When kidney qi is sufficiently strong and kidney essence is well nourished, fertility is then made possible.

(Li Qi-xin, Zhao Jin-song. Clinical Experience of Dr. Qi Guang-chong on Male Infertility without Identifiable Causes. *Liaoning Journal of Traditional Chinese Medicine*, 2001, 28 (7): 404)

6. Xu Fu-song: Clinical Experiences of Male Infertility

(1) Treatment of the Lung, Spleen and Stomach

In the treatment of male infertility, Dr. Xu recommends the use of medicinals that benefit the lung and stomach.

Select *mài dōng* (Radix Ophiopogonis), *shā shēn* (Radix Glehniae Littoralis), *sāng bái pí* (Cortex Mori) and *huáng qín* (Radix Scutellariae) to treat the lung, and *shí gāo* (Gypsum Fibrosum), *lú gēn* (Rhizoma Phragmitis), *zhú yè* (Folium bambusae) and *shān zhī* (Fruactus Gardenie) to treat the stomach. However, since infertility conditions are generally rooted in kidney deficiency, it is also essential to tonify the kidney with medicinals such as *shú dì* (Radix Rehmanniae Praeparata), *yú biào* (Piscis Vesica Aeris), *gǒu qǐ zǐ* (Fructus Lycii) and *zǐ hé chē* (Placenta Hominis).

The congenital essence relies on the nourishment provided by the acquired essence. Meanwhile, the production and transformation of acquired essence relies on the quality of the congenital essence. Because congenital essence produces the acquired essence, and acquired essence nourishes the congenital essence, one should treat the spleen and kidney together. While tonifying the kidney, it is also beneficial to add medicinals such as *dǎng shēn* (Radix Codonopsis), *fú líng* (Poria), *yì rén* (Semen Coicis) and *huáng jīng* (Rhizoma Polygonati).

Male reproductive conditions tend to become chronic, and patients will normally be required to take medicinals for an extended period. However, long-term medicinal applications often damage the spleen and stomach. For example, the excessive use of bitter and cold-natured medicinals can damage spleen and stomach yang, where the excessive use of yang-invigorating medicinals can damage spleen and stomach yin.

Taking prescriptions at improper or irregular times may cause stomach duct pain and diarrhea. According to Dr. Xu, the optimum times to take medicinals are at 9:30 each morning and evening. Also, overstimulation of the gastrointestinal tract may be avoided by taking medicinals with the stomach half-empty. These methods help to protect the spleen and stomach, while also maintaining a stable concentration of medicinals present in the blood.

(Xu Fu-song. Clinical Experience of Chinese Medicine Male Diseases. *National Journal of Andrology*, 1999, 5(4): 243)

(2) Male Infertility and Immunological Causes

An autoimmune response to sperm is a known cause of male infertility. Antisperm antibodies are found in about 10% of all male infertility patients, which accounts for about 3% of all infertility cases among couples. In normal conditions, the testes and male reproductive tract present a very strong immune barrier. The sperm antigen does not normally contact the immune system, and an immune response to the presence of sperm rarely occurs. The occurrence of an autoimmune response suggests that the sperm has penetrated the normal immune barrier, inducing an autoimmune response. Many of these conditions are caused by disorders which are easily identified, such as spermatic duct blockage that results in sperm antigen leakage. Any traumatic damage to the testicular blood-barrier may also lead to coagulation and sperm stoppage with positive AsAb.

There is no specific treatment for immune male infertility. Biomedical approaches usually include hormone therapy, but the typically large dosages needed often result in serious side effects. By seeking causes from the presenting pattern and determining treatment based on those causes, Chinese medicine associates this disease primarily with the liver and kidney, and secondly with the lung and spleen.

The root condition is associated with constitutional deficiency, while the branch pattern results from injury or infection. The pathomechanism here is deficiency of the upright leading to pathogens lodging internally. Deficiency here refers to insufficiencies of the liver, kidney, lung and spleen. Lodging of pathogens refers to patterns of damp-heat and static blood. Patterns of liver and kidney yin deficiency, damp-heat brewing internally, and disharmony of qi and blood can manifest with obstruction of the seminal duct.

Another cause may be related to lung and spleen qi deficiency, which is normally characterized by complaints of diarrhea and easily catching colds. This pattern can lead to pathogenic heat entering the nutrient-blood and essence chamber, also obstructing the seminal duct.

A. Liver and Kidney Yin Deficiency with Damp-heat

These patients usually present with a history of intemperate sexual activity, or reproductive tract injury or infection. Symptoms and signs include tidal fever in the afternoon, vexing heat in the five hearts, thirst with the desire to drink, aching lumbus and limp knees, yellow urine, constipation, and night sweating. The tongue appears red with a scant coating, and pulses are thin, wiry and rapid. The treatment principle here is to nourish yin, downbear fire, and clear damp-heat.

The recommended formula contains the following medicinals.

生地	shēng dì	12g	Radix Rehmanniae
泽泻	zé xiè	12g	Rhizoma Alismatis
丹皮	dān pí	10g	Cortex Moutan
碧桃干	bì táo gān	10g	Prunus persica (L.) Batsch
碧玉散（包）	Bì Yù Sǎn	15g	Bi Yu San (Be wrapt)
知母	zhī mǔ	6g	Rhizoma Anemarrhenae
茯苓	fú líng	10g	Poria
枸杞子	gǒu qǐ zǐ	10g	Fructus Lycii
车前子（包）	chē qián zǐ	10g	Semen Plantaginis (Be wrapt)
白芍	bái sháo	10g	Radix Paeoniae Alba

B. Lung and Spleen Qi Deficiency

These patients usually present a history of infection in the upper respiratory and digestive tracts. Symptoms and signs include frequent colds or flu, nasal congestion, sore throat, cough, poor appetite, diarrhea, abdominal pain or distention, nausea, dizziness, spontaneous sweating, and a dull facial complexion. The tongue appears pale with thin white coating and teeth marks. Pulses are thin and weak.

The treatment principle here is to tonify the lung, fortify the spleen, clear the intestines and purge heat.

The recommended formula contains the following medicinals.

人参	rén shēn	10g	Radix et Rhizoma Ginseng
白术	bái zhú	10g	Rhizoma Atractylodis Macrocephalae
茯苓	fú líng	10g	Poria
黄芪	huáng qí	12g	Radix Astragali
山药	shān yào	10g	Rhizoma Dioscoreae
木香	mù xiāng	6g	Radix Aucklandiae
砂仁（后下）	shā rén	2g	Fructus Amomi (Being decocted later)
黄连	huáng lián	2g	Rhizoma Coptidis

| 益元散（包） | yì yuán sǎn | 15g | Yi Yuan San (Be wrapt) |
| 芡实 | qiàn shí | 10g | Semen Euryales |

(Shan Shu-jian. *Clinical Experience of Ancient and Contemporary Experts: Male Diseases.* Beijing: China Press of Traditional Chinese Medicine, 1999: 207, 209)

7. Zhao Xi-wu: *Tiān Xióng Jiā Wèi Sǎn* in the Treatment of Male Infertility

(1) Male Infertility and Deficiency of the Kidney and Spleen

Male infertility typically appears with two main manifestations. The first shows increased numbers of abnormal sperm with low survival rates due to a pattern of clear and cold essence qi. The second is sexual dysfunction and impotence. Regarding the pattern of clear and cold essence qi, thin refers to the deficiency of essence, and cold refers to yang deficiency and decline of life gate fire. This pattern develops from a condition of physical debilitation, rather than as a result of other diseases. Kidney disorders usually affect the condition of the spleen, liver and heart, but in these cases, the spleen is particularly involved. The kidney is known as the congenital foundation, and it also functions to store essence and govern reproduction. The spleen is the acquired foundation, and it functions to transform and transport the refined essence of food to nourish the kidney. Therefore, exhaustion of kidney essence will not generally appear when the spleen is functioning properly. However, when the spleen and kidney become deficient, the presenting pattern may manifest with cold and thin semen. To tonify both kidney and spleen, modifications of *Tiān Xióng Sǎn* are recommended.

(2) *Tiān Xióng Jiā Wèi Sǎn* to Warm Yang and Replenish Essence

Tiān Xióng Sǎn (天雄散) was first mentioned in the '*Jīn Guì Yào Lüè*: Chapter Six, Blood *Bi* and Deficiency', in which the formula was presented without further explanation.

Tiān xióng (Aconiti Tuber Laterale Tianxiong) and *guì zhī* (Ramulus Cinnamomi) are selected primarily to warm yang. *Bái zhú* (Rhizoma Atractylodis Macrocephalae) is selected to strengthen the spleen, and *shēng lóng gǔ* (Os Draconis) to nourish yin and suppress hyperactive yang. This combination acts to invigorate the kidney and spleen, warm yang, and supplement essence.

According to Mo Mei-shi, *Tiān Xióng Sǎn* (天 雄 散) is an ancient family formula used mainly for the treatment of essence loss due to yang deficiency. However, classical literature generally associates essence loss with conditions of spermatorrhea, occurring either with or without dreams. The former pattern is caused by deficient cold and can thus be treated with *Tiān Xióng Sǎn* (天 雄 散). The latter condition is generally associated with the presence of unfulfilled desires.

The heart stores the spirit. Conditions associated with heart deficiency can be addressed with the addition of *Guì Zhī Tāng* (桂枝汤), which also acts to harmonize nutritive and defense. *Lóng gǔ* (Os Draconis) and *mǔ lì* (Concha Ostreae) are also added to consolidate essence. It should be noted that spermatorrhea is currently viewed as a normal physiological function.

Tiān xióng (Aconiti Tuber Laterale Tianxiong) is the chief medicinal in this formula. It acts to disperse cold and warm yang due to its pungent flavor and hot nature. *Fù zǐ* (Radix Aconiti Lateralis Praeparata) is a reasonably effective substitution, since availability is generally limited. Even though *tiān xióng* (Aconiti Tuber Laterale Tianxiong), *fù zǐ* (Radix Aconiti Lateralis Praeparata) and *wū tóu* (Radix Aconiti) are harvested from the same plant, their actions are actually quite different.

The first rhizome is referred to as *wū tóu* (Radix Aconiti), and the tuber attached to the center section is called *fù zǐ* (Radix Aconiti Lateralis Praeparata). A *wū tóu* (Radix Aconiti) rhizome may reach a length of 3-4 *cun,* in which case it is referred to as *tiān xióng* (Aconiti Tuber Laterale Tianxiong).

Fù zǐ (Radix Aconiti Lateralis Praeparata) is more effective at penetrating the channels; wheras *tiān xióng* (Aconiti Tuber Laterale Tianxiong) is less mobile in nature. *Wū tóu* has an empty core and so has a stronger influence on qi, wheras *tiān xióng* (Aconiti Tuber Laterale Tianxiong) has a solid core which more strongly influences essence. Qi is associated with dispersing, so *wū tóu* (Radix Aconiti) is selected used to disperse cold. Essence is associated consolidation and storage, so *tiān xióng* (Aconiti Tuber Laterale Tianxiong) is selected to warm the kidney and secure essence.

Tiān Xióng Sǎn is used to treat male infertility manifesting with cold and thin semen. Nourishing medicinals such as *ròu cōng róng* (Herba Cistanches), *gǒu qǐ zǐ* (Fructus Lycii), *bā jǐ tiān* (Radix Morindae Officinalis), *yín yáng huò* (Herba Epimedii), *dōng chóng xià cǎo* (Cordyceps), *dǎng shēn* (Radix Codonopsis) and *dāng guī* (Radix Angelicae Sinensis) are usually added to replenish essence and supplement qi.

Treatment of this condition requires a long-term course of therapy. Healthy dietary habits can enhance the tonifying effect of treatment, and cultivating a positive attitude can help avoid liver qi stagnation and mental depression. Sexual activity should also be restrained in order to avoid further depletion.

(Chan Shujian. *Clinical Experience of Ancient and Contemporary Experts: Male Diseases*. Beijing: China Press of Traditional Chinese Medicine, 1999: 165-167)

8. Luo Yuan-kai: Benefiting Kidney Yin for Low Sperm Counts, Warming Qi and Yang for High Sperm Mortality

Male infertility is most often associated with sexual dysfunctions such as impotence, premature ejaculation, and absent ejaculation.

Abnormalities of the semen include sperm count lower than 20×10^6/ml, reduced seminal fluid volume (less than 2.5 ml), low sperm motility (less than 60%), absence of viable sperm, abnormal sperm morphology (over 20%), and seminal non-liquefaction or poor liquefaction times. All of these conditions can contribute to the failure to conceive. If conception occurs when these conditions are present, embryonic development may be affected, which often leads to an early abortion.

Whether the condition manifests with impotence, premature ejection, or abnormal semen, kidney deficiency is always involved. In cases presenting with clear and cold essence qi or false heat due to yin deficiency, it is important to accurately differentiate patterns of yin and yang. The indiscriminate use of warming medicinals may damage kidney yin. Generally speaking, yin and yang should be supplemented together, with an emphasis on the more deficient of the two. It is said that when tonifying yin, one should never neglect yang, and when tonifying yang, one should never neglect yin. It is just as the ancient classics said, "A physician who can effectively tonify yang will seek yang within yin; the transformations become endless when yang is assisted by yin. A physician who can effectively tonify yin will seek yin from within yang; the resources become abundant when yin is invigorated by yang".

➤ With low sperm count, select *Zuǒ Guī Wán* (左归丸) or *Zuǒ Guī Yǐn* (左归饮) to primarily tonify kidney yin.

➤ With hyperactive fire due to yin deficiency, select *Zhī Bǎi Bā Wèi Wán* (知柏八味丸) to nourish yin and clear heat.

➤ With low sperm motility, *Yòu Guī Wán* (右归丸) or *Yòu Guī Yǐn* (右归饮) may be combined with *rén shēn* (Radix et Rhizoma Ginseng) and *huáng qí* (Radix Astragali) to warm yang and replenish qi.

➤ With absent ejaculation, psychological counseling should be provided to relieve the associated stress and anxiety. Methods which supplement essence and invigorate yang can improve sensitivity and promote ejaculation.

If these principles are correctly applied, the maximum treatment effect will be achieved with half the effort.

The empirical formula *Wēn Shèn Yì Jīng Tāng* (温肾益精汤) is also recommended.

炮天雄	*páo tiān xióng*	6~9g	Aconiti Tuber Laterale Tianxiong
熟地	*shú dì*	20g	Radix Rehmanniae Praeparata
菟丝子	*tù sī zǐ*	20g	Semen Cuscutae
怀牛膝	*huái niú xī*	20g	Radix Achyranthis Bidentatae
枸杞子	*gǒu qǐ zǐ*	20g	Fructus Lycii
炙甘草	*zhì gān cǎo*	6g	Radix et Rhizoma Glycyrrhizae Praeparata cum Melle
仙灵脾	*xiān líng pí*	10g	Herba Epimedii

For patients with prolonged erections caused by hyperactive fire due to yin deficiency, modifications of *Zhī Bǎi Bā Wèi Tāng* (知柏八味汤) can be used to nourish yin and purge ministerial fire. However, with inflammation due to prostatitis, treatment should first focus on the inflammation. Otherwise, tonification methods may prove ineffective.

(Chan Shu-jian. *Clinical Experience of Ancient and Contemporary Experts: Male Diseases*. Beijing: China Press of Traditional Chinese Medicine, 1999: 168-170)

9. CHEN WEN-BO: *SHĒNG JĪNG ZÀN YÙ WÁN* FOR BALANCED TONIFICATION

The etiologies of male infertility are quite complex. In summary, all of the following factors can disturb the essence chamber, deplete yin essence, and lead to essence qi deficiency: Six external pathogens invading, damage from the seven affects, excessive sexual activity, irregular diet, excessive taxation, organ deficiency, knocks and falls, phlegm congestion, kidney deficiency and essence cold, heat constraint in the essence chamber, stasis obstructing the essence vessel, damage from improper treatment, and the propagation of STD. Improper or delayed treatment can further deplete the true essence and lead to essence collapse, and even azoospermia. These factors often lead to temporary or even lifelong infertility.

An imbalance of kidney yin and kidney yang may result from external contraction of the six pathogens or internal conditions of wind, cold, damp, and fire due to dysfunction of the viscera. All of these may lead to infertility due to deficiency of the true essence. Liver stagnation and affect damage also leads to disordered free-coursing, which then results in disorders of qi, blood, yin, and yang. The resulting visceral dysfunction can manifest with impotence, premature ejaculation, and scant essence or essence exhaustion.

Excessive taxation can cause splenic failure of engendering and transformation, leading to grain qi failing to nourish the kidney. When the congenital essence is not sufficiently nourished by the acquired essence, oligospermia and infertility may result. Excessive drinking, smoking, and the consumption of sweet or greasy foods can engender fire heat, scorching the yin essence. Undescended testicles are associated with a deficiency of congenital essence, which can also result in azoospermia. Deficiencies of the viscera can also result in infertility due to oligospermia or weak sperm. Injury to the genital region or excessive masturbation can cause stagnation of the seminal duct. The improper application of Chinese medicinals or biomedicines can also affect sperm, causing oligospermia or weak sperm. Furthermore, sexually transmitted diseases, radiation, and congenital abnormalities may cause oligospermia, weak sperm, essence stagnation, and azoospermia.

Although the etiologies of male infertility may be complex, the pathomechanism generally involves manifestations of essence qi deficiency. These include oligospermia, immotile and non-viable sperm, stagnation of essence, abnormal sperm morphology, and excessively cold or hot essence. The major treatment principle here is to regulate yin and yang and engender essence. Other methods of treatment include rectifying qi, increasing humor, eliminating stasis, and nourishing, warming, clearing, and securing the kidney. It is very important to apply more than one single method throughout treatment, otherwise yin and yang may become more imbalanced and sperm counts may become further reduced.

For example, with oligospermia due to kidney yang insufficiency, the sperm count will generally increase after applying the method of warming the kidney. However, white blood cells may begin to appear in the semen. This indicates hyperactivity of the ministerial fire disturbing the essence chamber. If the same treatment method is continued, the sperm count will decrease and other disorders may appear.

A number of male infertility patients may meet two or more of the following criteria:

➢ Sperm counts lower than 20,000,000/ml
➢ Sperm mortality higher than 40%
➢ Sperm motility below medium
➢ Liquidation time over one hour
➢ Abnormal sperm morphology above 15%

In these cases, the following patterns are the three most commonly seen.

➢ **Kidney yang deficiency**: Symptoms and signs include impotence, premature ejaculation, low libido, bright-white facial complexion, aching pain of the lumbus and knees, and cold damp testes. The tongue appears pale with a thin white coating. Pulses are deep and slow, forceless at the *chi* position.

➢ **Yin essence deficiency**: Symptoms and signs include aching lumbus and limp knees, dizziness, tinnitus, profuse dreaming, night sweating, vexing heat in the five hearts, and a damp scrotum. The tongue appears red with white coating. Pulses are thin; and weak at the *chi* position.

➢ **Damp-heat in the essence chamber**: Symptoms and signs include aching lumbus and knees, distending pain or nodules of the testes, damp-heat sensations of the scrotum, and short voidings of yellowish urine. The tongue is red with a yellow slimy coating. Pulses are thin and wiry or slippery and slightly rapid, also weak at the *chi* position.

These three patterns may all be treated with modifications of *Shēng Jīng Zàn Yù Wán* (生精赞育丸).

The basic ingredients include *xiān líng pí* (Herba Epimedii), *ròu cōng róng* (Herba Cistanches), *shān yào* (Rhizoma Dioscoreae) and *gǒu qǐ zǐ* (Fructus Lycii).

【Modifications】

➢ With kidney yang deficiency, add *fù zǐ* (Radix Aconiti Lateralis Praeparata), *ròu guì* (Cortex Cinnamomi), *bā jǐ tiān* (Radix Morindae Officinalis) and *tù sī zǐ* (Semen Cuscutae).

➢ With yin essence deficiency, add *zhì hé shǒu wū* (Radix Polygoni Multiflori Praeparata cum Succo Glycines Sotae), *shú dì* (Radix Rehmanniae Praeparata), *nǚ zhēn zǐ* (Fructus Ligustri Lucidi) and *zhī mǔ* (Rhizoma Anemarrhenae).

➢ With damp-heat in the essence chamber, add *huáng bǎi* (Cortex Phellodendri Chinensis), *zhī mǔ* (Rhizoma Anemarrhenae), *lóng dǎn cǎo* (Gentianae Radix) and *yě jú huā* (Flos Chrysanthemi Indici).

➢ With stasis obstructing the seminal duct, add *dān shēn* (Radix et Rhizoma Salviae Miltiorrhizae), *hóng huā* (Flos Carthami) and *chì sháo* (Radix Paeoniae Rubra).

In this formula, *xiān líng pí* (Herba Epimedii) and *ròu cōng róng* (Herba Cistanches) tonify kidney yang, essence, and marrow. They are warm but not drying, so they will not damage yin. *Shān yào* (Rhizoma Dioscoreae) is sweet and neutral, tonifying both kidney and spleen. It supports the congenital foundation by strengthening the acquired foundation. *Gǒu qǐ zǐ* (Fructus Lycii) is neutral and sweet, nourishing both yin and essence. It also invigorates original yang while replenishing kidney essence and qi. These medicinals act together to promote fertility by benefiting both yin and yang.

Methods and precautions: Decoct one divided dose, to be taken twice daily.

The medicinals may also be prepared as 9g honey pills; two pills to be taken two or three times daily. Six months constitutes one course of treatment for patients with azoospermia, and three months for those with poor semen quality.

During treatment, special precautions should be taken to avoid catching cold. To protect the essence, sexual intercourse should ideally occur at a frequency of only two to four times each month. Patients with yin essence deficiency or damp-heat in the lower burner should also avoid smoking, alcohol, and acrid or spicy foods. For those patients with kidney yang deficiency, raw or cold-natured foods should also be avoided.

(Shan Shu-jian. *Clinical Experience of Ancient and Contemporary Experts: Male Diseases*. Beijing: China Press of Traditional Chinese Medicine, 1999: 171-174)

10. XIE HAI-ZHOU: TONIFYING KIDNEY AND ESSENCE WHILE ELIMINATING STASIS AND DISINHIBITING DAMPNESS

Generally speaking, male infertility is associated with patterns of kidney and essence deficiency. Patients presenting with oligospermia are easier to treat than those with azoospermia. The treatment method here should primarily emphasize tonification based on accurate pattern differentiation in order to effectively harmonize yin, yang, qi and blood.

Select kidney-warming and yang-invigorating medicinals that possess an affinity to flesh and animals, such as *Wŭ Zĭ Yăn Zōng Wán* (五 子衍宗丸), *Shēn Lù Sān Shèn Wán* (参鹿三肾丸), *Hé Chē Dà Zào Wán* (河 车大造丸) and *Qiān Jīn Jiŭ Zĭ Wán* (千金韭子丸).

There are three main precautions:

(1) Kidney tonification is primary. The kidney is the viscus of water and fire, and also the residence of both original yin and original yang. Yin and yang should both be reinforced, but we should also understand how to tonify fire within water. When composing prescriptions, select medicinals that nourish yin and replenish essence while also warming the kidneys and invigorating yang. When yang begins to arise, yin will begin to grow.

(2) For deficiency patterns, tonification is essential, but congestion may also occur. Therefore, add small amounts of acrid and aromatic medicinals, and also those which are stagnation-moving, blood-invigorating and collateral-freeing in nature. This is the approach of seeking yang within yin, which also seeks to tonify without causing stagnation. *Qiāng huó* (Rhizoma et Radix Notopterygii) is particularly effective for this purpose, due to its acrid, aromatic and mobile nature. It acts to disperse congestion and free stagnation while also tonifying.

(3) The root of infertility is the kidney, and the most commonly seen pattern is essence qi deficiency. However, excess patterns like damp-heat in the lower burner or essence obstruction may appear as part of complex patterns which involve both deficiency and excess.

Deficiency here refers to patterns that involve insufficiencies of kidney yin and kidney yang, where excess refers to patterns of damp-heat and stasis. Although it is relatively easy to treat deficiency conditions with tonification, eliminating pathogens and supporting the upright is much more challenging. Presentations involving damp-heat and stasis are often seen in the clinic, and simple tonification will only aggravate these conditions.

As the famous physician Zhang Jing-yue pointed out, "There is no fixed formula for the planting of seeds. Different medicinals are a suitable for different people. Apply warming medicinals for cold conditions, cooling medicinals for heat, astringent medicinals for efflux conditions, and tonifying medicinals for the deficient. Eliminate the imbalance so that yin and yang are restored to harmony; engendering and transformation will then take place." The results of improper treatment can become quite serious, especially in severe cases.

(Shan Shu-jian. *Golden Mirror of Treatment of Famous Doctors in Ancient and Modern Times: Male Diseases*. Beijing: China Press of Traditional Chinese Medicine, 1999: 175–176)

11. Xue Meng: Treating Male Infertility with *Zhù Yìng Zī Shēng Tāng* (助应资生汤) and *Qiáng Jīng Yì Shèn Wán* (强精益肾丸)

Male infertility conditions usually present with a combination of disorders including seminal emission, premature ejaculation, impotence, strangury-turbidity (prostatitis), and yin mounting (spermatitis, periorchitis, orchiopathy). The quality and quantity of seminal fluid is often affected. These conditions include reduced seminal fluid volume, low sperm counts, low sperm survival rates, asthenospermia, abnormal sperm morphology, azoospermia, ejaculatory incompetence, non-liquefaction of semen, and hemospermia. Whether yang deficiency or yin deficiency, the primary method is to tonify the kidney. This is because the kidney consists of two parts; the left kidney is known as the palace of essence and the right is known as the life gate. When the water and fire of the kidney fail to assist each another, yin will not remain calm and yang becomes unsound, so reproduction becomes impossible.

Liver stagnation with damp-heat pouring downward can result in an inhibited movement of essence through the orifices, and also kidney debilitation. In these cases, methods of freeing and tonification should be applied together. In this way, yin and yang will become balanced and the condition will improve. The therapeutic effect will be more obvious when the treatment includes counseling or psychotherapy. Sexual activities should remain moderate, and emotional stress must be avoided whenever possible.

Zhù Yìng Zī Shēng Tāng (助应资生汤) has been shown effective in cases of male infertility due to kidney debilitation. To reinforce the therapeutic effect, *Qiáng Jīng Yì Shèn Wán* (强精益肾丸) may also be applied.

(1) *Zhù Yìng Zī Shēng Tāng* (助应资生汤)

潼蒺藜	*tóng jí lí*	20g	Semen Astragali Complanati
枸杞子	*gǒu qǐ zǐ*	20g	Fructus Lycii
仙茅	*xiān máo*	20g	Rhizoma Curculiginis
菟丝子	*tù sī zǐ*	20g	Semen Cuscutae
薏米	*yì mǐ*	20g	Semen Coicis
清炙黄芪	*qīng zhì huáng qí*	30g	Radix Astragali Praeparata cum Melle
淫羊藿	*yín yáng huò*	30g	Herba Epimedii
当归	*dāng guī*	15g	Radix Angelicae Sinensis
胡芦巴	*hú lú bā*	15g	Semen Trigonellae
巴戟肉	*bā jǐ ròu*	15g	Radix Morindae Officinalis
韭菜子	*jiǔ cài zǐ*	15g	Semen Allii Tuberosi
北沙参	*běi shā shēn*	15g	Radix Glehniae
大蜈蚣	*dà wú gōng*	3 pieces	Scolopendra

(2) *Qiáng Jīng Yì Shèn Wán* (强精益肾丸)

潼蒺藜	*tóng jí lí*	60g	Semen Astragali Complanati
枸杞子	*gǒu qǐ zǐ*	60g	Fructus Lycii
仙茅	*xiān máo*	60g	Rhizoma Curculiginis
菟丝子	*tù sī zǐ*	60g	Semen Cuscutae

薏苡仁	yì yǐ rén	60g	Semen Coicis
清炙黄芪	qīng zhì huáng qí	90g	Radix Astragali Praeparata cum Melle
淫羊藿	yín yáng huò	90g	Herba Epimedii
北沙参	běi shā shēn	45g	Radix Glehniae
熟地	shú dì	60g	Radix Rehmanniae Praeparata
肉苁蓉	ròu cōng róng	45g	Herba Cistanches
阳起石	yáng qǐ shí	45g	Actinolitum
鱼鳔胶	yú biào jiāo	500g	Piscis Vesica Aeris
羊睾丸	yáng gāo wán	2 pairs	lamb testicles
猪脊髓	zhū jǐ suǐ	5 pieces	pig marrow
羊脊髓	yáng jǐ suǐ	5 pieces	sheep marrow
大蜈蚣	dà wú gōng	9 pieces	Scolopendra

Grind into fine powder and prepare honey-pills. 15g, twice daily. The powder may also be encapsulated; 15 pills twice daily. The dosage may be increased if needed. Smoking, alcohol, and acrid spicy foods are prohibited. Sexual activity should remain moderate.

(Shan Shu-jian. *Golden Mirror of Treatment of Famous Doctors in Ancient and Modern Times: Male Infertility.* Beijing: China Press of Traditional Chinese Medicine, 1999: 183–186)

12. YANG ZONG-MENG: REGULATING WOOD, CLEARING THE LIVER, RESOLVING CONSTRAINT AND INCREASING WATER

Oligospermia refers to sperm counts below $(2000\text{-}4000)\times10^4$/ml. The classic literature states that conditions manifesting with scant semen are generally associated with kidney qi deficiency and life gate fire debilitation, resulting in failure to engender essence. Essence cold is another principal cause. However, longstanding patterns of liver constraint also can transform into heat and lead to fire flaming upwards disturbing the heart. This fire can spread internally to invade the spleen, move downwards along with qi, and thus damage the kidney essence. This pattern is also associated with conditions of oligospermia and premature ejaculation.

These disorders often result from patterns of longstanding liver constraint transforming into heat and fire. Due to the free coursing function of the liver, pathogenic fire is then able to move upwards, downwards or transversely. This movement can result in dysfunctions of the heart, spleen and kidney. The kidney governs water, and is also known as the female viscus. So when the kidney becomes dysfunctional, essence will fail to be engendered. However, the primary treatment principle here is to clear liver heat.

Select *Dān Zhī Xiāo Yáo Sǎn* (丹栀逍遥散) with added *chì fú líng* (Poria Rubra), *zhú yè* (Folium bambusae), *chǎo yīn chén* (stir-fried Herba Artemisiae Scopariae) and *fáng fēng* (Radix Saposhnikoviae).

Chì fú líng (Poria Rubra), *zhú yè* (Folium bambusae), *dān pí* (Cortex Moutan) and *zhī zǐ* (Fructus Gardeniae) all enter the heart channel to purge heart heat. *Chǎo yīn chén* (stir-fried Herba Artemisiae Scopariae) is not as bitter or cold as *zhī zǐ* (Fructus Gardeniae), so it is able to clear heat without causing latent cold in the spleen and stomach. *Fáng fēng* (Radix Saposhnikoviae) acts to balance the liver and spleen. After several doses, the heart-spleen heat will downbear, and the sperm count will also increase.

At this point, select *Zhī Bǎi Dì Huáng Tāng* (知柏地黄汤) with added *qīng yán* (Halitum), *dān pí* (Cortex Moutan) and *chì fú líng* (Poria Rubra). *Qīng yán* (Halitum) acts to nourish the kidney, clear the liver, and purge ministerial fire. *Dān pí* (Cortex Moutan) and *chì fú líng* (Poria Rubra) are added to prevent the recurrence of heat entering the heart and spleen. These medicinals act in combination to regulate wood, increase water, nourish yin, and clear heat. When the liver and kidney become regulated, essence and blood will be engendered, and reproduction can be achieved.

(Shan Shu-jian. *Golden Mirror of Treatment of Famous Doctors in Ancient and Modern Times: Male Infertility*. Beijing: China Press of Traditional Chinese Medicine, 1999: 183–186)

13. LI PEI-SHENG: INFERTILITY AND THE KIDNEY, SPLEEN, AND LIVER.

The primary causes of male infertility include congenital deficiency, excessive masturbation, becoming sexually active too early, or an irregular lifestyle following serious disease. The pathomechanism is generally associated with the kidney. The five viscera function to store essential qi without discharging it, and the kidney governs hibernation and storage. The kidney also stores essence known as true yin, and the life fire known as true yang. True yin and true yang are normally constrained and not discharged. When the congenital or acquired constitution is weak, true yang or true yin becomes more easily depleted, and male infertility may occur.

(1) Kidney Yang Deficiency

Symptoms and signs include impotence, premature ejaculation, spontaneous emission, dizziness, blurred vision, pale complexion, cold limbs, aching lumbus with limp legs, and fatigue. The tongue body appears pale white. Pulses are deep and forceless, or faint and thin.

The true yang of the kidney is the life gate fire, which acts to invigorate kidney qi and strengthen sexual function. Impotence, premature ejaculation, or spontaneous emission may occur when the qi of the kidney becomes deficient. The lumbus is known as the residence of the kidney. Aching of the lumbus and limpness of the legs may occur when kidney yang becomes insufficient. When yang qi fails to nourish the upper body, dizziness and a pale complexion will appear. When yang qi fails to fulfill the exterior, the limbs become cold.

For patterns of deficient yang qi, the proper treatment principle is to tonify and warm the lower origin while invigorating kidney qi.

Select the formula *Yòu Guī Wán* (右归丸), which contains the medicinals *shú dì* (Radix Rehmanniae Praeparata), *shān yào* (Rhizoma Dioscoreae), *shān yú ròu* (Fructus Corni), *ròu guì* (Cortex Cinnamomi), *shú fù piàn* (Aconiti Tuber Laterale Conquitum), *dù zhòng* (Cortex Eucommiae), *gǒu qǐ zǐ* (Fructus Lycii), *dāng guī* (Radix Angelicae Sinensis), *lù jiǎo jiāo* (Colla Cornus Cervi), and *tù sī zǐ* (Semen Cuscutae).

Also, *Fù Zǐ Tāng* (附 子 汤) may be applied. It contains *shú fù piàn* (Aconiti Tuber Laterale Conquitum), *rén shēn* (Radix et Rhizoma Ginseng), *fú líng* (Poria), *bái zhú* (Rhizoma Atractylodis Macrocephalae), and *bái sháo* (Radix Paeoniae Alba). Add *ròu cōng róng* (Herba Cistanches), *yín yáng huò* (Herba Epimedii), *dù zhòng* (Cortex Eucommiae), *bā jǐ tiān* (Radix Morindae Officinalis), *tù sī zǐ* (Semen Cuscutae), and *gǒu qǐ zǐ* (Fructus Lycii).

Yang deficiency engenders cold, so when male infertility is associated with kidney yang deficiency, the tongue and pulse presentation will always indicate the presence of cold. The primary treatment principle is to tonify and warm true yang, because the transformation of yin is not possible without sufficient yang. However, yang cannot be engendered without yin, so it is also essential to select medicinals that foster yin, nourish humor, tonify essence, and engender marrow.

(2) Kidney Yin Deficiency

Symptoms and signs include impotence, premature ejaculation, spontaneous emission, dizziness, tinnitus, dry throat and mouth, vexation and insomnia, aching lumbus with limp legs, and fatigue. The tongue appears red or crimson. Pulses are thready and rapid.

Because the kidney stores essence, it is also considered to be the foundation of life. When kidney yin becomes deficient, the ministerial fire may easily become stirred. Impotence, premature ejaculation, or frequent spontaneous emission may occur and eventually lead to male infertility. Yin deficiency and humor dryness may result in deficiency heat engendering internally, which can manifest with dizziness and distending sensations of the head, blurred vision, tinnitus, and disturbed spirit.

The kidney also governs the bones and engenders marrow. When yin essence becomes insufficient, the bones and marrow will become malnourished. Aching of the lumbus and limpness of the legs with fatigue may occur. The pulses and tongue body will both display signs of hyperactive yin deficiency fire. The treatment principle here is to nourish yin, subdue yang, tonify the kidney, and engender essence.

The most commonly used formula for this pattern is *Guī Shèn Wán* (归肾丸), which contains *shú dì* (Radix Rehmanniae Praeparata), *shān yào* (Rhizoma Dioscoreae), *shān yú ròu* (Fructus Corni), *tù sī zǐ* (Semen Cuscutae), *dāng guī* (Radix Angelicae Sinensis), *fú líng* (Poria), *gǒu qǐ zǐ* (Fructus Lycii), and *dù zhòng* (Cortex Eucommiae).

Modifications include the addition of *guī bǎn jiāo* (Colla Carapax et Plastrum Testudinis), *guǎng yú biào jiāo* (Piscis Vesica Aeris), *yín yáng huò* (Herba Epimedii), *ròu cōng róng* (Herba Cistanches), *wǔ wèi zǐ* (Fructus Schisandrae Chinensis), and *sāng shèn zǐ* (Fructus Mori).

The treatment principle here is to primarily nourish kidney yin while also invigorating kidney water to restrain the brilliance of yang. However, when the ministerial fire becomes hyperactive, the fire must be suppressed in order to conserve yin humor. The proper application of these two methods is an important consideration during diagnosis and treatment.

Differentiation of kidney patterns begins with clinical presentations that indicate either kidney yang deficiency or kidney yin deficiency. But when it comes to more complex patterns of yin and yang dual deficiency, neutral tonification is required to nourish yin, invigorate yang, tonify essence, and boost qi. These methods aim to benefit the recovery of sexual function. Based on classical formulas, the empirical formulas *Shí Zǐ Yù Lín Tāng* (十子育麟汤) and *Shí Zǐ Yù Lín Gāo* (十子育麟膏) have been composed. The formula contains the following medicinals.

Gǒu qǐ zǐ (Fructus Lycii), *wǔ wèi zǐ* (Fructus Schisandrae Chinensis), *shé chuáng zǐ* (Fructus Cnidii), *sāng shèn zǐ* (Fructus Mori), *tù sī zǐ* (Semen Cuscutae), *fù pén zǐ* (Fructus Rubi), *chē qián zǐ* (Semen Plantaginis), *jīn yīng zǐ* (Fructus Rosae Laevigatae), *yì zhì rén* (Fructus Alpiniae Oxyphyllae), *chǎo bǔ gǔ zhī* (stir-fried Fructus Psoraleae), *hóng shēn* (Radix et Rhizoma Ginseng Rubra), *ròu cōng róng* (Herba Cistanches), *lù jiǎo jiāo* (Colla Cornus Cervi), *guī bǎn jiāo* (Testudinis Plastri Gelatinum), *dù zhòng* (Cortex Eucommiae), *yín yáng huò* (Herba Epimedii), *dāng guī* (Radix Angelicae Sinensis), *shú dì* (Radix Rehmanniae Praeparata), and *jú hóng* (Exocarpium Citri Rubrum). May be taken as a decoction, pills, or soft extract.

Even though the primary pathomechanism of male infertility is rooted in the kidney, patients presenting with liver constraint or weakness of the spleen may also display decreased reproductive function. These patterns can also contribute to male infertility.

If at first there are no physical symptoms, and impotence appears with asthenospermia, reproductive function can generally be recovered with proper treatment. For male infertility associated with congenital impotence and low libido, the treatment is more difficult. Significant therapeutic effects may not be achieved for several months, or sometimes even years. Patients should be advised to remain confident during long-term course of treatment, and to also restrain sexual activity.

Supporting yang qi is primary in cases of male infertility due to kidney yang deficiency, but we should also consider the fact that yang is rooted within yin. Therefore, yang-invigorating medicinals should generally be combined with medicinals that also nourish yin and replenish essence. Otherwise, chronic deficiency conditions may transform into patterns of hyperactive yang. Strong yang-invigorating minerals such as *yáng qǐ shí* (Actinolitum), *zhōng rǔ shí* (Stalactitum), and *liú huáng* (Sulphur) may display short-term effects when taken with alcohol. However, these medicinals should be used with caution because they will eventually damage true yin and also the true origin.

Dietary therapy is an effective complementary approach in the treatment of male infertility. "Insufficiency of essence may be supplemented with flavors." Medicinals with an affinity to flesh and blood are most recommended. This category of medicinals acts to strongly tonify essence, boost qi, nourish yin, and invigorate yang.

Shú fù kuài (Aconiti Tuber Laterale Conquitum) may be stewed with mutton. This medicinal recipe benefits patients with male infertility due to kidney yang deficiency. Other therapeutic foods include *guǎng yú biào jiāo* (Piscis Vesica Aeris), turtle meat, soft-shelled turtle, inkfish, sea slug, freshwater mussels, human placenta, and the testicles of oxen and dogs. *Lù róng* (Cornu Cervi Pantotrichum) and *hǎi gǒu shèn* (Callorhini Testes et Penis) should also be added to the daily diet.

(Shan Shu-jian. *Golden Mirror of Treatment by Famous Doctors in Ancient and Modern Times: Male Diseases*. Beijing: China Press of Traditional Chinese Medicine, 1999: 189–194)

14. Ban Xiu-wen: Necrospermia and Nourishing of the Liver and Kidney

In many cases of infertility, sexual intercourse and ejaculation are normal and both parties appear to be in good health. However, analysis of the seminal fluid may reveal reduced sperm counts with low survival rates and weak motility. If the proportion of non-viable sperm is greater than 2/3, this condition is referred to as necrospermia.

This syndrome can result from either congenital deficiency, or acquired malnourishment. Both conditions can manifest with patterns of true yin depletion and deficiency fire flaming internally, or life gate fire debilitation leading to internal yin exuberance and cold-damp accumulation. Conditions that display disliquefaction of semen and high numbers of non-viable sperm are caused by liver and kidney yin deficiency with water failing to assist fire. This results in deficiency fire stirring internally. The treatment principle here is to nourish yin and tonify the kidney while emolliating and nourishing liver yin.

The kidney stores essence. It is also known as the viscus of water and fire. It stores both true yin and original yang, and also serves as the foundation of reproduction. The liver stores blood and also governs orderly reaching. When the yin essence of the kidney is sufficient and the qi and blood of the liver are harmonious, normal sexual function and conception are possible. However, if the liver and kidney yin become deficient and essence and blood are depleted, water will then fail to assist fire. Deficient yang may become stirred, latent fire in the penetrating and conception channels will begin to flame, and scorching of the fluids and blood will occur. This further depletes the true essence, with manifestations of poor liquefaction and low sperm survival rates.

Select liver emolliating and nourishing medicinals such as *shǒu wū* (Radix Polygoni Multiflori), *sāng shèn zǐ* (Fructus Mori), and *gǒu qǐ zǐ* (Fructus Lycii), and liver soothing medicinals such as *hé huān huā* (Flos Albiziae), *sù xīn huā* (Flos Jasmini Officinalis), and *yù lán huā* (Flos Magnoliae).

Select formulas that nourish and tonify the kidney such as *Liù Wèi Dì Huáng Tāng* (六味地黄汤) and *Bā Xiān Cháng Shòu Wán* (八仙长寿丸) with added *dāng guī* (Radix Angelicae Sinensis) and *bái sháo* (Radix Paeoniae Alba).

With predominant yin deficiency, apply *Èr Zhì Wán* (二至丸), *Gān Mài Dà Zǎo Tāng* (甘麦大枣汤), *shǒu wū* (Radix Polygoni Multiflori) and *gǒu qǐ zǐ* (Fructus Lycii). Aromatic and neutral medicinals such as *sù xīn huā* (Flos Jasmini Officinalis), *hé huān huā* (Flos Albiziae) or *yù lán huā* (Flos

Magnoliae) may also be added.

Liù Wèi Dì Huáng Tāng (六味地黄汤) "treats diseases of all six channels, but particularly those of the kidney and liver. It is neither cold nor dry, but tonifies both qi and blood." (*Medical Formulas Collected and Analyzed* (医方集解, *Yī Fāng Jí Jiě*)).

Dāng guī (Radix Angelicae Sinensis), *bái sháo* (Radix Paeoniae Alba), *shŏu wū* (Radix Polygoni Multiflori), *gŏu qĭ zĭ* (Fructus Lycii), *Èr Zhì Wán* (二至丸) and *Gān Mài Dà Zăo Tāng* (甘麦大枣汤) may be applied to further tonify the kidney and liver while also nourishing yin and blood. *Sù xīn huā* (Flos Jasmini Officinalis), *hé huān huā* (Flos Albiziae) and *yù lán huā* (Flos Magnoliae) act to regulate, soothe, and promote the engendering of liver qi.

Neutral tonification of yin and yang may improve the prognosis at the late stage of treatment.

Select *Wŭ Zĭ Yăn Zōng Wán* (五子衍宗丸) with added *dāng guī* (Radix Angelicae Sinensis), *bái sháo* (Radix Paeoniae Alba), *tài zĭ shēn* (Radix Pseudostellariae), *shān yào* (Rhizoma Dioscoreae), *shān yú ròu* (Fructus Corni), and *nŭ zhēn zĭ* (Fructus Ligustri Lucidi).

Abnormal sperm morphology may result from patterns of yin deficiency with yang hyperactivity or yang debilitation with yin exuberance. Yin deficiency with yang hyperactivity leads to deficiency fire stirring and scorching true essence. This can result in the congealing of fluids and poor liquefaction of semen, or even necrospermia. Yang debilitation with yin exuberance can lead to damp obstruction and cold congealment. This may result in oligospermia, azoospermia, or low sperm survival rates. So treatments that nourish and warm should be clearly based on the presenting etiology, especially in cases which present yin essence depletion and ministerial fire moving frenetically.

(Shan Shu-jian. *Golden Mirror of Treatment of Famous Doctors in Ancient and Modern Times: Male Diseases*. Beijing: China Press of Traditional

Chinese Medicine, 1999: 197–200)

15. Liu Ming-han: Kidney Debilitation and Yì Jīng Líng (益精灵)

Reduced sperm counts, low survival rates, and high numbers of abnormal sperm are commonly seen in cases of male infertility. Normal production of semen relies on nourishment from the kidney yin, and also the warming function of kidney yang. Reproductive function also depends on the status of the true yin and true yang of the kidney. The original qi is associated with fire and yang, whereas semen belongs to water and yin. The secretions of the prostate and seminal vesicle are considered as "yin within yin", while the seminal fluid itself may be considered as "yang within yin". Furthermore, the sperm can also be divided into yin and yang aspects. The sperm body is "yin within yang", and the motility of sperm is "yang within yang"."Yang acts to transform qi, while yin acts to form shapes". The quantity of sperm is primarily associated with kidney yin, and motility is determined by the state of kidney yang.

In treatment, male infertility can be divided into three types:

➤ Basic type (sperm counts and survival rates both reduced)
➤ Kidney yin deficiency (low sperm counts)
➤ Kidney yang deficiency (low sperm survival rates).

Apply Yì Jīng Líng (益精灵) with modifications.

淫羊藿	yín yáng huò	500g	Herba Epimedii
锁阳	suǒ yáng	250g	Herba Cynomorii
巴戟天	bā jǐ tiān	250g	Radix Morindae Officinalis
熟地	shú dì	250g	Radix Rehmanniae Praeparata
山萸肉	shān yú ròu	90g	Fructus Corni
附片	fù piàn	90g	Aconiti Tuber Laterale
肉苁蓉	ròu cōng róng	200g	Herba Cistanches
枸杞子	gǒu qǐ zǐ	150g	Fructus Lycii

黄芪	*huáng qí*	250g	Radix Astragali
当归	*dāng guī*	90g	Radix Angelicae Sinensis
韭菜子	*jiŭ cài zĭ*	60g	Semen Allii Tuberosi
车前子	*chē qián zĭ*	60g	Semen Plantaginis
菟丝子	*tù sī zĭ*	150g	Semen Cuscutae
桑椹子	*sāng shèn zĭ*	150g	Fructus Mori
龟板胶	*guī bǎn jiāo*	100g	Testudinis Plastri Gelatinum
鹿角胶	*lù jiǎo jiāo*	100g	Colla Cornus Cervi
茺蔚子	*chōng wèi zĭ*	150g	Fructus Leonuri
甘草	*gān căo*	100g	Radix et Rhizoma Glycyrrhizae

Infuse the medicinals with distilled spirits containing 60% alcohol for 7 to 15 days. Take 25 to 50 ml three times daily, before or with meals. The medicinals may be infused twice if needed.

Decoction: The dosage of *yín yáng huò* (Herba Epimedii) is reduced to 30g, with all other medicinals reduced to one-tenth of the above amounts. Decoct to 300-400 ml as one divided dose, taken three times daily.

【Modifications】

(1) For kidney yang deficiency with normal sperm counts with low survival rates, inhibited ejaculation, frequent or dribbling urination, impotence, premature ejaculation, dream emission, and cold painful lumbus and knees, large dosages of *huáng qí* (adix Astragali), *ròu guì* (Cortex Cinnamomi), and *fù piàn* (Aconiti Tuber Laterale) may be added to the basic formula.

The following medicinals may also be added.

党参	*dăng shēn*	20g	Radix Codonopsis
黄精	*huáng jīng*	30g	Rhizoma Polygonati
阳起石	*yáng qĭ shí*	30g	Actinolitum
仙茅	*xiān máo*	20g	Rhizoma Curculiginis
海狗肾	*hăi gǒu shèn*	1 piece	Callorhini Testes et Penis
金樱子	*jīn yīng zĭ*	30g	Fructus Rosae Laevigatae

(2) For kidney yin deficiency with low seminal fluid volume, reduced sperm count, normal survival rate, aching lumbus with limp knees, tinnitus, and poor memory, large dosages of *shú dì* (Radix Rehmanniae Praeparata), *shān yú ròu* (Fructus Corni), *gǒu qǐ zǐ* (Fructus Lycii) and *sāng shèn zǐ* (Fructus Mori) may be added to the basic formula.

The following medicinals may also be added.

首乌	*shǒu wū*	30g	Radix Polygoni Multiflori
桑寄生	*sāng jì shēng*	30g	Herba Taxilli
女贞子	*nǚ zhēn zǐ*	30g	Fructus Ligustri Lucidi

The above dosages apply to decocted formulas. Dosages may be increased by ten times for alcohol infusions. The largest dosage for any single medicinal is 300g, or 30g when decocted.

The formula *Yì Jīng Líng* (益 精 灵) contains medicinals that can improve the overall quality of sperm. *Yín yáng huò* (Herba Epimedii) "governs male infertility due to yang expiration" (*Materia Medica of Ri Hua-zi* (日华子诸家本草 , *Rì Huá Zǐ Zhū Jiā Běn Cǎo*)). *Suǒ yáng* (Herba Cynomorii), *bā jǐ tiān* (Radix Morindae Officinalis), *fù piàn* (Aconiti Tuber Laterale), *ròu guì* (Cortex Cinnamomi), *ròu cōng róng* (Herba Cistanches), *jiǔ cài zǐ* (Semen Allii Tuberosi), *tù sī zǐ* (Semen Cuscutae), and *chōng wèi zǐ* (Fructus Leonuri) benefit the kidney and invigorate yang. *Guī jiāo* (Testudinis Plastri Gelatinum), *lù jiāo jiāo* (Colla Cornus Cervi), *shú dì* (Radix Rehmanniae Praeparata), *gǒu qǐ zǐ* (Fructus Lycii), *sāng shèn zǐ* (Fructus Mori) and *shān yú ròu* (Fructus Corni) nourish yin and replenish essence. *Huáng qí* (Radix Astragali) and *dāng guī* (Radix Angelicae Sinensis) tonify qi and blood. *Gān cǎo* (Radix et Rhizoma Glycyrrhizae) acts to harmonize the middle and fortify the spleen. *Chē qián zǐ* (Semen Plantaginis) acts to free the water passage so as to promote ejaculation.

This formula applies the principle, "Yin cannot become engendered without yang; yang cannot grow without yin." The formula also acts to nourish yin, invigorate yang, and tonify qi and blood while freeing the essence passage. These actions strongly benefit the essence to promote fertility.

During the course of treatment, sexual activity should be restrained with a maximum frequency of 1-2 times per week. Some patients may experience slight abdominal distention, diarrhea, and reduced food intake at first, but those symptoms will usually resolve after 1 or 2 days. Sperm quality generally improves dramatically during treatment, but then declines when the medicinal are discontinued. Alcohol preparations and decoctions are equally effective.

(Shan Shu-jian. *Golden Mirror of Treatment of Famous Doctors in Ancient and Modern Times: Male Diseases*. Beijing: China Press of Traditional Chinese Medicine, 1999: 201–203)

16. JIN WEI-XIN: NON-LIQUEFACTION OF SEMEN AND YÈ HUÀ SHĒNG JĪNG TĀNG (液化升精汤)

Non-liquefaction of semen is a primary cause of male infertility. Delayed liquefaction results in semen that remains relatively motionless in the vaginal canal. Congealed seminal fluid leads not only to increased rates of sperm mortality, but also hinders the semen from successfully passing through the uterine neck. This condition is often associated with other infertility factors including low sperm counts and reduced sperm survival rates.

Associated patterns include effulgent kidney fire scorching the fluids, which results in thickening of the seminal fluid. Kidney yang deficiency or original yang insufficiency may also lead to coldness of the essence palace, and abnormal qi transformation. Patterns of damp-turbidity or damp-heat pouring downwards into the bladder can result in turbidity mixing with the clear, which manifests with thick semen and also non-liquefaction. In some cases, phlegm-damp may obstruct the essence orifices and also lead to disliquefaction.

Yè Huà Shēng Jīng Tāng (液化升精汤) has been shown very effective for treatment of these clinical presentations.

The formula contains the following medicinals.

丹皮	*dān pí*	9g	Cortex Moutan
地骨皮	*dì gǔ pí*	9g	Cortex Lycii
白芍	*bái sháo*	9g	Radix Paeoniae Alba
赤芍	*chì sháo*	9g	Radix Paeoniae Rubra
生地	*shēng dì*	12g	Radix Rehmanniae
麦冬	*mài dōng*	15g	Radix Ophiopogonis
玄参	*xuán shēn*	12g	Radix Scrophulariae
生牡蛎	*shēng mǔ lì*	30g	Concha Ostreae Cruda
浙贝母	*zhè bèi mǔ*	12g	Bulbus Fritillariae Thunbergii
枸杞子	*gǒu qǐ zǐ*	12g	Fructus Lycii
丹参	*dān shēn*	15g	Radix et Rhizoma Salviae Miltiorrhizae
山萸肉	*shān yú ròu*	9g	Fructus Corni
金银花	*jīn yín huā*	18g	Flos Lonicerae Japonicae
连翘	*lián qiào*	9g	Fructus Forsythiae
夏枯草	*xià kū cǎo*	9g	Spica Prunellae
柴胡	*chái hú*	9g	Radix Bupleuri
竹叶	*zhú yè*	9g	Lophatheri Folium
茯苓	*fú líng*	9g	Poria
淫羊藿	*yín yáng huò*	12g	Herba Epimedii

Dān pí (Cortex Moutan), *dì gǔ pí* (Cortex Lycii), *bái sháo* (Radix Paeoniae Alba), *shēng dì* (Radix Rehmanniae Recens) and *fú líng* (Poria) are the main ingredients of *Qīng Jīng Tāng* (清经汤). This formula was originally used to treat advanced or profuse menstruation with its actions of clearing heat and cooling the blood. It eliminates heat and preserves yin by gently clearing fire without excessively purging water. When used for non-liquefaction of semen, it can clear kidney fire, nourish yin, and preserve fluids while also eliminating deficiency heat and engendering yin humor.

Xuán shēn (Radix Scrophulariae), *shēng mǔ lì* (Concha Ostreae Cruda) and *zhè bèi mǔ* (Bulbus Fritillariae Thunbergii) are the main ingredients of *Xiāo Luǒ Wán* (消瘰丸). This formula acts to clear heat, transform phlegm, soften hardness, and dissipate binding. It promotes liquefaction while also preserving liver and kidney yin.

Shēng dì (Radix Rehmanniae Recens), *mài dōng* (Radix Ophiopogonis) and *xuán shēn* (Radix Scrophulariae) are the main ingredients of *Zēng Yè Tāng* (增液汤). This formula acts to increase humor and moisturize dryness.

Shān yú ròu (Fructus Corni) is used to tonify the liver and kidney while astringing. It also acts to regulate yin and yang with a slightly warm nature. *Jīn yín huā* (Flos Lonicerae Japonicae), *lián qiào* (Fructus Forsythiae) and *xià kū cǎo* (Spica Prunellae) clear heat, resolve toxin, soften hardness, and dissipate binding. *Chì sháo* (Radix Paeoniae Rubra) and *dān shēn* (Radix et Rhizoma Salviae Miltiorrhizae) clear heat and cool the blood while also invigorating blood and transforming stasis. *Chái hú* (Radix Bupleuri) is used to course the liver and rectify qi. *Fú líng* (Poria) can fortify the spleen with bland percolation and also disinhibit pathogenic damp. *Zhú yè* (Folium bambusae) clears the upper and penetrates the lower. It is used to clear heat, disinhibit dampness, and eliminate vexation. *Gǒu qǐ zǐ* (Fructus Lycii) is sweet, neutral and moist, and so used to nourish the liver and kidney. Sweet and warm *Yín yáng huò* (Herba Epimedii) acts to tonify kidney yang.

This formula is a combination of *Qīng Jīng Tāng* (清经汤), *Xiāo Luǒ Wán* (消瘰丸), *Zēng Yè Tāng* (增液汤) and *Liù Wèi Dì Huáng Wán* (六味地黄丸). The principles of tonification and purging are perfectly combined in this formula. It not only tonifies the liver, kidney and spleen yin, but it also acts to warm deficient kidney yang. Furthermore, it can clear heat, disinhibit dampness, transform phlegm, disperse hardness, invigorate blood, and move static stagnation.

This formula is primarily indicated for patterns of kidney yin and yang dual deficiency. Symptoms and signs include thick sperm with poor liquefaction, aching lumbus and limp knees, dizziness, tinnitus, vexing heat in the five hearts, aversion to cold, cold limbs, fatigue, lack of strength, insomnia, profuse dreaming, and dry mouth without the desire to drink. The tongue appears pale or red with little coating. Pulses are thin and weak, or thin and rapid.

Precautions: This formula is specifically indicated for yin and yang dual deficiency. Modifications are required when predominant patterns of kidney yin or kidney yang deficiency appear.

(Shan Shu-jian. *Golden Mirror of Treatment by Famous Doctors in Ancient and Modern Times: Male Diseases*. Beijing: China Press of Traditional Chinese Medicine, 1999: 210–213)

17. YAN DE-XIN: ABSENT EJACULATION AND *Xuè Fǔ Zhú Yū Tāng* (血府逐瘀汤)

In clinic, ejaculatory incompetence is generally treated by tonifying the kidney and invigorating yang, or freeing the collaterals. Cases presenting with damp-heat in the liver channel may be treated with *Lóng Dǎn Xiè Gān Tāng* (龙胆泻肝汤), where other patterns may require coursing the liver and resolving constraint. In fact, patterns of deficiency are seen only in a minority of cases.

The kidney stores essence and engenders marrow. The brain is known as the sea of marrow, so it is closely associated with kidney function as well as the central nervous system. When kidney deficiency patterns in younger patients manifest with impotence, premature ejaculation, ejaculatory incompetence, and oligospermia, proper treatment should also address the the brain. It is seldom effective to simply warm the kidney and tonify yang. To effectively treat the brain, treatment of the heart is also required since the heart controls the blood vessels, also known as the residence of blood. Methods of invigorating blood and transforming stasis are also required to achieve a therapeutic effect, and *Xuè Fǔ Zhú Yū Tāng* (血府逐瘀汤) is an effective formula for this purpose.

Many practitioners will prescribe large doses of *rén shēn* (Radix et Rhizoma Ginseng) and *lù róng* (Cornu Cervi Pantotrichum) at the first sight of ejaculatory incompetence, or even testosterone or gonadotrophic hormones. However, this kind of treatment can aggravate the excess patterns of stasis and stagnation, and also result in an inhibition of the qi dynamic. Treatment with *Zhú Yū Tāng* (逐瘀汤) can effectively reverse this condition.

Signs and symptoms of blood stasis patterns include dry mouth with no desire to drink, purple tongue and lips, rough skin with purple spots, alopecia, inhibited movement of the limbs, fluctuating emotions, profuse dreaming, and even confused thinking. Pulses may appear rough, tight, deep, or slow. A correct diagnosis requires the presence of only one or two of these symptoms. It is essential in these cases to properly apply the stasis-eliminating method.

(Shan Shu-jian. *Golden Mirror of Treatment of Famous Doctors in Ancient and Modern Times: Male Diseases*. Beijing: China Press of Traditional Chinese Medicine, 1999: 217–219)

18. Lin Shi-xin: Ejaculatory Incompetence and the Liver

Medicinals and formulas that primarily tonify the kidney and invigorate yang are not usually effective in the treatment of male functional ejaculatory incompetence. For patients with constitutional yang deficiency, warming yang is essential. However, the typical patient complaining of ejaculatory incompetence is usually in good physical condition, but also presenting with signs of a liver pattern, including excess pulses images and an often irascible temper. Treating with the method of purging liver wood very often results in fertility.

The recommended formula contains the following medicinals.

柴胡	chái hú	10g	Radix Bupleuri
赤芍	chì sháo	10g	Radix Paeoniae Rubra
炒枳实	chǎo zhǐ shí	10g	Fructus Aurantii Immaturus (dry-fried)
甘草梢	gān cǎo shāo	5g	Radix et Rhizoma Glycyrrhizae
穿山甲	chuān shān jiǎ	10g	Squama Manis
王不留行	wáng bù liú xíng	20g	Semen Vaccariae
川牛膝	chuān niú xī	10g	Radix Cyathulae
黑白丑	hēi bái chǒu	10g	Semen Pharbitidis
石菖蒲	shí chāng pú	10g	Rhizoma Acori Tatarinowii
滑石粉	huá shí fěn	10g	Pulvis Talci

Four decoctions per week. Three weeks constitute one course of treatment.

Although the engendering and storage of semen relies mainly on the kidney, the function of free-coursing depends on the liver, since the liver likes orderly reaching. When the orderly reaching of liver qi is normal, blood becomes effulgent, qi is well distributed throughout the sinews, and free-coursing becomes timely. When orderly reaching fails, dispersing becomes inhibited, and dysfunctions of ejaculation may appear. This presentation is quite different from those conditions resulting from kidney depletion.

In this formula, *Sì Nì Sǎn* (四逆散) is applied to course the liver qi. *Chuān shān jiǎ* (Squama Manis) and *wáng bù liú xíng* (Semen Vaccariae) are essential medicinals to promote lactation in females. In this formula, they act to course the liver qi in order to disinhibit the free-coursing of essence. *Huá shí* (Talcum) and *niú xī* (Radix Achyranthis Bidentatae) move downward to disinhibit the orifices. *Shí chāng pú* (Rhizoma Acori Tatarinowii) is used to open the orifices and disperse depression. *Hēi bái chǒu* (Semen Pharbitidis) acts to free the passage of water, grain and essence, so this is added to guide the medicinals to the seminal duct. These medicinals act together to regulate the qi dynamic and also promote the free-coursing of semen.

(Shan Shu-jian. *Golden Mirror of Treatment of Famous Doctors in Ancient and Modern Times: Male Diseases*. Beijing: China Press of Traditional Chinese Medicine, 1999: 219–220)

19. YANG QIAN-QIAN: *HUÁNG QÍ HUÁ SHÍ TĀNG* (黄芪滑石汤) IN THE TREATMENT OF FUNCTIONAL EJACULATORY INCOMPETENCE

Functional ejaculatory incompetence is commonly seen in clinic. It may be divided into three patterns: Qi deficiency, damp-heat obstructing the orifices, and yin-essence insufficiency. However, complex patterns may present signs of both deficiency and excess, and all three patterns may be seen in the same patient. The treatment principle here is to benefit qi, nourish yin, tonify the kidney, replenish essence, clear and disinhibit damp-heat, and open the orifices.

The empirical formula *Huáng Qí Huá Shí Tāng* (黄芪滑石汤) is known to be very effective for this condition.

Huáng Qí Huá Shí Tāng (黄芪滑石汤) contains the following medicinals.

黄芪	*huáng qí*	17g	Radix Astragali
滑石	*huá shí*	15g	Talcum
甘草	*gān cǎo*	5g	Radix et Rhizoma Glycyrrhizae
楮实子	*chǔ shí zǐ*	9g	Fructus Broussonetiae
茯苓	*fú líng*	15g	Poria
车前子	*chē qián zǐ*	27g	Semen Plantaginis
菟丝子	*tù sī zǐ*	15g	Semen Cuscutae
肉苁蓉	*ròu cōng róng*	10g	Herba Cistanches
南豆花	*nán dòu huā*	9g	Flos Dolichoris Album
穿山甲	*chuān shān jiǎ*	9g	Squama Manis
王不留行	*wáng bù liú xíng*	9g	Semen Vaccariae

In *Corrections of Mistakes in the Medical Profession* (医林改错 , *Yī Lín Gǎi Cuò*), Qing dynasty physician Wang Qing-ren recorded a case of treating an elderly man with longstanding painful urination with *Huáng Qí Gān Cǎo Tāng* (黄芪甘草汤). Since semen and urine share the same orifice in males, *Huáng Qí Huá Shí Tāng* (黄芪滑石汤) was composed. *Huáng qí* (Radix Astragali) is sweet and slightly warm. It is an essential medicinal for tonifying qi. It is also recorded that *huáng qí* (Radix Astragali) can tonify deficiency in men, while also disinhibiting both yin qi and urine. Modern research has shown that *huáng qí* (Radix Astragali) displays excitatory effects on the central nervous system, thus a most appropriate sovereign medicinal.

Ejaculatory incompetence is generally associated with yin qi deficiency, so *tù sī zǐ* (Semen Cuscutae), *ròu cōng róng* (Herba Cistanches) and *chǔ shí zǐ* (Fructus Broussonetiae) are employed as ministers to tonify yin essence. *Chǔ shí zǐ* (Fructus Broussonetiae) and *ròu cōng róng* (Herba Cistanches) act to both tonify and free. *Huá shí* (Talcum), *fú líng* (Poria) and *chē qián zǐ* (Semen Plantaginis) disinhibit water and free the essence orifice. *Nán dòu huā* (Flos Lablab) acts to aromatically eliminate dampness, while opening the upper and freeing the lower. *Chuān shān jiǎ* (Squama Manis) frees the orifices, and *wáng bù liú xíng* (Semen Vaccariae) disinhibits urine. Both medicinals are mobile in nature, and so employed as assistants. As the envoy, *gān cǎo* (Radix et Rhizoma Glycyrrhizae) acts to harmonize the formula while also disinhibiting urine.

Huáng Qí Huá Shí Tāng (黄芪滑石汤) is very effective, even if all of the ingredients are unavailable. Decoct with three bowls of water until one bowl remains; take on an empty stomach. Decoct the dregs once again at bedtime. One daily dose, with seven days constituting one treatment course. Discontinue use with colds or flu with fever, cough, or sore throat.

For patients with predominant yin essence deficiency manifesting with dizziness, palpitation, tinnitus, and aching lumbus; the following medicinals may be added.

柏子仁	bǎi zǐ rén	12g	Semen Platycladi
女贞子	nǚ zhēn zǐ	12g	Fructus Ligustri Lucidi
杜仲	dù zhòng	9g	Cortex Eucommiae

Bǎi Hé Liù Wèi Dì Huáng Tāng (百合六味地黄汤) may also be selected. The patient may also be advised to consume fish soup as a dietary therapy.

With predominant damp-heat obstructing the orifices manifesting with a bitter taste in the mouth, slimy tongue coating, yellow urine, and genital pain; the following medicinals may be added.

蒲公英	pú gōng yīng	9g	Herba Taraxaci
土茯苓	tǔ fú líng	9g	Rhizoma Smilacis Glabrae
鸡蛋花	jī dàn huā	12g	Flos Plumeriae Acutifoliae

With predominant qi deficiency manifesting with impotence, reduced sex drive, and fatigue with weak pulses; the following medicinals may be added.

| 党参 | dǎng shēn | 17g | Radix Codonopsis |
| 巴戟天 | bā jǐ tiān | 12g | Radix Morindae Officinalis |

Sān Rén Tāng (三仁汤) with quail eggs, or pigeon stewed with *rén shēn* (Radix et Rhizoma Ginseng) and *lù róng* (Cornu Cervi Pantotrichum) may also be applied.

(Shan Shu-jian. *Golden Mirror of Treatment of Famous Doctors in Ancient and Modern Times: Male Diseases*. Beijing: China Press of Traditional Chinese Medicine, 1999: 220–223)

20. Liu Ming-han: *Tōng Jīng Líng* (通精灵) for Absent Ejaculation

Although the functional absence of ejaculation is commonly seen in clinic, little relevant information has been recorded in the classical literature. As a result, few practitioners are very familiar with this disorder. Since seminal emission is commonly seen along with accompanying symptoms, practitioners tend to believe that the patient's essence gate is insecure, and that chronic disease has lead to a condition of deficiency. The deficiency is then treated with with tonification in order to secure the essence and check emission. However, as tonification is applied, seminal emission increases, and normal ejaculation becomes impossible. In fact, deficiency is not the main cause, since dream emission is rather due to "spillage due to fullness", and the absence of ejaculation is a result of dysfunction of the essence gate. Based on this pathomechanism, the treatment principle here must free the essence and check emission, that is, a combination of methods which both free and tonify. The following methods have been chosen to address the variety of possible clinical manifestations: warm the kidney and free the gate, nourish the kidney and free the gate, resolve constraint and free the gate, and transform dampness, clear heat, free the gate and check emission. *Tōng Jīng Líng* (通 精灵) modifications I through V are selected respectively.

(1) Kidney Yang Deficiency

This pattern is mostly seen in patients over the age of 40, particularly in those who have lead a sexually active lifestyle for the previous 10 to 20 years. These patients often present with patterns of kidney yang deficiency due to the frequent loss of semen.

Symptoms and signs include aching lumbus and limp legs, dream emission, white or somber gray facial complexion, long voidings of clear urine, frequent nighttime urination, decreased sex drive, incomplete erection, and reduced duration of sexual intercourse. The tongue appears pale with a thin white or moist coating, or tender and enlarged with teethmarks. Pulses are deep and thin. The treatment principle here is to warm the kidney and free the gate.

Select *Tōng Jīng Líng Yī Hào Fāng* (通精灵一号方). In this formula, *fù piàn* (Aconiti Tuber Laterale), *ròu guì* (Cortex Cinnamomi), *xiān líng pí* (Herba Epimedii) and *yáng qǐ shí* (Actinolitum) act to warm the kidney and assist yang. *Shēng dì* (Radix Rehmanniae), *shú dì* (Radix Rehmanniae Praeparata) and *shān yú ròu* (Fructus Corni) tonify kidney yin. *Má huáng* (Herba Ephedrae) is acrid in flavor and warm in nature. It acts to open the gate and free blockage.

Modern research has found that ephedrine can stimulate the central nervous system and promote ejaculation. *Wú gōng* (Scolopendra) is known as the "fastest and most powerful medicinal for promoting movement. It effectively opens qi and blood congestion of the organs, channels and collaterals." It may be combined with *quán xiē* (Scorpio), *dì lóng* (Pheretima), and *jiāng cán* (Bombyx Batryticatus) to course the collaterals and promote ejaculation. *Dāng guī* (Radix Angelicae Sinensis) nourishes blood. *Bái sháo* (Radix Paeoniae Alba) acts to tonify and emolliate the liver, as well as nourishing the ancestral sinew. This emolliating nature can help to balance the relatively harsh actions of *chóng* based medicinals. *Niú xī* (Achyranthes Bidentata) enters the kidney and promotes the downward movement of the other medicinals, and *jiǔ cài zǐ* (Semen Allii Tuberosi) acts to assist yang. Acting together, these medicinals can effectively warm the kidney and free the gate.

(2) Kidney Yin Deficiency

This pattern is usually appears in yin-blood deficient individuals with a history of frequent masturbation. Seminal emission typically occurs 3 to 4 times each week, and in severe cases it may even occur during the daytime. The sea of marrow becomes empty, and symptoms of heart blood deficiency may also appear.

Symptoms and signs include dizziness, tinnitus, lack of strength, heat in the center of the palms and soles, insomnia, seminal emission, seminal efflux, clear scant semen, and low sperm counts with reduced motility. The tongue appears red with scant coating. Pulses are deficient and wiry or slightly rapid. The treatment principle here is to nourish the kidney and free the gate. Select *Tōng Jīng Líng Èr Hào Fāng* (通精灵二号方).

Zhī mǔ (Rhizoma Anemarrhenae) and *huáng bǎi* (Cortex Phellodendri Chinensis) nourish yin and clear the ministerial fire. *Shēng dì* (Radix Rehmanniae Recens), *nǔ zhēn zǐ* (Fructus Ligustri Lucidi) and *gǒu qǐ zǐ* (Fructus Lycii) nourish kidney yin. *Guī jiāo* (Colla Carapax et Plastrum Testudinis) and *lù jiǎo jiāo* (Colla Cornus Cervi) replenish essence and tonify marrow. *Chì sháo* (Radix Paeoniae Rubra) and *dān shēn* (Radix et Rhizoma Salviae Miltiorrhizae Miltiorrhizae) nourish blood. *Hàn lián cǎo* (Herba Ecliptae Prostratae) acts to clear heat and nourish yin. *Dì lóng* (Pheretima) frees the orifices and invigorates blood. *Liú jì nú* (Herba Artemisiae Anomalae), *wáng bù liú xíng* (Semen Vaccariae), *lù lù tōng* (Fructus Liquidambaris), and *chuān pò shí* (Radix Vanieriae Caulis seu) are used to clear heat, purge fire, free the orifices, and promote ejaculation.

For those with extremely frequent seminal emission, *Zhī Bǎi Dì Huáng Wán* (知柏地黄丸) or *Guī Pí Yǎng Xīn Wán* (归脾养心丸) may be applied at the same time. The daily diet may also be supplemented with soy milk and stewed pork with seaweed.

(3) Stasis Obstructing the Seminal Duct

Signs and symptoms include dizziness, intermittent low-pitched tinnitus, itching or numbness, painful skin of the genital region, erectile dysfunction, or erections appearing without stimulation. Stabbing pains may also be present in the kidney area, heels, soles, testicles, and lower abdomen. The symptoms generally become aggravated following rest and improve with activity. The tongue appears with static spots at the margin. Pulses are wiry and slippery or rough. Seminal fluid appears sticky and with poor liquefaction. Examination may also reveal inflammation, conglutination, and swelling of the ejaculatory duct.

Medicinals that primarily tonify the kidney and replenish essence will have no observable effect in treatment, because the proper treatment principle here is to transform stasis and free the gate. Select *Tōng Jīng Líng Sān Hào Fāng* (通精灵三号方).

Ancient Chinese physicians have always attributed chronic and difficult cases to conditions of phlegm and stasis. In this formula, *táo rén* (Semen Persicae), *hóng huā* (Flos Carthami), *dāng guī* (Radix Angelicae Sinensis), *dān shēn* (Radix et Rhizoma Salviae Miltiorrhizae Miltiorrhizae), and *sān qī* (Radix et Rhizoma Notoginseng) are selected to nourish and invigorate blood, transform stasis, and engender the new. Meanwhile, *bái jiè zǐ* (Semen Brassicae Albae) is used to eliminate phlegm. *Fú líng* (Poria) and *chén pí* (Pericarpium Citri Reticulatae) fortify the spleen, percolate dampness, rectify qi, and transform phlegm. *Mù tōng* (Caulis Akebiae) moves water and frees the semen passage. *Shí chāng pú* (Rhizoma Acori Tatarinowii) is acrid and warm, and so acts to "open the heart and disinhibit the nine orifices". *Bīng piàn* (Borneolum Syntheticum) opens the orifices with its aromatic quality. These medicinals act effectively together to transform the turbid and open the orifices. *Guì zhī* (Ramulus Cinnamomi) warms and frees the vessels. *Guì zhī* (Ramulus Cinnamomi) is also known to promote ejaculation by increasing muscle strength at the lower aspect of the pelvic cavity.

(4) Obstruction Due to Stagnation of Liver Qi

This pattern usually results from longstanding emotional depression that often includes a continuing loss of self-confidence. These patients report previously persistent erections that have gradually become incomplete or absent along with diminishing sexual desire. Other signs and symptoms include irritability, distending hypochondriac pain, and a frequent desire to sigh. The tongue appears light red with a thin white coating. Pulses are wiry. Treatment here should resolve constraint and open the gate. Select *Tōng Jīng Líng Sì Hào Fāng* (通精灵四号方).

In this formula, *chái hú* (Radix Bupleuri) acts to course the liver and resolve constraint. *Bái sháo* (Radix Paeoniae Alba), *chuān xiōng* (Rhizoma Chuanxiong) and *dāng guī* (Radix Angelicae Sinensis) are used to harmonize the nutrient aspect while nourishing and invigorating blood. *Zhǐ qiào* (Fructus Aurantii) and *xiāng fù* (Rhizoma Cyperi) are used to soothe the liver and rectify qi. *Yù jīn* (Radix Curcumae) can resolve constraint, loosen the chest, and disperse qi stagnation. *Shēng dì* (Radix Rehmanniae Recens) and *shú dì* (Radix Rehmanniae Praeparata) are used to nourish and tonify the liver and kidney. *Jiǔ cài zǐ* (Semen Allii Tuberosi) and *chē qián zǐ* (Semen Plantaginis) invigorate sexual function and disinhibit the lower orifices. *Chuān pò shí* (Radix Vanieriae Caulis seu), *biē jiǎ* (Carapax Trionycis), and *chuān shān jiǎ* (Squama Manis) can break concretion, disperse binding, and free the essence gate.

(5) Damp-heat Obstruction

Signs and symptoms include dizziness, generalized heaviness, acute lower abdominal distention, aching lumbus and limp knees, sagging and distending sensations of the perineum, short voidings of reddish or yellow urine, bitter taste, vexation, irascibility, persistent erection, frequent dream emission, and thick sticky and occasionally bloody semen. The tongue appears red with a thin yellow or yellow slimy coating. Pulses are wiry and slippery, or slippery and rapid. Examination may reveal the presence of pyocyte, erythrocyte (red blood cells), leukocyte (white blood cells), low sperm count, and high numbers of non-viable sperm. These patients often suffer from prostatitis or seminal vesiculitis. The treatment principle here is to transform dampness, clear heat, free the gate, and check emission. Select *Tōng Jīng Líng Wǔ Hào Fāng* (通精灵五号方).

In this formula, *lóng dǎn cǎo* (Gentianae Radix) is used to purge excess fire in the liver and bladder and eliminate damp-heat in the lower burner. *Huáng qín* (Radix Scutellariae) and *shān zhī* (Fruactus Gardenie) purge fire. *Zé xiè* (Rhizoma Alismatis) and *chē qián zǐ* (Semen Plantaginis) are used to clear heat and disinhibit dampness. *Shēng dì* (Radix Rehmanniae Recens), *dāng guī* (Radix Angelicae Sinensis) and *dān pí* (Cortex Moutan) are used to clear heat, cool the blood, and nourish yin-blood. *Chái hú* (Radix Bupleuri) acts to course the liver and rectify qi by seeking upbearing within downbearing. *Chái hú* (Radix Bupleuri) maintains orderly reaching while effectively purging excess fire in the liver channel. *Bì xiè* (Rhizoma Dioscoreae Hypoglaucae) and *yì yǐ rén* (Semen Coicis) act to fortify the spleen and disinhibit dampness. *Shí chāng pú* (Rhizoma Acori Tatarinowii) frees the orifices and resolves turbidity. *Liú jì nú* (Herba Artemisiae Anomalae) is used to resolve concretion and disperse binding to help free the essence.

Some patients display patterns that can not be clearly differentiated. In these cases, careful observation of the tongue and pulse, physical constitution, and personality must be combined with a clear investigation into the medical etiology. The numerous signs and symptoms listed here are intended only as a guideline, with the main presenting symptoms and pulse images being the true basis of formula selection. Various combinations of pulse and symptoms appear in different patterns, and in some patients the original presentation may change. Therefore, proper treatment should not be limited to one simple formula or method, and the appropriate formula modifications must also be applied in a timely manner.

(Shan Shu-jian. *Clinical Experience of Ancient and Contemporary Experts: Male Diseases*. Beijing: China Press of Traditional Chinese Medicine, 1999: 223-226)

PERSPECTIVES OF INTEGRATIVE MEDICINE

Rather than being associated with any specific disease, male infertility is generally associated with multiple pathogenic factors, sometimes including structural disorders of the reproductive organs. It is impossible to rely on one specific drug or therapeutic method, since the pathogenesis is so often varied. To achieve ideal therapeutic effects, an integrated approach to treatment method may be required. Chinese medicinals, acupuncture, immune therapies, anti-inflammatory medicines, and even surgical techniques are most effective when applied according to accurate syndrome differentiation.

Challenges and Solutions

CHALLENGE #1: DETERMINING PATHOGENESIS AND PATHOLOGY

Male infertility may occur as a result of many different factors, and it may also be classified in a number of ways. When classified according to the viability of sperm, the condition may be divided into absolute infertility (azoospermia), and relative infertility (oligospermatism). When classified according to pathology, the condition may be divided into primary infertility (the female has never conceived), and secondary infertility (with a previous pregnancy). When classified according to the condition of the reproductive organs, it can be divided into pre-testicular, testicular and post-testicular types.

50 to 80 million people suffer with infertility, and this number continues to increase by two million each year. Male infertility is characterized by a continuous decline of seminal fluid quality. This condition is certainly a sensitive issue for most men.

Major risk factors include drug and alcohol abuse, smoking, environmental toxins, and sexually transmitted disease. The long-term use of pharmaceutical medications may also exhibit side effects that influence the healthy production of sperm.

To effectively treat male infertility, a proper diagnosis is essential from the beginning. Physical examination and laboratory testing should be performed, and a thorough medical history must be taken. Detailed questions about marriage, sexual habits, and reproductive health are necessary during the interview. A complete medical history of the couple, including present medications, is essential. Also inquire about family history, living arrangements, and sexual habits. Physical examination must be performed to evaluate the genital organs and male sexual characteristics. Significant findings include genital abnormalities such as tubercle of the epididymis or spermatic duct, redundant prepuce or phimosis, varicocele, eczema, or obvious asymmetry of the testes. Laboratory testing is necessary to evaluate the seminal fluid, including the presence of sperm antibodies. On occasion, genetic examination is indicated. When associated disorders are found present, these should be treated concurrently. It is also essential that the female receive a thorough GYN examination.

CHALLENGE #2: AZOOSPERMATISM

For azoospermatism due to testicular disease, artificial insemination may become the only recourse. But with obstructive azoospermia, relatively good therapeutic effects can be obtained with proper treatment. For this condition, there are two key aspects in diagnosis and treatment.

First, azoospermatism due to epididymitis must be properly diagnosed. Azoospermia refers to the absence of sperm, and this condition generally manifests in one of two ways.

A. Testicular sperm production is normal, but ejaculation is impossible due to obstruction of the spermatic duct. This condition is referred to as obstructive azoospermia.

B. Dysfunction of testicular sperm production. This condition is referred to as secretory azoospermia.

According to statistics, 55% of azoospermia related conditions are associated with obstructive factors. This fact suggests that epididymitis may be one of the major causes of obstructive azoospermia. The epididymal duct is easily obstructed by inflammatory and deciduous cells of the epithelium. Furthermore, the spermatic duct is composed of many structures, and pathology of any these structures may lead to azoospermatism.

To properly diagnose azoospermatism due to epididymitis, a detailed medical history is required. In addition to apparent swelling and pain of the scrotum, or epididymitis of the testicles, a medical history of tuberculosis, venereal disease or trauma is also very significant. However, azoospermatism due to epididymitis can not be ruled out even without a medical history of acute inflammation. Physical examination is also essential for making a correct diagnosis. Bilateral indurations of the epididymis may reveal pain upon palpation.

Secondary sex characteristics, testicular size, and the spermatic duct will all appear normal in cases where epididymitis alone is the cause of azoospermatism. Libido and sexual activity also remains unaffected in these patients.

Evaluation of endocrine function is also indicated. Azoospermia due to lesions of the CNS (particularly of the hypothalamus and pituitary) may be ruled out if FSH, LH, and testosterone blood levels remain within normal ranges.

Even when testicular palpation reveals hard and painful nodules on both sides, azoospermatism due to epididymitis still cannot be confirmed. A definite diagnosis is not usually possible until testicular biospy and examination of the spermatic duct are performed. However, biopsy is not necessary when laboratory findings reveal reduced testosterone levels, and FSH levels three times higher than the normal value. In that case, the diagnosis is azoospermatism due to testicular lesion.

Seminal fluid will normally test positive for fructose. If fructose tests negative, and seminal fluid reveals an absence of sperm, this suggests obstruction or agenesis of the seminal vesicle. Levels of sperm plasma carnitine, α-glycuronide, and glycerophosphoryl choline may also be measured. Any obvious decline in these levels also suggests obstruction of the epididymis. Direct contrast examination of the spermatic duct can reveal the precise location, but the contrast agent can cause inflammation. Other diagnostic methods include catheterization, aspiration of the seminal vesicle, or ultrasonography.

The next step is to determine the correct treatment approach according to pattern differentiation. Obstruction of epididymis is generally associated with inflammatory hyperplasia and also fibrosis of the surface tissues. Chinese medicine considers these conditions as patterns of phlegm and blood stasis, so the correct treatment principle is to invigorate blood, eliminate stasis, and transform phlegm.

Epididymal induration is a secondary change due to chronic epididymitis, and also a primary cause of obstructive azoospermatism. Some patients report no discomfort, while others experience a dull pain. An exterior contraction of cold-damp may lead to cold congealing in the channels, causing damage to the testicles. Liver qi stagnation due to emotional depression may also result in local qi stagnation and blood stasis.

Chinese medicinals that invigorate blood and eliminate stasis should be used in the treatment of induration. Their application is most effective when be applied at the earliest stage of its formation, and also immediately following the acute stage.

Selected medicinals may include *dān shēn* (Radix et Rhizoma Salviae Miltiorrhizae Miltiorrhizae), *chì sháo* (Radix Paeoniae Rubra), *jī xuè téng* (Caulis Spatholobi), *chuān xiōng* (Rhizoma Chuanxiong), *zé lán* (Herba Lycopi), *máo dōng qīng* (Radix Ilicis pubescentis), *jiāng huáng* (Rhizoma Curcumae Longae), *sū mù* (Lignum Sappan), *wǔ líng zhī* (Faeces Togopteri), *chuān shān jiǎ* (Squama Manis), *pú huáng* (Pollen Typhae), *sān qī* (Radix et Rhizoma Notoginseng) and *yán hú suŏ* (Rhizoma Corydalis).

When obvious induration is accompanied by chronic inflammation, select medicinals that break blood and disperse stasis.

These include *táo rén* (Semen Persicae), *hóng huā* (Flos Carthami), *xuè jié* (Sanguis Draconis), *rŭ xiāng* (Olibanum), *mò yào* (Myrrha), *sān léng* (Rhizoma Sparganii), *é zhú* (Rhizoma Curcumae), *zhè chóng* (Eupolyphaga seu Oposthoplatia), *shuĭ zhì* (Hirudo) and *méng chóng* (Tabanus).

Modern pharmacological research has found that Chinese medicinals that invigorate blood and eliminate stasis can also inhibit fibroblast hyperplasia, promote the decomposition of collagenous tissue, and accelerate absorption of hyperplastic lesions. These medicinals enhance phagocytic function, inhibit inflammation, and reduce inflammatory exudation while also promoting its absorption.

Insight from Empirical Wisdom

1. PATTERN DIFFERENTIATION OF MALE INFERTILITY AND CHRONIC PROSTATITIS

When male infertility is combined with chronic prostatitis, changes in sperm quality will occur. Asthenospermia, poor liquefaction times, and an increase of white blood cells may appear in the seminal fluid. There may be no obvious physical symptoms, so diminishing the inflammation while also engendering essence may prove to be difficult. There is no definite conclusion as to whether chronic prostatitis effects reproduction. However, since the prostate is the largest secondary sex gland in the human body, and its secretions enter the seminal fluid, an inflammatory lesion will certainly affect the components of semen. Clinical experience shows that the activity and function of sperm can easily become disturbed. In fact, the seminal fluids of patients with chronic prostatitis usually display a number of physical and chemical changes. Bacterium and baceriotoxins can consume the nutritive components of seminal plasma, change pH values, disturb enzyme activity, and also increase the viscosity of seminal plasma. They can also affect fertility by reducing sperm motility and stimulating the production of sperm antibodies. Practical experience shows that after chronic prostatitis becomes relieved, semen quality is improved and pregnancy often occurs.

In patients with chronic prostatitis, the inflammation should be identified as infectious or non-infectious. With infectious inflammation, it is necessary to differentiate whether the condition is specific or non-specific, and to also identify the specific pathogenic bacteria. Most cases of chronic prostatitis are caused by non-bacterial inflammation. However, for many patients with definable etiologies, a specific treatment plan is still necessary. For patients with non-infective prostatitis, the treatment plan should be based on Chinese pattern differentiation. Even though we advocate integrative approaches, it is at present quite difficult to accurately correlate pattern differentiation with the biomedical diagnosis. At the same time, there is sufficient evidence to suggest that improved therapeutic effects can be obtained when the choice of treatment is informed by pattern differentiation.

Cases of prostatitis can present with patterns of deficiency, heat, dampness, and stasis. There are also obvious differences in the manifestations of deficiency heat versus excess heat. If the application of cold and cooling medicinals that clear heat and disinhibit dampness is too excessive, not only will the inflammation remain, but the upright qi will also become damaged. Similarly, patterns of kidney deficiency will also manifest differently depending on the presence of qi deficiency, yin deficiency, or yang deficiency. Pathogens may linger internally with the excessive use of medicinals that warm and tonify kidney yang, or those which tonify the kidney and replenish essence. General speaking, if the decline of seminal quality is caused by prostatitis; the primary treatment principle should be to eliminate the pathogen while supporting the upright. This approach aims to diminish inflammation and improve the quality of the sperm and seminal plasma. In some cases, conception may occur even before the inflammation is resolved. Clinical reports show that significant improvement of sperm quality can result from the application of medicinals that clear heat, disinhibit damp, course the liver, and resolve constraint.

Lifestyle modification is also very important. This includes refraining from masturbation, and also from withholding ejaculation during sexual intercourse. Sexual activity should be neither too frequent nor too restrained, but should be properly regulated according to the physical condition and mental status of the individual. With non-infectious prostatitis, sexual activity once every 1 or 2 weeks is appropriate. If the prostate secretions show the presence of bacteria, patients should use condoms or refrain from sexual activity until the culture becomes negative. Refraining from sexual activity is particularly important with the presence of any sexually transmitted disease.

In daily life, the patient should be advised to maintain a regular sleep schedule, avoid taxation, and also to take steps to avoid catching cold. Sitting, driving, or riding bicycles for extended periods are also inadvisable. Cold and damp places are to be generally avoided. Professional drivers, cooks and others who work with high temperatures should do their best to consume enough water to increase the output of urine, and to also take frequent outdoor walks.

2. VARICOCELE AND SPERM QUALITY

In Chinese medicine, varicocele is associated with patterns of static blood obstruction, also referred to as "sinew tumor". It has been said that "latent yang exists within static blood". This means that local obstruction of blood and qi frequently transforms into heat and engenders fire, thus increasing the local temperature. Heat constraint brewing internally will damage fluids and scorch essence, causing patterns of deficiency fire to become more exuberant. Patterns of yin deficiency and fluid damage give way to one another. In addition to qi stagnation and blood stasis, yin deficiency with internal heat is also a key pathomechanism. Therefore, nourishing yin and clearing heat are very important principles in the treatment this condition.

Current research shows that Chinese medicinals that tonify the kidney and nourish yin may also act to promote and regulate reproductive hormones. These include *shēng dì huáng* (Radix Rehmanniae Recens), *biē jiǎ* (Carapax Trionycis), *nǚ zhēn zǐ* (Fructus Ligustri Lucidi), *hé shǒu wū* (Radix Polygoni Multiflori), *hàn lián cǎo* (Herba Ecliptae), *sāng jì shēng* (Herba Taxilli), *cì wǔ jiā* (Radix et Rhizoma seu Caulis Acanthopanacis Senticosi), *tù sī zǐ* (Semen Cuscutae) and *dōng chóng xià cǎo* (Cordyceps).

Blood-invigorating medicinals can also assist in the repair of damaged tissues. *Dān shēn* (Radix et Rhizoma Salviae Miltiorrhizae Miltiorrhizae) and *chì sháo* (Radix Paeoniae Rubra) both improve blood microcirculation, and they also display anti-inflammatory effects. *Táo rén* (Semen Persicae) and *hóng huā* (Flos Carthami) act to promote the absorption of inflammatory secrections while also improving blood circulation. The combined application of these medicinals may also improve sperm production.

3. Differentiation of Deficiency and Excess Patterns

Although male infertility presents a variety of clinical etiologies and symptoms, deficiency and excess patterns must first be clearly differentiated. Deficiency here refers to essence qi insufficiency and yin and yang dual deficiency of the kidney. Excess patterns manifest with phlegm turbidity, static blood, or damp-heat obstructing the spermatic duct. Complex presentations manifesting with both deficiency and excess are also common.

Impotence, clear and cold semen, seminal emission, premature ejaculation, aching lumbus, dizziness, and tinnitus all indicate insufficiency of kidney qi.

A history of acute or chronic disease, physical injury, oligospermia, azoospermia, painful ejaculation, ejaculatory incompetence, encrusted skin lesions, hypertonicity of the lesser abdomen, and a dark facial complexion can indicate static blood obstruction.

Abnormalities of sperm quantity and quality, forceless erection, fatigue with no desire to speak, glomus and oppression in the chest and stomach duct, and obesity can indicate internal brewing of phlegm turbidity.

Inhibited ejaculation, bloody semen, fullness in the chest and rib-side, dribbling urination, scorching pain in the penis, and a bitter taste and sliminess in the mouth usually indicates damp-heat pouring downwards.

Secondly, differentiate seminal cold and seminal heat. Seminal cold refers to clear and cold semen with ejaculation. It usually results from insufficiency of the life gate fire. Seminal heat manifests with a heat sensation in the female's uterus at ejaculation. This usually indicates kidney water deficiency and hyperactivity of the ministerial fire.

Thirdly, differentiate between insufficient semen and seminal loss. Insufficient semen refers to low seminal fluid volume, usually due to essence qi deficiency. Seminal loss refers to incontinence or excessive efflux of semen. This usually results from kidney qi deficiency and failure to storing essence.

Also differentiate patterns of bloody semen and seminal turbidity. Bloody semen results from kidney qi taxation. However, turbidity may appear white or red in color. Other manifestations of seminal turbidity include secretion from the external urethral orifice, and itching or pain of the penis.

Typical patterns associated with infertility include the following pulse images.

➢ Deep pulses at the *chi* position indicate kidney deficiency.

➢ Thready and rough pulses indicate essence and blood deficiency.

➢ Weak pulses indicate qi and blood dual deficiency.

➢ Thin pulses indicate deficiency taxation.

➢ Rough pulses indicate static blood stagnation and obstruction of the spermatic duct.

Summary

There are a number of causative factors that may be involved with onset of male infertility. The pathogenic factors involved are not completely understood, and many patients will present with an absence obvious clinical symptoms. Diagnosis and differentiation it is most difficult in the early stages, especially when relying only upon the traditional four examinations. For this reason, the diagnostic methods of Chinese medicine are often combined with modern biomedical methods.

Most cases of oligospermatism, asthenospermia, oligospermia and non-liquefaction of sperm can be effectively treated with methods of Chinese medicine, as well as conditions of immune infertility. Chinese medicine not only reduces the side effects of hormone therapy, but also eliminates the antibody over a longer period of time, which results in lower rates of recurrence.

The chance of conception may be improved in patients who present with moderate or severe varicocele. In cases that display inflammation of the secondary sex organs, Chinese medicinals are commonly applied in combination with high spermatic vein ligation. With non-specific inflammation of the secondary sex organs, treatments based on syndrome differentiation can significantly improve sperm quality in most patients.

Although azoospermatism is one of the most challenging infertility conditions, proper pattern differentiation and treatment often results in a satisfactory therapeutic effect. Chinese medicinals may also display significant inductive or differential effects on spermatogonial stem cells. Recent developments in reproductive technology offer new hope for many patients, especially the application of intracytoplasmic sperm injection, or ICSI. The growth and maturation of sperm cells are significantly enhanced when Chinese medicinals are applied in combination with ICSI. Furthermore, the risk of hereditary defects may be reduced with the resulting improvement in sperm quality. Chinese medicinal treatments can certainly improve the rates of conception when applied according to accurate syndrome differentiation.

SELECTED QUOTES FROM CLASSICAL TEXTS

Plain Questions 1: Treatise of Heavenly Truth from Remote Antiquity (素问 · 上古天真论篇第一 , *Sù Wèn · Shàng Gǔ Tiān Zhēn Lùn Piān Dì Yī*):

丈夫八岁,肾气实,发长齿更。二八,肾气盛,天癸至,精气溢泻,阴阳和,故能有子。……五八,肾气衰,发堕齿槁。六八,阳气衰竭于上,面焦,发鬓颁白。七八,肝气衰,筋不能动。八八,天癸竭,精少,肾脏衰,形体皆极,则齿发去。肾者主水,受五脏六腑之精而藏之,故五脏盛乃能泻。今五脏皆衰,筋骨解堕,天癸尽矣,故发鬓白,身体重,行走不正,而无子耳。

"In the male at age eight, kidney qi becomes replete, hair begins to grow, and the teeth change. At age sixteen, kidney qi becomes exuberant, *tian gui* arrives, the essential qi flows forth, yin and yang are in harmony, and conception becomes possible. At age forty, kidney qi debilitates, the hair falls out, and the teeth wither. At age forty-eight, yang qi debilitates in the upper body, the face appears scorched, and the hair at the temples becomes white. At age fifty-six, liver qi debilitates and the sinews are unable to move freely. At age sixty-four, *tian gui* becomes exhausted, essence diminishes, the kidney debilitates, the physique loses it tone, and the teeth and hair fall out. The kidney governs water and also stores the essence from the five viscera and six bowels, so when the five viscera are exuberant, the kidney is able to discharge. When all five viscera are debilitated, the sinews and bones deteriorate, *tian gui* is exhausted, the hair at the temples is white, the body feels heavy, one cannot walk straight, and conception is impossible."

Essential Prescriptions of the Golden Coffer (金匮·血痹虚劳病脉证并治第六 , *Jīn Guì · Xuè Bì Xū Láo Bìng Mài Zhèng Bìng Zhì*):
男子脉浮弱而涩，为无子，精气清冷。

"Floating, weak and rough pulses among males indicate infertility due to clear and cold essence qi."

The Origin and Indicators of Disease (诸病源候论·虚劳病诸候上 , *Zhū Bìng Yuán Hòu Lùn · Xū Láo Bìng Zhū Hòu Shàng*):
虚劳无子候，丈夫无子者，其精清如水，冷如冰铁，皆为无子之候。又泄精，精不射出，但聚于阴头亦无子。无此之候，皆有子。交会当用阳时，阳时从夜半至禺中是也。以此时有子，皆聪明长寿。勿用阴时，阴时从午至亥。有子皆顽暗而短命。切宜详审之。

"The indications for infertility due to deficiency taxation: In men, the semen is as clear as water and icy cold. This sign indicates infertility. When the semen is not ejaculated with force, but gathers at the head of the penis, this may also lead to infertility. Without these indications, fertility is generally possible. Sexual intercourse should occur during the time period corresponding to yang, which is from midnight until eleven in the morning. Women that conceive during this period give birth to children who display both wisdom and longevity. The time corresponding to yin occurs between noon and eleven in the evening. Women that conceive during this time give birth to children who are mischievous and dull, with short lifespans. These facts should be carefully considered."

A Thousand Gold Pieces Emergency Formulary (备急千金要方·求子论 , *Bèi Jí Qiān Jīn Yào Fāng · Qiú Zǐ Lùn*):

凡人无子，当为夫妻俱有五劳七伤，虚羸百病所致，故有绝嗣之殃。

"Infertility is commonly seen when both the husband and wife suffer the five taxations and seven damages, or other various diseases caused by deficiency. This can lead to breaking of the family bloodline."

Compendium of Good Remedies for Women (妇人大全良方·求嗣门 , *Fù Rén Dà Quán Liáng Fāng · Qiú Sì Mén*):

凡欲求子，当先察夫妇有无劳伤痛疾，而依方调治，使内外和平，则有子矣。

"To seek fertility, first observe if the couple displays taxation, damage or any painful disease. Treat accordingly, harmonize the internal and external, and conception will occur."

Four Essentials on Life Cultivation (养生四要·却痰 , *Yǎng Shēng Sì Yào · Què Tán*):

凡丈夫无子者有二病焉，一曰禀赋不足，二曰色欲太过，所以阳道痿弱，精气衰冷。

"Male infertility results from two kinds of male disease. One is weakness of the congenital constitution, and the other is associated with excessive sexual activity. Both lead to wilting and weakening of the yang passage, with debilitation and coldness of essence qi."

Widely Inherited Guiding Principles (广嗣纪要·择配篇 , *Guǎng Sì Jì Yào· Zé Pèi Piān*):

纵欲无度则精竭，精竭则少而不多，精竭于内则阳衰于外，痿而不举，举而不坚，坚而不久，隐曲且不得，况欲输其精乎？是则肾肝俱损，不惟无子，而且有难状之疾矣。

"Excessive sexual activities certainly lead to essence exhaustion, which means that only a small amount of essence remains, rather than a great deal. Essence which is exhausted internally will cause yang to debilitate externally, manifesting with wilting and absent erection, unfirm erection, or erection that is firm but not longlasting. When sexual activities become impossible, how can essence be transported? When the kidney and liver both become damaged, not only will infertility appear, but also other difficult to describe diseases."

Jĭng Yuè's Complete Compendium (景岳全书·妇人规, *Jĭng Yuè Quán Shū · Fù Rén Guī*):

凡饮食之类，则人之脏气各有所宜，似不必过为拘执。惟酒多者为不宜。盖胎种先天之气，极宜清楚，极宜充实。而酒性淫热，非为乱性，亦且乱精。精为酒乱，则湿热其半，真精其半耳。精不充实，则胎元不固；精多湿热，则他日痘疹、惊风、脾败之类，率已受造于此矣。故凡欲择期布种者，必宜先有所慎。

"Different kinds of food and drink correspond with different kinds of visceral qi, so there are no strict rules or prohibitions here. However, alcohol should not be consumed excessively. The qi of earlier heaven is planted within the fetus, so it needs to remain clear and abundant. The nature of alcohol is excessively hot. It not only affects one's behavior, but also the essence. Once essence becomes corrupted by alcohol, it will then consist of half true essence, and half damp-heat. When essence becomes insufficient, the fetal origin becomes insecure. When damp-heat is contained in the essence, pediatric poxes, fright wind, and splenic failure will eventually occur. Those people wanting to select a date for planting the seed should therefore be cautious."

Secret Records of the Stone Chamber (石室秘录·子嗣论, *Shí Shì Mì Lù · Zĭ Sì Lùn*):

男子不生子，有六因……一精寒也，一气衰也，一痰多也，一相火或也，一精少也，一气郁也。

"There are six causes of male infertility, and they are referred to as cold-essence, qi debilitation, excessive phlegm, ministerial fire, insufficient essence, and qi depression."

Records on Pattern Identification (辨证录 , *Biàn Zhèng Lù*):

男子身体肥大，必多痰涎，往往不能生子。此精中带湿，流入子宫而仍出也。夫精必贵纯，湿气杂于精中，则胎多不育⋯⋯凡人饮食，原该化精而不化痰，⋯⋯多痰之人，饮食虽化为精，而湿多难化，遂乘精气入肾之时，亦同群共入，正以遍身俱是痰气，肾欲避湿而不能也。湿既入肾、是精非纯粹之精，安得育麟哉？治法必须化痰为先。然徒消其痰，而痰不易化，盖痰之生本于肾气之寒，痰之多由于胃气之弱。⋯⋯故治痰必当治肾胃之二经，健其胃气而痰可化，补其肾气而痰可消矣。

"Obese males usually present with excessive phlegm-drool and also infertility. Infertility here is caused by dampness combining with essence, which then flows through the female uterus. However, the essence needs to be pure. When damp-qi becomes mixed with essence, even if conception occurs, it will not last for long. The food and drink that people consume are normally transformed into essence, rather than phlegm. For those presenting with excessive phlegm, even though food and drink are transformed into essence, the dampness remains difficult to be transformed. Thus, dampness enters the kidney along with the essence-qi. When phlegm-qi is generally present, the kidney cannot avoid being affected by dampness. After dampness enters the kidney, the essence will become impure, and fertility will become impossible. The primary treatment principle here is to transform phlegm. However, it is difficult to simply transform phlegm, because the generation of the phlegm is rooted in the cold condition of the kidney qi, and phlegm may also continue to increase due to weakness of the stomach qi. So to treat phlegm effectively, the kidney and stomach channels must both be treated. Fortifying the stomach qi can transform phlegm, where tonifying the kidney qi can disperse phlegm."

男子有面色萎黄不能生子者，乃血少之故也。……世人生子动曰父精母血，不知父亦有血也。夫血气足而精亦足，血气全而精亦全……唯是血不能速生，必补其气，盖血少者由于气衰。

"When a male with a withering-yellow facial complexion presents with infertility, this is due to blood insufficiency. It is common knowledge that fertility results from the father's essence and the mother's blood. However, the father also has blood. Blood and qi must be both sufficient and wholesome; only then can the essence become sufficient and wholesome. Yet, the engenderment of blood does not happen quickly. The qi must be tonified first, since blood deficiency appears as a result of qi debilitation."

Official Medical Record on Reproduction (医学正印种子篇 , *Yī Xué Zhèng Yìn Zhòng Zǐ Piān*):

生子专责在肾，但一经之病易治，有病在别经而移疾于肾者，有一人而兼数病，因而无子者，其治法颇难，其立方不易。

"The kidney governs reproduction. Diseases of only one channel are easy to treat, but many conditions are first located in one channel and only later pass to the kidney. Many people contract diseases which will later manifest as infertility. In these cases, treatment will be difficult and the formula will be a challenge to properly compose."

Treasured Private Copy of a Rare Book on Reproduction (秘本种子金丹 , *Mì Běn Zhòng Zǐ Jīn Dān*):

疾病之关于胎孕者，男子则在精，女子则在血，无非不足而然。男子不足，则有精滑、精清、精冷或临事不坚或流而不射，或梦遗频频、或小便淋漓，或好女色以致阴虚，阴虚腰肾痛惫，或好男风以致阳极，阳极则亢而亡阴，……或素患阴疝，阴疝则脾肾乘离。此外，或以阳衰，阳衰则多寒，或能阴虚，阴虚则多热，皆男子之病，不行尽诿之妇人也。不得其源而医之，则事无济也。

"For men, diseases related to reproduction are rooted in the essence, whereas for women they are rooted in the blood. Men with insufficiency patterns may present with seminal efflux, seminal cold, clear semen, impotence, difficult ejaculation, dream emission, or stranguric urination. Overindulgence in sexual activities with women lead to yin deficiency, which manifests as aching and exhaustion of the lumbus and kidney. Overindulgence in sexual activities with men lead to yang becoming extreme. Extreme yang becomes hyperactive, which then leads to the collapse of yin. Long-standing yin mounting will cause the spleen and kidney to become disconnected. Furthermore, yang debilitation causes excessive cold, yin deficiency causes excessive heat, and these are all male diseases. Do not always place the blame of infertility on the woman. Treating disease without understanding its true source is useless."

Prescriptions for Rescuing Lives (济生方·求子, *Jì Shēng Fāng · Qiú Zǐ*):

论曰，素问云：夫天地者，万物之父母也；阴阳者，血气之男女也。夫有夫妇，则有父子。婚姻之后，则有生育。生育者，人伦之本也。……男女婚姻贵乎及时，夫妇贵乎强壮，则易于受形也。且父少母老生女必羸，母壮父衰生男必弱，诚有斯理。或男子真精气不浓，妇女血衰而气旺，是谓夫病妇疹，皆使人无子。治疗之法，女子当养血抑气，以减喜怒，男子益肾生精，以节嗜欲，依方调治，阴阳和平，则妇人乐有子矣。

"*Plain Questions* states that heaven and earth are the parents of the ten thousand things, and that yin and yang together represent man; whose source is blood and qi. When there is a couple, parenthood is inevitable. After marriage, there will be reproduction. Reproduction is the root of human relations."

"Time is essential to a marriage, and a good physical condition is essential to pregnancy. A young father with an older mother or a strong mother with a weak father will definitely produce weak children. This theory is in fact true. When the true essence qi of a man becomes thin, and the women's blood is debilitated but her qi is effulgent, this is known as "a sick husband and a wife with papules".

This situation leads to infertility. The treatment for the women is to nourish blood and restrain qi, thus reducing her emotion. For the man, treatment must benefit the kidney to engender essence, thus controlling his desire. When yin and yang become peaceful following regular treatment, the woman will become happy and pregnant."

The Gateway to Medicine (医学入门 · 杂病分类 · 内伤类 · 虚类 · 求嗣 , *Yī Xué Rù Mén·Zá Bìng Fēn Lèi·Nèi Shāng Lèi·Xū Lèi·Qiú Sì*):

求嗣之理非玄微: 山无不草木, 人无不生育, 妇人要经调, 男子要神足。男子阳精微薄, 虽遇血海虚静, 流而不能直射子宫, 多不成胎。皆因平时嗜欲不节, 施泄太多所致。宜补精元, 兼用静功存养, 无令妄动, 候阳精充实, 依时而合, 一举而成矣。女人阴血衰弱, 虽投其精, 不能摄入子宫, 虽交而不孕, 虽孕而不育。是以男女配合, 必当其年。未笄之女, 阴气未完; 欲盛之妇, 所生多女。性行和者, 经调易挟; 性行妒者, 月水不匀。相貌恶者, 刑重; 颜容媚者, 福薄。太肥, 脂满子宫, 不能受精; 太瘦, 子宫无血, 精不能聚, 俱不宜子, 不可不知。

"The approach to seeking fertility is not so mysterious. Just as few mountains exist without grass and trees; it is also unreasonable that people cannot produce children. Women require regular menstruation, and men require sufficient spirit. If the yang essence of men is sparse and thin, even when the sea of blood is peaceful, the essence will be unable to reach the uterus and thus the fetus cannot be formed. The root cause of this condition is intemperate sexuality. Tonify the essence and origin, while peacefully reserving and nourishing the essence without disturbing it. By waiting until yang essence becomes replete, and having relations at the proper time, there will be success. When the yin-blood of a woman becomes debilitated and weak, essence cannot be obtained by the uterus. Intercourse will not lead to pregnancy, and pregnancy will not lead to delivery. Therefore, a man and woman should only join when they are both at the appropriate age. Immature girls do not possess complete yin qi. Women with exuberant desire always give birth to females. Good-tempered women display regular menstruation, and are thus easily impregnated. The jealous types present irregular menstruation. The ugly ones have terrible disasters. Those women who are too good-looking have little luck. In those too obese, the uterus becomes congested and thus unable to accept the essence. When too thin, the uterus lacks blood and the essence cannot gather. These women are unfit to have children."

MODERN RESEARCH

Some sources state that sexual or reproductive dysfunction in the male is involved in nearly 50% of all infertility cases. In recent years, improved research methods have resulted in a number of new developments in the Chinese medical approach to the treatment of male infertility. The following research reports from China illustrate some of the most relevant advances in the field of reproductive medicine.

Clinical Research

1. PATTERN DIFFERENTIATION AND TREATMENT

Although there are a variety of Chinese medical approaches to the treatment of male infertility, diagnosis and treatment based on pattern differentiation is still the primary method.

Dr. Zhen treated 180 cases of oligospermatism based on pattern differentiation. For oligospermatism due to yin deficiency, modified *Liù Wèi Dì Huáng Tāng* (六味地黄汤) was administered. For yang deficiency, modified *Yòu Guī Wán* (右归丸) was administered. After one to three months of treatment, results showed that the above formulas were effective for temporary oligospermatism. Sperm counts became normal in 80% and 20% of type I (sperm count > 10×10^6/ml) and type II (sperm count < 10×10^6/ml) cases respectively. The sperm count significantly increased in 13.3% and 70% of type I and type II cases respectively. [1]

Dr. Lu treated 82 patients with dysspermia according to three types: Kidney yang deficiency, kidney yin deficiency, and damp-heat. The results showed that 28 subjects became pregnant with a pregnancy rate of 34.15%. In the control group of 76 cases, 23 spouses became pregnant with a pregnancy rate of 30.26%. However, in 30 cases treated only with clomifene, 3 spouses became pregnant, with an overall pregnancy rate of 10% [2].

Dr. Qiu applied *Wŭ Zĭ Bŭ Shèn Wán* (五子补肾丸) and *Huán Jīng Jiān* (还精煎) in the treatment of 66 subjects with poor sperm quality and patterns of kidney deficiency. 50 cases recovered at a rate of 75.75%, and the total effective rate reached 98.5% [3].

Dr. Bai divided 49 cases of male infertility into three types: yang deficiency of the spleen and kidney, kidney yin deficiency, and damp-heat of lower burner.

Modified *Shēng Yù Tāng* (生育汤) consisting of *yín yáng huò* (Herba Epimedii), *ròu cōng róng* (Herba Cistanches), *gŏu qĭ zĭ* (Fructus Lycii), *biē jiă* (Carapax Trionycis), *shān yào* (Rhizoma Dioscoreae) and *niú xī* (Radix Achyranthis Bidentatae) was administered. 19 subjects became pregnant with a pregnancy rate of 38.78% [4].

Dr. Chen divided 25 cases of male infertility into yang deficiency of the spleen and kidney, and kidney essence insufficiency. Modifications of *shān zhū yú* (Fructus Corni), *tù sī zĭ* (Semen Cuscutae), *dăng shēn* (Radix Codonopsis), *shān yào* (Rhizoma Dioscoreae), *shú dì huáng* (Radix Rehmanniae Praeparata), *bái zhú* (Rhizoma Atractylodis Macrocephalae), *dāng guī* (Radix Angelicae Sinensis), *yín yáng huò* (Herba Epimedii) and *suŏ yáng* (Herba Cynomorii) were administered. 23 cases were recovered and 2 cases shown ineffective [5].

Dr. Zhang treated 400 cases of male infertility based on pattern differentiation.

For kidney yin deficiency and seminal cold, *tù sī zĭ* (Semen Cuscutae) 15g, *gŏu qĭ zĭ* (Fructus Lycii) 15g, *fù pén zĭ* (Fructus Rubi) 15g, and *yín yáng huò* (Herba Epimedii) 30g were administered.

For kidney yin and yang dual deficiency, medicinals such as *shú dì huáng* (Radix Rehmanniae Praeparata) 25g, *chăo shān yào* (Rhizoma Dioscoreae)(stir-fried) 15g, *shān zhū yú* (Fructus Corni) 15g, *dāng guī* (Radix Angelicae Sinensis) 15g, *bā jĭ tiān* (Radix Morindae Officinalis) 15g, *tù sī zĭ* (Semen Cuscutae) 15g, *dăng shēn* (Radix Codonopsis) 15g, *yín yáng huò* (Herba Epimedii) 10g, *zhì huáng qí* (Radix Astragali Praeparata cum Melle) 20g, *jīn yīng zĭ* (Fructus Rosae Laevigatae) 25g, *lóng gŭ* (Os Draconis) 30g, *mŭ lì* (Concha Ostreae) 30g, *lù jiăo piàn* (Cornu Cervi) 30g, *xiān máo* (Rhizoma Curculiginis) 12g, *shú fù zĭ* (Radix Aconiti Lateralis Praeparata) 7g and *ròu guì* (Cortex Cinnamomi) 5g were applied.

For decline of the life gate fire and essence and blood deficiency, *huáng qí* (Radix Astragali) 15g, *jīn yīng zĭ* (Fructus Rosae Laevigatae) 15g, *gŏu qĭ zĭ* (Fructus Lycii) 15g, *shú dì huáng* (Radix Rehmanniae Praeparata) 15g, *dān shēn* (Radix et Rhizoma Salviae Miltiorrhizae) 15g, *bā jĭ tiān* (Radix Morindae Officinalis) 10g, *yín yáng huò* (Herba Epimedii) 10g, *tù sī zĭ* (Semen Cuscutae) 10g, *nŭ zhēn zĭ* (Fructus Ligustri Lucidi) 10g, *shān zhū yú* (Fructus Corni) 10g, *huái niú xī* (Radix Achyranthis Bidentatae) 10g and *sān qī* (Radix et Rhizoma Notoginseng) 5g were used. Additionally, two pairs of *gé jiè* (Gecko) and *lù róng* (Cornu Cervi Pantotrichum) 20g were ground into fine powder. 2g was administered with yellow rice wine every night before bedtime.

For kidney deficiency and damp-heat obstruction, *dù zhòng* (Cortex Eucommiae) 10g, *gŏu qĭ zĭ* (Fructus Lycii) 10g, *bì xiè* (Rhizoma Dioscoreae

Hypoglaucae) 10g, *yì yǐ rén* (Semen Coicis) 10g, *fú líng* (Poria) 10g, *zhè chóng* (Eupolyphaga seu Opisthoplatia) 10g, *zǎo rén* (Semen Ziziphi Spinosae) 10g, *huáng bǎi* (Cortex Phellodendri Chinensis) 10g, *huò xiāng* (Herba Pogostemonis) 15g and *mù tōng* (Caulis Akebiae) 6g were decocted. Taken 3 times daily.

For hyperactive fire due to yin deficiency, *gǒu qǐ zǐ* (Fructus Lycii) 20g, *tù sī zǐ* (Semen Cuscutae) 20g, *fù pén zǐ* (Fructus Rubi) 20g, *bái sháo* (Radix Paeoniae Alba) 20g, *shú dì huáng* (Radix Rehmanniae Praeparata) 20g, *shān yào* (Rhizoma Dioscoreae) 20g, *tiān mén dōng* (Radix Asparagi) 20g, *mài mén dōng* (Radix Ophiopogonis) 20g, *nǚ zhēn zǐ* (Fructus Ligustri Lucidi) 20g, *chē qián zǐ* (Semen Plantaginis) 10g, *wǔ wèi zǐ* (Fructus Schisandrae Chinensis) 10g, *chái hú* (Radix Bupleuri) 10g, *zhǐ shí* (Fructus Aurantii Immaturus) 10g, *hàn lián cǎo* (Ecliptae Prostratae) 10g, *táo rén* (Semen Persicae) 6g, *hóng huā* (Flos Carthami) 3g, *wú zhū yú* (Fructus Evodiae) 5g and *gān cǎo* (Radix et Rhizoma Glycyrrhizae) 5g were used. One dose every three days. Sexual activity is forbidden during the treatment course.

300 cases were recovered, 80 cases shown effective and 20 cases ineffective. The total effective rate reached 95% [6].

Dr. Jin divided male immune infertility into three types: yin deficiency of the liver and kidney, internal stagnation of toxic heat, and qi stagnation with blood stasis.

➢ For yin deficiency of the liver and kidney, *shēng dì huáng* (Radix Rehmanniae Recens) 10g, *gǒu qǐ zǐ* (Fructus Lycii) 10g, *huáng qí* (Radix Astragali) 10g, *bái sháo* (Radix Paeoniae Alba) 10g, *dǎng shēn* (Radix Codonopsis) 10g, *chē qián zǐ* (Semen Plantaginis) 10g, *fú líng* (Poria) 10g, *sāng jì shēng* (Herba Taxilli) 10g, *pú huáng* (Pollen Typhae) 10g, *jī xuè téng* (Caulis Spatholobi) 10g and *mài mén dōng* (Radix Ophiopogonis) 10g were administered.

➢ For internal stagnation of toxic heat, *dāng guī* (Radix Angelicae

Sinensis) 10g, *chì sháo* (Radix Paeoniae Rubra) 10g, *huáng lián* (Rhizoma Coptidis) 10g, *hé shǒu wū* (Radix Polygoni Multiflori) 10g, *tuō lì cǎo* (Herba Agrimoniae) 10g, *bǎn lán gēn* (Radix Isatidis) 10g, *chuān xiō*ng (Rhizoma Chuanxiong) 10g, *yì yǐ rén* (Semen Coicis) 10g, *jīn yín huā* (Flos Lonicerae Japonicae) 10g, *bái huā shé shé cǎo* (Herba Hedyotis) 10g and *pú gōng yīng* (Herba Taraxaci) 10g were administered.

➢ For qi stagnation and blood stasis, *xiāng fù* (Rhizoma Cyperi) 10g, *yì yǐ rén* (Semen Coicis) 10g, *hòu pò* (Cortex Magnoliae Officinalis) 10g, *qīng pí* (Pericarpium Citri Reticulatae Viride) 10g, *chén pí* (Pericarpium Citri Reticulatae) 10g, *shēng pú huáng* (Pollen Typhae) 10g, *sāng zhī* (Ramulus Mori) 10g, *fú líng* (Poria) 10g, *biě táo gān* (Prunus persica (L.) Batsch) 10g, *sī guā luò* (Retinervus Luffae Fructus) 10g, and *Bì Yù Sǎn* (碧玉散) 10g were administered.

Decoct in water and take one dose per day. Three months constitute one treatment course. After one or two treatment courses, antisperm antibodies in 45 cases tested negative, among which 27 spouses became pregnant. 12 cases were shown ineffective [7].

Dr. Yan Zhen-jun divided 109 cases of male infertility into six types: kidney yin deficiency, kidney yang deficiency, kidney yin and yang dual deficiency, liver depression transforming into fire, heart-spleen depletion and downpouring of damp-heat. *Chun Fu Shi Capsules* I to VI were administered. 24, 32 and 40 cases were shown effective, among which 11, 18, and 29 spouses became pregnant after one, two, and three treatment courses respectively. 58 spouses became pregnant in 109 cases, with a total effective rate of 80% [8].

Dr. Yang studied a group of patients with spleen qi deficiency who also presented with oligospermia, thin sperm, unwillingness to speak, abdominal distention, loose stools, fatigue, pale complexion, poor appetite, a pale tongue with a moist white coating and faint or deficient pulses.

The empirical formula *Jiàn Pí Yì Qì Tián Jīng Tāng* (健脾益气填精汤) consists of *bái zhú* (Rhizoma Atractylodis Macrocephalae) 15g, *fú líng* (Poria) 15g, *tù sī zǐ* (Semen Cuscutae) 15g, *dāng guī* (Radix Angelicae Sinensis) 15g, *fù pén zǐ* (Fructus Rubi) 15g, *biǎn dòu* (Semen Lablab Album) 15g, *dǎng shēn* (Radix Codonopsis) 12g, *chén pí* (Pericarpium Citri Reticulatae) 12g, *zǐ hé chē* (Placenta Hominis) 10g, *zhì shēng má* (Rhizoma Cimicifugae Praeparata cum Melle) 10g, *huáng qí* (Radix Astragali) 30g, *shān yào* (Rhizoma Dioscoreae) 30g and *zhì gān cǎo* (Radix et Rhizoma Glycyrrhizae Praeparata cum Melle) 3g.

➤ For impotence, *xiān líng pí* (Herba Epimedii) and *xiān máo* (Rhizoma Curculiginis) were added.

➤ For lassitude in the loin and legs, *dù zhòng* (Cortex Eucommiae) and *xù duàn* (Radix Dipsaci) were added.

➤ For insomnia and profuse dreaming, *yuǎn zhì* (Radix Polygalae) and *suān zǎo rén* (Semen Ziziphi Spinosae) were added.

➤ For poor appetite, *chǎo shān zhā* (Fructus Crataegi), *chǎo shén qū* (Massa Medicata Fermentata), *chǎo mài yá* (Fructus Hordei Germinatus) and *lái fú zǐ* (Semen Raphani) were added.

Decoct in water, divide into 2 doses and take once in the morning and night for three months. 56 cases were recovered, 8 cases shown effective and 4 cases ineffective. The total effective rate was 94% [9].

Dr. Cai divided 98 male infertility patients into five groups: kidney yang deficiency, kidney yin deficiency, phlegm-damp brewing internally, liver qi stagnation and blood stasis, and complex patterns. Semen analysis and hormone levels were evaluated. Results showed the density and survival rates of sperm in kidney yang deficiency and liver qi stagnation and blood stasis groups were lower than those in the kidney yin deficiency group. As compared with the kidney yang deficiency group, the levels of testosterone in the kidney yin deficiency, phlegm-damp brewing internally, and liver qi stagnation and blood stasis groups were higher. The levels of LH and FSH in the kidney yin deficiency group were lower than those in the kidney yang deficiency group. This suggests a relationship between Chinese medicine patterns and sperm quality, sperm survival rates, and hormone levels in cases of male infertility [10].

Dr. Wang treated 100 cases of male infertility due to nonliquefaction of semen by dividing subjects into three groups: yin deficiency, yang deficiency and damp-heat.

➢ For yin deficiency, symptoms and signs included nonliquefaction of semen, dizziness, tinnitus, feverish sensation in the chest, profuse dreaming, night sweating, weakness of the loins and legs, a red and dry tongue with a thin yellow coating, and thready and rapid or deep and thready pulses.

➢ For yang deficiency, they included nonliquefaction of semen, coldness of the body and limbs, lassitude, pale complexion, pale red tongue with a thin white coating, and deep slow and weak pulses.

➢ For damp-heat, they included nonliquefaction of semen, bitter taste in the mouth, poor appetite, moist scrotum, frequent urination, heat sensation with urination, a moist red tongue with a white or yellow greasy coating, and slippery and rapid pulses.

88 cases were shown effective, 12 cases ineffective, and the total effective rate reached 88%. This indicates that treatment based on pattern differentiation is effective for male infertility due to nonliquefaction of semen. [11]

2. Specific Formulas

(1) Male Immune Infertility

According to statistics, 10% to 20% of male infertility cases are related to immune factors. Therefore, increasing attention is being given to the study of infertility associated with antisperm antibodies (AsAb).

Antibiotics, immunosuppressants, and artificial insemination are used in the treatment of male infertility. However, these methods cannot be widely applied due to their limited therapeutic effects and numerous side-effects. Further research into Chinese medicinal approaches is therefore warranted.

Dr. Mi treated 64 cases of immune male infertility with the empirical formula *Yi Qì Bǔ Shèn Jiě Dú Tāng* (益气补肾解毒汤) consisting of *huáng qí* (Radix Astragali), *bái zhú* (Rhizoma Atractylodis Macrocephalae), *shān yào* (Rhizoma Dioscoreae), *dāng guī* (Radix Angelicae Sinensis), *shú dì huáng* (Radix Rehmanniae Praeparata), *gǒu qǐ zǐ* (Fructus Lycii), *yín yáng huò* (Herba Epimedii), *bái huā shé shé cǎo* (Herba Hedyotis), *bàn zhī lián* (Herba Scutellariae Barbatae) and *gān cǎo* (Radix et Rhizoma Glycyrrhizae). 24 cases were considered recovered with an overall recovery rate of 37.50%. The total effective rate reached 90.63% [12].

Dr. Huang treated 35 male infertility patients testing positive for AsAb with the empirical formula *Zhuǎn Yīn Tāng* (转阴汤) consisting of *fēng fáng* (Nidus Vespae), *yín yáng huò* (Herba Epimedii), *dāng guī* (Radix Angelicae Sinensis), *tù sī zǐ* (Semen Cuscutae), *gǒu qǐ zǐ* (Fructus Lycii), *ròu cōng róng* (Herba Cistanches), *dān shēn* (Radix et Rhizoma Salviae Miltiorrhizae), *mài yá* (Fructus Hordei Germinatus), *shuǐ zhì* (Hirudo) and *huáng qí* (Radix Astragali). AsAb tested negative in 28 cases at a total rate of 80% [13].

Dr. Wang treated 30 cases of immune male infertility with modified *Yù Píng Fēng Sǎn* (玉屏风散) consisting of *zhì huáng qí* (Radix Astragali Praeparata cum Melle) 25g, *chǎo bái zhú* (Rhizoma Atractylodis Macrocephalae) (stir-fried) 15g, *dāng guī* (Radix Angelicae Sinensis) 15g, *fáng fēng* (Radix Saposhnikoviae) 9g, and *shú dì huáng* (Radix Rehmanniae Praeparata) 20g.

➢ For kidney yang deficiency, *tù sī zǐ* (Semen Cuscutae) was added.

➢ For liver-kidney yin dual deficiency, *shú dì huáng* (Radix Rehmanniae

Praeparata) was replaced with *shēng dì huáng* (Radix Rehmanniae Recens), and *huáng jīng* (Rhizoma Polygonati) and *nǚ zhēn zǐ* (Fructus Ligustri Lucidi) were added.

➤ For liver channel damp-heat, *mǔ dān pí* (Cortex Moutan), *zé xiè* (Rhizoma Alismatis) and *huáng bǎi* (Cortex Phellodendri Chinensis) were added.

➤ For liver qi stagnation, *chén pí* (Pericarpium Citri Reticulatae) and *xiāng fù* (Rhizoma Cyperi) were added.

Decocted in water and taken with prednisone 5mg once daily. One month constituted one treatment course. After one to three courses, AsAb in 30 cases tested negative and one case was shown ineffective. The effective rates and pregnancy rates reached 96.8% and 36.2% respectively [14].

Dr. Dai treated 48 immune male infertility patients with hyperactivity of fire due to yin deficiency with the empirical formula *Miǎn Yì II* (免疫 II 号) consisting of *zhī mǔ* (Rhizoma Anemarrhenae) 10g, *huáng bǎi* (Cortex Phellodendri Chinensis) 10g, *shēng dì huáng* (Radix Rehmanniae Recens) 10g, *shān zhū yú* (Fructus Corni) 10g, *shān yào* (Rhizoma Dioscoreae) 10g, *dān shēn* (Radix et Rhizoma Salviae Miltiorrhizae) 10g, *fú líng* (Poria) 10g, *chì sháo* (Radix Paeoniae Rubra) 10g, *chái hú* (Radix Bupleuri) 5g, *shēng dà huáng* (Radix et Rhizoma Rhei) 5g, *pú gōng yīng* (Herba Taraxaci) 20g, *jīn yín huā* (Flos Lonicerae Japonicae) 20g and *mǔ lì* (Concha Ostreae) 20g. Decocted in water and taken once daily.

After AsAb levels tested negative, *Yù Lín I* (毓麟 I 号) was administered, consisting of *Wǔ Zǐ Yǎn Zōng Wán* (五子衍宗丸) and *Dāng Guī Sháo Yào Sǎn* (当归芍药散). 30 subjects in the control group were given prednisone 5mg. Antibiotics were applied in cases with inflammation. Three months constituted one treatment course. After three courses, the effective rate in the treatment group was superior to that of control (*p*<0.01). Sperm quality in the treatment group was also markedly improved (*p*<0.01) [15].

Dr. Xu considers the liver and kidney as the main disease location, and secondarily the spleen and lung. The fundamental pathogenesis involves kidney deficiency, while damp-heat and stasis blood patterns are secondary. Random parallel testing was applied to observe the efficacy and safety of the empirical formula *Jīng Tài Lái* (精泰来), consisting of *shēng dì* (Radix Rehmanniae Recens), *zé xiè* (Rhizoma Alismatis), *yě jú huā* (Flos Chrysanthemi Indici), *pú gōng yīng* (Herba Taraxaci), *shēng pú huáng* (Pollen Typhae), *yì mǔ cǎo* (Herba Leonuri), *tiān huā fěn* (Radix Trichosanthis) and *chì sháo* (Radix Paeoniae Rubra).

198 subjects were randomly and equally divided into a *Jīng Tài Lái* group and a prednisone group. Six months constituted on course of treatment.

AsAb tested negative 83.2% and 64.8% in the *Jīng Tài Lái* group and prednisone group, respectively. Pregnancy rates were 48.7% and 18.0%. Significant differences were found between the two treatment groups ($p<0.05$). Also, the respective incidence rates of adverse reactions were 15.1% and 20.4% [16].

Dr. He Yian-ping treated 46 cases of male immune infertility with *Guī Shèn Wán* (归肾丸) consisting of *shú dì huáng* (Radix Rehmanniae Praeparata) 30g, *tù sī zǐ* (Semen Cuscutae) 30g, *nǚ zhēn zǐ* (Fructus Ligustri Lucidi) 15g, *shān yào* (Rhizoma Dioscoreae) 15g, *gǒu qǐ zǐ* (Fructus Lycii) 20g, *hé shǒu wū* (Radix Polygoni Multiflori) 20g, *sāng jì shēng* (Herba Taxilli) 20g, *shān zhū yú* (Fructus Corni) 10g and *yín yáng huò* (Herba Epimedii) 10g.

➤ With blood stasis, *sān qī* (Radix et Rhizoma Notoginseng) 15g and *dān shēn* (Radix et Rhizoma Salviae Miltiorrhizae) 30g were added.

➤ With qi deficiency, *dǎng shēn* (Radix Codonopsis) 15g and *huáng qí* (Radix Astragali) 30g were added.

➤ When combined with inflammation of the genital tract, *pú gōng yīng* (Herba Taraxaci) 30g and *rěn dōng téng* (Caulis Lonicerae Japonicae)

30g were added.

The recovery and total effective rates reached 21.74% and 89.13%, with rates of 10% and 70% in the control group [17].

Dr. Yue treated 62 cases of immune male infertility with the empirical formula *Kàng Miǎn Cù Yù Wán* (抗免促育丸) consisting of *shú dì huáng* (Radix Rehmanniae Praeparata), *gǒu qǐ zǐ* (Fructus Lycii), *nǚ zhēn zǐ* (Fructus Ligustri Lucidi), *tù sī zǐ* (Semen Cuscutae), *yín yáng huò* (Herba Epimedii), *hé shǒu wū* (Radix Polygoni Multiflori), *huáng qí* (Radix Astragali), *dāng guī* (Radix Angelicae Sinensis), *hóng huā* (Flos Carthami), *chuān xiōng* (Rhizoma Chuanxiong), *dān shēn* (Radix et Rhizoma Salviae Miltiorrhizae), *táo rén* (Semen Persicae), *bái zhú* (Rhizoma Atractylodis Macrocephalae), *yì yǐ rén* (Semen Coicis), *chē qián zǐ* (Semen Plantaginis), *hǔ zhàng* (Rhizoma et Radix Polygoni Cuspidati) and *bái huā shé shé cǎo* (Herba Hedyotis).

The presence of AsAb was observed after treatment, with 90.32% testing negative. 41 subjects conceived within one year, with a pregnancy rate of 66.13%. This study suggests that *Kàng Miǎn Cù Yù Wán* (抗免促育丸) may be effective for immune male infertility due to AsAb[18].

Dr. He treated 35 cases of immune male infertility with the empirical formula *Guī Shèn Wán* (归肾丸) consisting of *shú dì huáng* (Radix Rehmanniae Praeparata) 30g, *tù sī zǐ* (Semen Cuscutae) 30g, *nǚ zhēn zǐ* (Fructus Ligustri Lucidi) 15g, *shān yào* (Rhizoma Dioscoreae) 15g, *gǒu qǐ zǐ* (Fructus Lycii) 20g, *sāng jì shēng* (Herba Taxilli) 20g, *shān zhū yú* (Fructus Corni) 10g and *yín yáng huò* (Herba Epimedii) 10g. The seminal plasma level of IL-6, activity rates and forward movement indexes of sperm were observed before and after treatment.

After treatment the level of IL-6 dropped from (68.2±8.5) pg/ml to (42.9±5.9) pg/ml with significant differences than before treatment (*p*<0.01). This suggests that *Guī Shèn Wán* (归肾丸) can obviously decrease the level of IL-6 in seminal plasma, which may explain the mechanism of this formula in the treatment of male immune infertility. [19].

Dr. Chen Qi-hua randomly divided 72 cases of immune male infertility into two groups. Prednisone was given to 32 subjects in the control group. The treatment group was administered the empirical formula *Yì Qì Chú Shī Tāng* (益气除湿汤), consisting of *huáng qí* (Radix Astragali) 30g, *rén shēn* (Radix et Rhizoma Ginseng) 10g, *ròu cōng róng* (Herba Cistanches) 10g, *huáng bǎi* (Cortex Phellodendri Chinensis) 10g, *lóng dǎn cǎo* (Gentianae Radix) 5g, *chē qián zǐ* (Semen Plantaginis) 10g, *shān yào* (Rhizoma Dioscoreae) 15g, *shēng dì huáng* (Radix Rehmanniae Recens) 10g and *gān cǎo* (Radix et Rhizoma Glycyrrhizae) 5g.

The recovery and total effective rates of the treatment group reached 52.5% and 90%, with rates of only 19% and 69% in the control group.[20]

Dr. Zou Qiang treated 50 cases of male infertility due to positive AsAb with *Hǔ Zhàng Dān Shēn Yǐn* (虎杖丹参饮) consisting of *hǔ zhàng* (Rhizoma et Radix Polygoni Cuspidati) 15g, *pú gōng yīng* (Herba Taraxaci) 15g, *zǐ cǎo* (Radix Arnebiae) 15g, *huáng qí* (Radix Astragali) 15g, *dān shēn* (Radix et Rhizoma Salviae Miltiorrhizae) 15g, *chì sháo* (Radix Paeoniae Rubra) 15g, *dāng guī* (Radix Angelicae Sinensis) 15g, *hé shǒu wū* (Radix Polygoni Multiflori) 15g, *nǚ zhēn zǐ* (Fructus Ligustri Lucidi) 15g, *shēng dì huáng* (Radix Rehmanniae Recens) 15g, *yín yáng huò* (Herba Epimedii) 15g and *hóng huā* (Flos Carthami) 10g.

➢ With severe damp-heat, *bài jiàng cǎo* (Herba Patriniae) 20g and *huáng bǎi* (Cortex Phellodendri Chinensis) 9g were added.

➢ With severe blood stasis, *sān qī fěn* (Radix et Rhizoma Notoginseng) 3g was added.

➢ With severe kidney deficiency, *bā jǐ tiān* (Radix Morindae Officinalis) 15g was added.

Prednisone was given to 35 cases in the control group.

AsAb tested negative in 41 cases in the treatment group with a rate of 82.0%, as compared with 19 cases with a rate of 54.3% in the control group (P < 0.05)[21].

(2) Male Infertility due to Abnormal Sperm

The incidence of male infertility due to abnormal sperm morphology is relatively high. Chinese medicine shows a satisfactory therapeutic effect in the treatment of this condition.

A. Azoospermatism

A number of currently clinical reports indicate that Chinese medicine can effectively treat azoospermatism caused by blockage of the spermatic duct. Most patients display kidney qi deficiency along with spermatic duct obstruction. The main treatment principle here is to tonify kidney qi while dredging the spermatic duct.

Modified combinations of *Shēng Jīng Sǎn* (生 精 散) and *Táo Hóng Sì Nì Sǎn* (桃红四逆散) may be applied. Medicinals include *wǔ wèi zǐ* (Fructus Schisandrae Chinensis), *gǒu qǐ zǐ* (Fructus Lycii), *tù sī zǐ* (Semen Cuscutae), *fù pén zǐ* (Fructus Rubi), *chē qián zǐ* (Semen Plantaginis), *chuān shān jiǎ* (Squama Manis), *wáng bù liú xíng* (Semen Vaccariae), *lù lù tōng* (Fructus Liquidambaris), *guì zhī* (Ramulus Cinnamomi), *táo rén* (Semen Persicae) and *hóng huā* (Flos Carthami) [22].

Dr. Ye treated 40 cases of azoospermatism with *Shēng Jīng Tōng Guān Tāng* (生精通关汤) consisiting of *shēng dì huáng* (Radix Rehmanniae Recens) 30g, *shú dì huáng* (Radix Rehmanniae Praeparata) 30g, *tù sī zǐ* (Semen Cuscutae) 30g, *shí chāng pú* (Rhizoma Acori Tatarinowii) 30g, *shé chuáng zǐ* (Fructus Cnidii) 30g, *gǒu qǐ zǐ* (Fructus Lycii) 20g, *cì wǔ jiā* (Radix et Rhizoma seu Caulis Acanthopanacis Senticosi) 15g, *yín yáng huò* (Herba Epimedii) 15g, *wáng bù liú xíng* (Semen Vaccariae) 15g, *jiǔ cài zǐ* (Semen Allii Tuberosi) 15g, *lù lù tōng* (Fructus Liquidambaris) 15g, *dāng guī* (Radix Angelicae Sinensis) 15g, *chì sháo* (Radix Paeoniae Rubra) 10g and *bái sháo* (Radix Paeoniae Alba) 10g.

> With yin deficiency, *zhī mǔ* (Rhizoma Anemarrhenae), *mài mén*

dōng (Radix Ophiopogonis), *hé shǒu wū* (Radix Polygoni Multiflori) and *sāng shèn zǐ* (Fructus Moriare) were added.

➢ With yang deficiency, *shú fù zǐ* (Radix Aconiti Lateralis Praeparata), *xì xīn* (Radix et Rhizoma Asari), *lù jiǎo jiāo* (Colla Cornus Cervi) and *bā jǐ tiān* (Radix Morindae Officinalis) were added.

When combined with blood stasis, *dān shēn* (Radix et Rhizoma Salviae Miltiorrhizae), *chuān xiōng* (Rhizoma Chuanxiong), *chuān shān jiǎ* (Squama Manis) and *hóng huā* (Flos Carthami) were added.

Results showed 30 cases recovered, 6 with excellent effect, and 4 ineffective [23].

Dr. Wang treated 25 cases of azoospermatism with *Shēng Jīng Dān* (生精丹) consisting of *yín yáng huò* (Herba Epimedii) 6g, *tù sī zǐ* (Semen Cuscutae) 6g, *gǒu qǐ zǐ* (Fructus Lycii) 6g, *bā jǐ tiān* (Radix Morindae Officinalis) 6g, *yú biào jiāo* (Piscis Vesica Aeris) 6g, *shān yáng gāo wán* (testicle of goat) 6g, *xiōng cán é* (male silk moth) 6g, *zǐ hé chē* (Placenta Hominis) 6g, *ròu cōng róng* (Herba Cistanches) 6g, *jiǔ cài zǐ* (Semen Allii Tuberosi) 6g, *hóng shēn* (Radix et Rhizoma Ginseng Rubra) 5g, *shú dì huáng* (Radix Rehmanniae Praeparata) 5g, *hé shǒu wū* (Radix Polygoni Multiflori) 5g, *xiān máo* (Rhizoma Curculiginis) 5g, *lù róng* (Cornu Cervi Pantotrichum) 4g, *bǔ gǔ zhī* (Fructus Psoraleae) 4g, *ròu guì* (Cortex Cinnamomi) 3g, *shú fù zǐ* (Radix Aconiti Lateralis Praeparata) 3g, *dāng guī* (Radix Angelicae Sinensis) 3g and *dān shēn* (Radix et Rhizoma Salviae Miltiorrhizae) 3g. 12g was taken twice daily, with three months as one treatment course. Smoking, drinking and cottonseed oil were forbidden during treatment.

Results showed 7 cases recovered, 13 cases improved, and 5 with no result [24].

Dr. Zhao treated 46 cases of obstructive and inflammatory azoospermatism with *Huà Yū Tián Jīng Tāng* (化瘀填精汤) consisting of *sān léng* (Rhizoma Sparganii) 40g, *é zhú* (Rhizoma Curcumae) 40g, *wáng bù liú xíng* (Semen

Vaccariae) 12g, *huáng qí* (Radix Astragali) 30g, *dāng guī* (Radix Angelicae Sinensis) 30g, *shú dì* (Radix Rehmanniae Praeparata) 30g and *sāng jì shēng* (Herba Taxilli) 30g.

After treatment for 60 days, 10 cases recovered (the spouse became pregnant) at a rate of 21.74%. 7 cases showed excellent effect (the sperm index became normal) with a rate 15.22%. 18 cases were shown effective (sperm present in the seminal fluid) at 39.13%. 11 cases were shown ineffective, with a proportion of 23.91%. The total effective rate reached 76.09%[25].

Dr. Ji Hong-xia treated 13 cases of azoospermatism with *Bǔ Shèn Shēng Jīng Sǎn* (补肾生精散) consisting of *tù sī zǐ* (Semen Cuscutae), *gǒu qǐ zǐ* (Fructus Lycii), *jiǔ cài zǐ* (Semen Allii Tuberosi), *jīn yīng zǐ* (Fructus Rosae Laevigatae), *ē jiāo* (Colla Corii Asini), *lù jiǎo jiāo* (Colla Cornus Cervi) and *gǒu jǐ* (Rhizoma Cibotii). Andriol was given to 9 subjects in the control group.

Results in the treatment group showed 4 cases were recovered, 5 cases with excellent effect, 2 cases effective and 2 cases ineffective. The total effective rate of treatment group was 88.5%, which was superior to 45% in the control group (*p*<0.05) [26].

Dr. Hu Bing-de treated 36 cases of azoospermatism with the empirical formula *Shēng Jīng Tāng* (生精汤) consisting of *bàn zhī lián* (Herba Scutellariae Barbatae) 20g, *jiāng cán* (Bombyx Batryticatus) 15g, *jí xìng zǐ* (Semen Impatientis) 12g, *shuǐ zhì* (Hirudo) 5g, *lù lù tōng* (Fructus Liquidambaris) 9g, *wáng bù liú xíng* (Semen Vaccariae) 15g, *wú gōng* (Scolopendra) 2g, *yáng gāo wán* (sheep testicle) 1 pair, *chì sháo* (Radix Paeoniae Rubra) 9g, *zhǐ shí* (Fructus Aurantii Immaturus) 10g, *chái hú* (Radix Bupleuri) 9g, *táo rén* (Semen Persicae) 10g, *chuān shān jiǎ* (Squama Manis) 15g, *niú xī* (Radix Achyranthis Bidentatae) 10g, *zào jiǎo cì* (Spina Gleditsiae) 10g, *sān léng* (Rhizoma Sparganii) 10g, *é zhú* (Rhizoma Curcumae) 10g and *gǒu qǐ zǐ* (Fructus Lycii) 15g.

➢ With kidney yin deficiency, *shú dì huáng* (Radix Rehmanniae Praeparata), *shān zhū yú* (Fructus Corni), *nǚ zhēn zǐ* (Fructus Ligustri Lucidi), *zhī mǔ* (Rhizoma Anemarrhenae) and *guī bǎn jiāo* (Colla Carapax et Plastrum Testudinis) were added.

➢ With kidney yang deficiency, *fù zǐ* (Radix Aconiti Lateralis Praeparata), *yín yáng huò* (Herba Epimedii), *bā jǐ tiān* (Radix Morindae Officinalis) and *lù jiǎo jiāo* (Colla Cornus Cervi) were added.

➢ With spleen deficiency, *bái zhú* (Rhizoma Atractylodis Macrocephalae) and *fú líng* (Poria) were added.

When combined with seminal emission or premature ejaculation, *jīn yīng zǐ* (Fructus Rosae Laevigatae) and *qiàn shí* (Semen Euryales) were added.

For severe downpouring of damp-heat, *lóng dǎn cǎo* (Gentianae Radix) and *huáng qín* (Radix Scutellariae) were added.

31 cases were recovered and 5 cases shown ineffective, with an overall recovery rate of 86% [27].

Dr. Han Xiao-feng treated 86 cases of azoospermatism with the empirical formula *Sì Jūn Shēng Jīng Tāng* (四君生精汤) consisting of *rén shēn* (Radix et Rhizoma Ginseng) 20g, *fú líng* (Poria) 15g, *bái zhú* (Rhizoma Atractylodis Macrocephalae) 15g, *gān cǎo* (Radix et Rhizoma Glycyrrhizae) 5g, *shú dì huáng* (Radix Rehmanniae Praeparata) 50g, *shān yào* (Rhizoma Dioscoreae) 10g, *bái sháo* (Radix Paeoniae Alba) 10g, *gǒu qǐ zǐ* (Fructus Lycii) 25g, *dāng guī* (Radix Angelicae Sinensis) 30g, *fù zǐ* (Radix Aconiti Lateralis Praeparata) 10g, *zé xiè* (Rhizoma Alismatis) 10g, *chái hú* (Radix Bupleuri) 10g and *mǔ dān pí* (Cortex Moutan) 10g.

When combined with distending pain of the lower abdomen, *yán hú suǒ* (Rhizoma Corydalis) 12g and *bái zhǐ* (Radix Angelicae Dahuricae) 12g were added.

When combined with lassitude in the loin and legs, *dù zhòng* (Cortex Eucommiae) 12g and *niú xī* (Radix Achyranthis Bidentatae) 12g were added.

> With severe qi deficiency, *huáng qí* (Radix Astragali) 30g was added.

> With excess ministerial fire due to yin deficiency of the liver and kidney, *guī bǎn* (Carapax et Plastrum Testudinis) 24g and *mǔ lì* (Concha Ostreae) 30g were added.

> With disharmony between the heart and kidney and excessive fire due to liver deficiency, *suān zǎo rén* (Semen Ziziphi Spinosae) 24g, *cháo bǎi zǐ rén* (Semen Platycladi) 9g, *gōu téng* (Ramulus Uncariae Cum Uncis) 9g, *shēng lóng chǐ* (Dens Dragonis) 9g and *dǎn nán xīng* (Arisaema cum Bile) 9g were added.

Results showed 62 cases with excellent effect, 18 cases effective and 6 cases ineffective, with a total effective rate of 93.02% [28].

B. Oligospermatism and Abnormal Sperm Morphology

In Chinese medicine, conditions of oligospermatism and abnormal sperm morphology are associated with scant semen, cold semen, and thin semen. The main pathogenesis involves kidney qi deficiency or qi and blood dual deficiency. The treatment principles include tonifying the kidney, assisting yang and boosting essence, and supplementing qi and nourishing blood. Chinese Medicine approaches display significant therapeutic effects in the treatment of male infertility secondary to oligospermatism.

Bǔ Zhōng Yì Qì Tāng (补中益气汤) was given to 55 subjects with male infertility due to oligospermatism or asthenospermia. Results showed increased sperm counts in 37 cases and sperm vitality improved in 42 cases with 13 women achieving pregnancy [29].

Microscopic studies performed by Dr. Wang revealed that *Wáng Shì Shēng Jīng Tāng* (王氏生精汤), displays an ability to alter the membranous structure of pathological sperm. The formula contains the medicinals *huáng jīng* (Rhizoma Polygonati), *hé shǒu wū* (Radix Polygoni

Multiflori), and *yín yáng huò* (Herba Epimedii) [30].

Dr. Jin evaluated the curative effects of the empirical preparation *Yùn Yù Dān Capsules* (孕育丹胶囊). The formula consists of *shú dì huáng* (Radix Rehmanniae Praeparata) 20g, *tù sī zǐ* (Semen Cuscutae) 20g, *nǚ zhēn zǐ* (Fructus Ligustri Lucidi) 15g, *yín yáng huò* (Herba Epimedii) 15g and *hé chē fěn* (Placenta Hominis) 2g. 10 capsules were taken daily. 30 days constituted one course of treatment. After treatment, 31 women became pregnant. Significant differences in sperm volume, sperm density, sperm vitality, grade II and III sperm, follicule-stimulating hormone (FSH), luteotropic hormone (LH) and testosterone also appeared after treatment ($p<0.001$) [31].

Dr. Zhang treated 85 cases of oligospermaism with *Shēng Jīng Tāng* (生精汤) consisting of *tù sī zǐ* (Semen Cuscutae) 15g, *gǒu qǐ zǐ* (Fructus Lycii) 15g, *huáng qí* (Radix Astragali) 15g, *huáng jīng* (Rhizoma Polygonati) 15g, *bài jiàng cǎo* (Herba Patriniae) 15g, *shān zhū yú* (Fructus Corni) 6g, *yín yáng huò* (Herba Epimedii) 10g, *dāng guī* (Radix Angelicae Sinensis) 10g, *chuān niú xī* (Radix Cyathulae) 10g, *huáng bǎi* (Cortex Phellodendri Chinensis) 10g and *shēng dì huáng* (Radix Rehmanniae Recens) 20g.

➤ With severe kidney yin deficiency, *sāng gēn* (radix Mori), *nǚ zhēn zǐ* (Fructus Ligustri Lucidi) and *fù pén zǐ* (Fructus Rubi) were added.

➤ With kidney yang deficiency, *xiān máo* (Rhizoma Curculiginis), *bā jǐ tiān* (Radix Morindae Officinalis) and *suǒ yáng* (Herba Cynomorii) were added.

➤ With severe blood stasis, *chuān xiōng* (Rhizoma Chuanxiong), *yù jīn* (Radix Curcumae), *táo rén* (Semen Persicae), *hóng huā* (Flos Carthami), *sān léng* (Rhizoma Sparganii) and *é zhú* (Rhizoma Curcumae) were added.

➤ With prostatitis, *hóng tēng* (Caulis Sargentodoxae) and *bì xiè* (Rhizoma Dioscoreae Hypoglaucae) were added.

➤ With epididymal induration, *jú hé* (Semen Citri Reticulatae), *lì zhī hé* (Semen Litchi), *zhì rǔ xiāng* (Olibanum)(stir-fried) and *zhì mò yào*

(Myrrha)(stir-fried) were added.

Decocted once daily, with 30 days as one treatment course.

Results showed 44 cases recovered, 30 cases with excellent effect, 6 cases effective, and 5 cases ineffective. The total effective rate reached 94.1% [32].

Dr. Wang treated 986 cases of oligospermatism and asthenospermia with the empirical formula *Yú Piāo Shēng Jīng Tāng* (鱼鳔生精汤) consisting of *gǒu qǐ zǐ* (Fructus Lycii) 12g, *yú biào mò* (Piscis Vesica Aeris) 12g, *shā yuàn zǐ* (Semen Astragali Complanati) 20g, *dǎng shēn* (Radix Codonopsis) 20g, *yín yáng huò* (Herba Epimedii) 20g, *hǎi gǒu shèn fěn* (Callorhini Testes et Penis) powder 3g, *tù sī zǐ* (Semen Cuscutae) 15g, *dù zhòng* (Cortex Eucommiae) 15g, *shān yào* (Rhizoma Dioscoreae) 25g, *fù pén zǐ* (Fructus Rubi) 10g and *gān cǎo* (Radix et Rhizoma Glycyrrhizae) 9g.

➤ With kidney yang deficiency, *lù hán cǎo* (Herba Evolvuli), *hǎi mǎ* (Hippocampus), *ròu guì* (Cortex Cinnamomi) and *bā jǐ tiān* (Radix Morindae Officinalis) were added.

➤ With kidney yin deficiency, *lù jiǎo jiāo* (Colla Cornus Cervi), *biē jiǎ* (Carapax Trionycis), *nǚ zhēn zǐ* (Fructus Ligustri Lucidi), *shú dì huáng* (Radix Rehmanniae Praeparata) and *huáng jīng* (Rhizoma Polygonati) were added.

➤ With downpouring of damp-heat, *xuán shēn* (Radix Scrophulariae), *jīn yín huā* (Flos Lonicerae Japonicae), *yú xīng cǎo* (Herba Houttuyniae), *qī yè yī zhī huā* (Rhizoma Paridis) and *huáng bǎi* (Cortex Phellodendri Chinensis) were added.

➤ With qi stagnation and blood stasis, *táo rén* (Semen Persicae), *hóng huā* (Flos Carthami), *chuān shān jiǎ* (Squama Manis), *chuān xiōng* (Rhizoma Chuanxiong) and *lì zhī hé* (Semen Litchi) were added.

Decocted in water and taken once daily. Three months were considered as one treatment course. Smoking, alcohol, tea, and cottonseed oil were prohibited. Sexual intercourse was also restricted to once every

5 to 7 days. After 1 to 2 treatment courses, 508 subjects were recovered, with 312 cases showing excellent effect, 104 cases effective, and 62 cases ineffective. The total effective rate reached 93.7% [33].

Dr. Liu treated 98 male infertility patients with *Sàn Yù Tāng* (散郁汤) consisting of *chái hú* (Radix Bupleuri), *bái sháo yào* (Radix Paeoniae Alba), *dāng guī* (Radix Angelicae Sinensis), *chuān xiōng* (Rhizoma Chuanxiong), *xiāng fù* (Rhizoma Cyperi), *chén pí* (Pericarpium Citri Reticulatae), *cì jí lí* (Fructus Tribuli), *ròu cōng róng* (Herba Cistanches), *bā jǐ tiān* (Radix Morindae Officinalis), *zhǐ qiào* (Fructus Aurantii), *hé shǒu wū* (Radix Polygoni Multiflori), *gǒu qǐ zǐ* (Fructus Lycii), *jīn yín huā* (Flos Lonicerae Japonicae) and *bái huā shé shé cǎo* (Herba Hedyotis).

100 cases in the control group recieved vitamin E 100mg and Theragran tablets once daily. Indolmixin 50mg, erythromycin 0.25g, Vitamin A 25,000 U and Vitamin C 200mg were taken three times each day. 20 days constituted one treatment course. Treatment continued for five courses or until pregnancy occurred.

In the treatment group, results showed 53 cases recovered, 15 cases effective and 30 ineffective, with a total effective rate of 69.39%. In the control group, results showed 19 cases recovered, 22 cases effective and 59 cases ineffective, with a total effective rate of 41%. Significant differences between the two groups were observed ($p<0.01$) [34].

Dr. Zeng treated 180 male infertility patients with *Shǒu Wū Huán Jīng Capsules* (首乌还精胶囊) consisting of *hé shǒu wū* (Radix Polygoni Multiflori), *huáng qí* (Radix Astragali), *yín yáng huò* (Herba Epimedii), *tù sī zǐ* (Semen Cuscutae) and *zǐ hé chē* (Placenta Hominis). 5 capusles; taken 3 times daily. (Each capsule is equal to 1.2g of the crude medicinal) 3 months constituted one course of treatment, with an interval of 5 to 10 days between courses. All subjects were treated for 1 to 3 courses.

Results showed 54 cases recovered, 82 cases with excellent effect, 33 cases effective and 11 cases ineffective, with a total effective rate of

93.89%. Significant differences in sperm volume, hormone levels, and zinc appeared after treatment ($p<0.01$ or $p<0.05$). *Shǒu Wū Huán Jīng Capsules* also appears to improve sperm motility rates [35].

Dr. Li treated 120 male infertility patients with the empirical formula *Shēng Jīng Zhù Yù Tāng* (生精助育汤) consisting of *shēng dì huáng* (Radix Rehmanniae Recens), *huáng qí* (Radix Astragali), *xiān máo* (Rhizoma Curculiginis), *yín yáng huò* (Herba Epimedii), *nǚ zhēn zǐ* (Fructus Ligustri Lucidi), *fú líng* (Poria), *mǔ dān pí* (Cortex Moutan), *dān shēn* (Radix et Rhizoma Salviae Miltiorrhizae Miltiorrhizae), *shān yào* (Rhizoma Dioscoreae), *rén shēn* (Radix et Rhizoma Ginseng), *ē jiāo* (Colla Corii Asini) and *fù pén zǐ* (Fructus Rubi). 2 months constituted one treatment course. After one course, examination suggested that *Shēng Jīng Zhù Yù Tāng* can obviously improve sperm motility as well as morphological characteristics ($p<0.01$). After one course of treatment, 16 women also became pregnant [36].

Dr. Zhu Yu-fen studied 158 cases of oligospermatism by dividing them into five treatment groups.

➢ With kidney yang deficiency, treatment involved medicinals that warm the kidney and replenish essence. Modified *Wǔ Zǐ Yǎn Zōng Wán* (五子衍宗丸) consisting of *tù sī zǐ* (Semen Cuscutae) 15g, *gǒu qǐ zǐ* (Fructus Lycii) 12g, *fù pén zǐ* (Fructus Rubi) 10g, *wǔ wèi zǐ* (Fructus Schisandrae Chinensis) 10g, *chē qián zǐ* (Semen Plantaginis) 10g, *yín yáng huò* (Herba Epimedii) 15g, *chuān xù duàn* (Radix Dipsaci) 12g, *ròu cōng róng* (Herba Cistanches) 10g, *zào jiǎo cì* (Squama Manis)15g, *dāng guī* (Radix Angelicae Sinensis)10g, *dǎng shēn* (Radix Codonopsis) 12g and *huáng qí* (Radix Astragali) 18g was used.

➢ With erectile dysfunction, *yáng qǐ shí* (Actinolitum) and *xiān máo* (Rhizoma Curculiginis) were added.

➢ With combined with seminal emission, *jīn yīng zǐ* (Fructus Rosae Laevigatae), *lóng gǔ* (Os Draconis) and *mǔ lì* (Concha Ostreae) were added.

➤ With kidney yin deficiency, treatment involved medicinals that enrich the kidney, replenish essence and nourish the blood. Modified *Liù Wèi Dì Huáng Tāng* (六味地黄汤) consisting of *shú dì huáng* (Radix Rehmanniae Praeparata) 10g, *shān zhū yú* (Fructus Corni) 12g, *shān yào* (Rhizoma Dioscoreae) 15g, *zé xiè* (Rhizoma Alismatis) 10g, *fú líng* (Poria) 12g, *gǒu qǐ zǐ* (Fructus Lycii) 15g, *tù sī zǐ* (Semen Cuscutae) 12g, *bái sháo* (Radix Paeoniae Alba) 12g, *hé shǒu wū* (Radix Polygoni Multiflori) 12g, *dǎng shēn* (Radix Codonopsis)12g, *huáng qí* (Radix Astragali) 18g and *zào jiǎo cì* (Spina Gleditsiae) 15g was used.

➤ When combined with insomnia and profuse dreaming, *yè jiāo téng* (Polygoni Multiflosi Caulis) and *chǎo suān zǎo rén* (Semen Ziziphi Spinosae) (stir-fried) were added.

➤ With qi and blood dual deficiency, treatment involved medicinals that supplement the spleen, boost qi, nourish the blood, supplement the kidney, and replenish essence. Modified combinations of *Sì Jūn Zǐ Tāng* (四君子汤) and *Wǔ Zǐ Yǎn Zōng Wán* (五子衍宗丸) were used. The medicinals included *dǎng shēn* (Radix Codonopsis) 15g, *huáng qí* (Radix Astragali) 15g, *fú líng* (Poria) 12g, *bái zhú* (Rhizoma Atractylodis Macrocephalae) 12g, *gān cǎo* (Radix et Rhizoma Glycyrrhizae) 6g, *yín yáng huò* (Herba Epimedii) 12g, *gǒu qǐ zǐ* (Fructus Lycii) 15g, *shān yào* (Rhizoma Dioscoreae) 20g, *bái sháo* (Radix Paeoniae Alba) 15g, *dāng guī* (Radix Angelicae Sinensis) 10g, *zào jiǎo cì* (Squama Manis) 15g, *shú dì huáng* (Radix Rehmanniae Praeparata) 10g, *zǐ hé chē* (Placenta Hominis) 15g and *tù sī zǐ* (Semen Cuscutae) 12g.

➤ With qi stagnation and blood stasis, treatment involved medicinals that course the liver, rectify qi, invigorate the blood, and transform stasis. Modified *Chái Hú Shū Gān Sǎn* (柴胡疏肝散) was used. The medicinals included *chái hú* (Radix Bupleuri) 9g, *chì sháo* (Radix Paeoniae Rubra) 9g, *bái sháo* (Radix Paeoniae Alba) 9g, *dāng guī* (Radix Angelicae Sinensis) 15g, *zhǐ qiào* (Fructus Aurantii) 6g, *chuān xiōng* (Rhizoma of Chuangxiong) 10g, *xiāng fù* (Rhizoma Cyperi) 10g, *chén pí* (Pericarpium Citri Reticulatae) 6g, *táo rén* (Pericarpium Citri Reticulatae) 9g, *hóng huā* (Flos Carthami) 15g, *mǔ dān pí* (Cortex Moutan) 6g, *gān cǎo* (Radix et Rhizoma Glycyrrhizae) 6g, *gǒu qǐ zǐ* (Fructus Lycii) 10g, *chuān xù duàn* (Radix Dipsaci) 12g, *hé shǒu wū* (Radix Polygoni Multiflori) 15g and *zào jiǎo cì* (Spina Gleditsiae) 15g.

➢ With downpouring of damp-heat, treatment involved medicinals that clear heat, eliminate damp, supplement the kidney and replenish essence. Modified *Dǎo Chì Sǎn* (导 赤 散) was used. The medicinals included *shēng dì huáng* (Radix Rehmanniae Recens) 15 to 30g, *chì sháo* (Radix Paeoniae Rubra) 15 to 30g, *zhū líng* (Polyporus) 15 to 30g, *fú líng* (Poria) 15 to 30g, *mù tōng* (Caulis Akebiae) 6g, *zhú yè* (Folium bambusae) 10g, *chē qián zǐ* (Semen Plantaginis) 10g, *zé xiè* (Rhizoma Alismatis) 10 to 20g, *dān shēn* (Radix et Rhizoma Salviae Miltiorrhizae) 10 to 20g, *gān cǎo shāo* (Radix et Rhizoma Glycyrrhizae) 5g, *huáng bǎi* (Cortex Phellodendri Chinensis) 6g, *zào jiǎo cì* (Spina Gleditsiae) 15g, *gǒu qǐ zǐ* (Fructus Lycii) 15g, *shān zhū yú* (Fructus Corni) 12g and *shān yào* (Rhizoma Dioscoreae) 15g.

Results showed 125 cases recovered, 28 cases effective and 5 cases ineffective with a total effective rate of 96.8% [37].

Dr. Chen Lei treated 46 male patients with infertility due to abnormal sperm with *Èr Xiān Tāng* (二 仙 汤). The medicinals included *yín yáng huò* (Herba Epimedii) 30g, *xiān máo* (Rhizoma Curculiginis) 15g, *shú dì huáng* (Radix Rehmanniae Praeparata) 30g, *guī bǎn* (Carapax et Plastrum Testudinis) 30g, *tù sī zǐ* (Semen Cuscutae) 20g, *zhī mǔ* (Rhizoma Anemarrhenae) 15g, *ròu cōng róng* (Herba Cistanches) 15g, *bā jǐ tiān* (Radix Morindae Officinalis) 15g, *táo rén* (Semen Persicae) 10g and *hóng huā* (Flos Carthami) 10g.

➢ With spleen deficiency and exuberant dampness, *xiāng fù* (Rhizoma Cyperi) 15g, *zhì bàn xià* (Rhizoma Pinelliae) 15g, *chuān xiōng*

(Rhizome Chuangxiong) 5g, *shēng dì huáng* (Radix Rehmanniae Recens) 20g and *fú líng* (Poria) 30g were added.

➢ With spleen and kidney dual deficiency, *fú líng* (Poria) 10g, *shān zhū yú* (Fructus Corni) 15g, *mǔ dān pí* (Cortex Moutan) 10g, *chái hú* (Radix Bupleuri) 10g, *huáng bǎi* (Cortex Phellodendri Chinensis) 10g, *zé xiè* (Rhizoma Alismatis) 10g and *shuǐ niú jiǎo fěn* (Cornu Bubali) 50g were added.

➢ With qi stagnation and blood stasis, *dān shēn* (Radix et Rhizoma Salviae Miltiorrhizae Miltiorrhizae) 15g, *é zhú* (Rhizoma Curcumae) 15g, *niú xī* (Radix Achyranthis Bidentatae) 10g, and *dāng guī* (Radix Angelicae Sinensis) 10g were added.

After two courses of treatment, results showed 9 cases recovered, 18 cases with excellent effect, 13 cases effective and 6 cases ineffective with a total effective rate of 86.96% [38].

Dr. Zhuang Tian-qu treated 40 cases of azoospermia by supplementing the kidney and coursing the liver. Medicinals included *yín yáng huò* (Herba Epimedii) 30g, *shú dì huáng* (Radix Rehmanniae Praeparata) 30g, *gǒu qǐ zǐ* (Fructus Lycii) 15g, *huáng jīng* (Rhizoma Polygonati) 15g, *hé shǒu wū* (Radix Polygoni Multiflori) 15g, *chái hú* (Radix Bupleuri) 10g and *fó shǒu* (Fructus Citri Sarcodactylis) 10g.

Results showed 8 cases with excellent effect, 24 cases effective and 8 cases ineffective. Grade A sperm, grade B sperm, and motility rates were significantly improved after treatment ($p<0.05$).

Dr. Gao Hong-shou treated 43 subjects with azoospermia using modified *Wǔ Wèi Xiāo Dú Yǐn* (五味消毒饮) consisting of *jīn yín huā* (Flos Lonicerae Japonicae) 15g, *jú huā* (Flos Chrysanthemi) 10g, *pú gōng yīng* (Herba Taraxaci) 20g, *zǐ huā dì dīng* (Herba Violae) 15g, *dān shēn* (Radix et Rhizoma Salviae Miltiorrhizae Miltiorrhizae) 25g, *huáng qín* (Radix Scutellariae) 12g, *niú bàng zǐ* (Fructus Arctii) 15g, *zhì dà huáng* (Radix et Rhizoma Rhei)(stir-fried) 3g and *gān cǎo* (Radix et Rhizoma

Glycyrrhizae) 3g.

> With yang deficiency, *jīn yín huā* (Flos Lonicerae Japonicae), *jú huā* (Flos Chrysanthemi) and *huáng qín* (Radix Scutellariae) were removed, and *yín yáng huò* (Herba Epimedii) and *bā jǐ tiān* (Radix Morindae Officinalis) were added.

> With kidney yin deficiency, *nǚ zhēn zǐ* (Fructus Ligustri Lucidi) and *hàn lián cǎo* (Herba Ecliptae) were added.

> With seminal emission, *jīn yīng zǐ* (Fructus Rosae Laevigatae), *qiàn shí* (Semen Euryales) and *wǔ wèi zǐ* (Fructus Schisandrae Chinensis) were added.

Evaluation of motility rates showed 21 cases recovered, 17 cases markedly increased, and 5 cases ineffective. The total effective rate reached 88.4% [39].

Dr. He Yi-xin treated 168 cases of male infertility due to asthenospermia with *Huó Jīng Zhòng Zǐ Tāng* (活精种子汤) consisting of *huáng qí* (Radix Astragali) 30g, *shān zhū yú* (Fructus Corni) 12g, *tù sī zǐ* (Semen Cuscutae) 15g, *gǒu qǐ zǐ* (Fructus Lycii)15g, *ròu cōng róng* (Herba Cistanches) 12g, *sāng shèn zǐ* (Fructus Mori) 30g, *xiān máo* (Rhizoma Curculiginis) 15g, *yín yáng huò* (Herba Epimedii) 30g, *shuǐ zhì* (Hirudo) 5g, *lù jiǎo jiāo* (Colla Cornus Cervi) 15g and *gān cǎo* (Radix et Rhizoma Glycyrrhizae) 10g.

> With hyperactivity of fire due to yin deficiency, *lù jiǎo jiāo* (Colla Cornus Cervi), *xiān máo* (Rhizoma Curculiginis) and *yín yáng huò* (Herba Epimedii) were removed while *zhī mǔ* (Rhizoma Anemarrhenae) 10g, *huáng bǎi* (Cortex Phellodendri Chinensis) 15g, *guī bǎn jiāo* (Colla Carapax et Plastrum Testudinis) 15g, *hàn lián cǎo* (Ecliptae Prostratae) 30g and *nǚ zhēn zǐ* (Fructus Ligustri Lucidi) 30g were added.

> With damp-heat, *lù jiǎo jiāo* (Colla Cornus Cervi), *yín yáng huò* (Herba Epimedii) and *xiān máo* (Rhizoma Curculiginis) were removed while *tǔ fú líng* (Rhizoma Smilacis Glabrae) 30g and *bài jiàng cǎo* (Herba Patriniae) 30g were added.

➤ With varicocele, *zĭ dān shēn* (Radix et Rhizoma Salviae Miltiorrhizae) 30g, *chì sháo* (Radix Paeoniae Rubra) 12g and *shēn sān qī* (Radix et Rhizoma Notoginseng) 10g were added.

After 1 to 3 treatment courses, 61 women conceived. Results showed 82 cases recovered, 14 cases effective, and 11 cases ineffective. The total effective rate reached 93.4% [40].

Dr. Qu Xi-cai studied 82 subjects with abnormal due to mycoplasma infection by dividing them into three treatment groups.

➤ For damp-heat brewing and binding, medicinals were applied to clear heat, resolve toxin, transform dampness and disinhibit urine. *Wŭ Lín Săn* (五 淋 散) was applied with modifications. The medicinals included *chì fú líng* (Poria Rubra) 24g, *chì sháo yào* (Radix Paeoniae Rubra) 12g, *zhī zĭ* (Fructus Gardeniae)10g, *shēng gān căo* (Radix et Rhizoma Glycyrrhizae) 6g, *huáng băi* (Cortex Phellodendri Chinensis) 12g, *zé xiè* (Rhizoma Alismatis) 10g, *zĭ huā dì dīng* (Herba Violae) 15g and *dāng guī* (Radix Angelicae Sinensis) 10g.

➤ With kidney yin deficiency, medicinals were applied to nourish yin, clear heat, resolve toxin, and disinhibit urine. *Zhī Băi Dì Huáng Wán* (知柏地黄丸) was applied with modifications. Medicinals included *shú dì huáng* (Radix Rehmanniae Praeparata) 18g, *shān zhū yú* (Fructus Corni) 12g, *shān yào* (Rhizoma Dioscoreae) 15g, *mŭ dān pí* (Cortex Moutan) 12g, *fú líng* (Poria)12g, *zé xiè* (Rhizoma Alismatis) 10g, *zhī mŭ* (Rhizoma Anemarrhenae) 10g, *huáng băi* (Cortex Phellodendri Chinensis) 10g, *zĭ huā dì dīng* (Herba Violae)15g and *zhī zĭ* (Fructus Gardeniae) 10g.

➤ With kidney qi deficiency, medicinals were applied to nourish the kidney, replenish essence, warm yang and boost qi. *Wú Bĭ Shān yào Wán* (无比山药丸) was applied with modifications. Medicinals included *shān zhū yú* (Fructus Corni) 12g, *zé xiè* (Rhizoma Alismatis) 10g, *shú dì huáng* (Radix Rehmanniae Praeparata) 18g, *fú líng* (Poria) 12g, *bā jĭ tiān* (Radix Morindae Officinalis) 12g, *huái niú xī* (Radix Achyranthis Bidentatae) 10g, *chì shí zhī* (Halloysitum Rubrum) 6g, *shān yào* (Rhizoma Dioscoreae) 12g, *dù zhòng* (Cortex Eucommiae) 10g, *tù sī zǐ* (Semen Cuscutae) 10g, *ròu cōng róng* (Herba Cistanches) 15g, *wǔ wèi zǐ* (Fructus Schisandrae Chinensis) 6g and *huáng qí* (Radix Astragali) 15g.

Oral antibiotics were also administered to all subjects.

Results showed 48 cases with excellent effect (32 pregnancies), 23 cases effective, and 11 cases ineffective. The total effective rate reached 86.6% [41].

Dr. Ouyang Hong-gen treated 50 cases of oligospermatism with empirical formula *Shēng Jīng Fāng* (生精方) consisting of *shú dì huáng* (Radix Rehmanniae Praeparata) 15g, *hé shǒu wū* (Radix Polygoni Multiflori) 30g, *zǐ hé chē* (Placenta Hominis) 3g, *shā yuàn zǐ* (Semen Astragali Complanati) 30g, *huáng jīng* (Rhizoma Polygonati) 15g, *gǒu qǐ zǐ* (Fructus Lycii) 15g, *fú líng* (Poria) 15g and *yín yáng huò* (Herba Epimedii) 10g.

➢ With severe damp-heat, *huáng bǎi* (Cortex Phellodendri Chinensis) 9g, *lóng dǎn cǎo* (Gentianae Radix) 4g and *pú gōng yīng* (Herba Taraxaci) 15g were added.

➢ With kidney yin deficiency, *shēng dì huáng* (Radix Rehmanniae Recens) 15g and *guī bǎn* (Carapax et Plastrum Testudinis) 15g were added.

➢ With kidney yang deficiency, *bā jǐ tiān* (Radix Morindae Officinalis) 12g and *tù sī zǐ* (Semen Cuscutae) 15g were added.

➢ With severe blood stasis, *dān shēn* (Radix et Rhizoma Salviae Miltiorrhizae) 15g, *chì sháo* (Radix Paeoniae Rubra) 15g and *yì mǔ cǎo* (Herba Leonuri) 20g were added.

30 subjects in the control group were administered clomiphenein.

Results in the treatment group showed 40 cases recovered and 6 cases improved with a total effective rate of 92.0%. The control group showed 19 cases recovered and 4 cases improved with a total effective rate of 76.7%. Significant differences were observed between the two groups

(p<0.01).[42]

Dr. Li randomly and equally divided 120 cases of male infertility into two groups. For the treatment group, *Bǔ Fèi Zhuàng Jīng Tāng* (补肺壮精汤) consisting of *huáng qí* (Radix Astragali), *sāng bái pí* (Cortex Mori), *tiān dōng* (Radix Asparagi), *sāng piāo xiāo* (Oötheca Mantidis), *zhǐ qiào* (Fructus Aurantii), *tù sī zǐ* (Semen Cuscutae), *shā yuàn zǐ* (Semen Astragali Complanati), *zhì hé shǒu wū* (Radix Polygoni Multiflori Praeparata cum Succo Glycines Sotae), *sāng yè* (Folium Mori) and *fú líng* (Poria) was used. The control group recieved *Wǔ Zǐ Yǎn Zōng Tāng* (五子衍宗汤) consisting of *tù sī zǐ* (Semen Cuscutae), *fù pén zǐ* (Fructus Rubi), *gǒu qǐ zǐ* (Fructus Lycii), *chē qián zǐ* (Semen Plantaginis) and *wǔ wèi zǐ* (Fructus Schisandrae Chinensis). One month constituted one treatment course. The overall clinical effect, sperm vitality and α-glycosidase levels were observed before and after treatment.

Treatment group results showed 18 cases with excellent effect, 38 cases effective and 4 cases ineffective with a total effective rate of 93.3%. In the control group, 9 subjects showed excellent effect, 28 cases effective and 23 cases ineffective with a total effective rate of 61.7%. A significant difference in the total effective rates between the two groups were observed (p<0.01). Sperm vitality and levels of α-glycosidase were also obviously improved in the treatment group (p<0.01), with no obvious changes in the control group (p>0.05). This suggests that *Bǔ Fèi Zhuàng Jīng Tāng* can improve sperm vitality and epididymal function.[43]

Dr. Zhu Tong randomly divided 44 cases of spontaneous oligospermatism into two groups. 30 subjects in the treatment group were administered *Shēng Jīng Capsules* (生精胶囊) consisting of *shú dì huáng* (Radix Rehmanniae Praeparata) 20g, *ròu cōng róng* (Herba Cistanches) 20g, *yín yáng huò* (Herba Epimedii) 20g, *rén shēn* (Radix et Rhizoma Ginseng) 10g, *bái zhú* (Rhizoma Atractylodis Macrocephalae) 10g, *tù sī zǐ* (Semen Cuscutae) 30g, *fù pén zǐ* (Fructus Rubi)15g, *wǔ wèi zǐ* (Fructus Schisandrae Chinensis) 10g, *huáng qí*

(Radix Astragali) 30g, *xù duàn* (Radix Dipsaci) 15g, *jiǔ cài zǐ* (Semen Allii Tuberosi) 10g, *bā jǐ tiān* (Radix Morindae Officinalis) 10g, *dù zhòng* (Cortex Eucommiae) 10g, *lù róng* (Cornu Cervi Pantotrichum) 2.5g, *fú líng* (Poria) 15g, *gǒu qǐ zǐ* (Fructus Lycii) 20g, *chén pí* (Pericarpium Citri Reticulatae) 5g, *chuān xiōng* (Rhizoma Chuanxiong) 5g, *qiāng huó* (Rhizoma et Radix Notopterygii) 5g, *chē qián zǐ* (Semen Plantaginis) 20g and *gān cǎo* (Radix et Rhizoma Glycyrrhizae) 5g. 14 subjects in the control group were administered oral clomiphene.

The recovery and total effective rates were 50% and 90.0% in the treatment group, and 28.6% and 71.4% in the control group.[44]

C. Necrospermia

Necrospermia is often associated with inflammation of the epididymis, seminal vesicle or prostate. The pathogenesis may involve kidney qi deficiency, dual qi and blood deficiency, or hyperactivity of fire due to yin deficiency and internal static blood obstruction due to longstanding disease. The treatment principles are to supplement the kidney, replenish essence, tonify qi, nourish blood, enrich yin, clear heat, quicken the blood and resolve stasis.Proper treatment can also relieve inflammation of the seminal vesicle and epididymis.

Dr. Li holds that necrospermia caused by inflammation of the genital duct is mainly associated with hyperactivity of fire due to yin deficiency and blood stasis with heat bind. Treatment involves enriching yin, downbearing fire, clearing heat and transforming stasis. The empirical formula *Sǐ Jīng Zǐ No. 1* (死精子 1 号方) has been shown very effective.

Medicinals include *jīn yín huā* (Flos Lonicerae Japonicae), *dān shēn* (Radix et Rhizoma Salviae Miltiorrhizae Miltiorrhizae), *pú gōng yīng* (Herba Taraxaci), *shēng dì huáng* (Radix Rehmanniae Recens), *dāng guī* (Radix Angelicae Sinensis), *zhī mǔ* (Rhizoma Anemarrhenae), *huáng bǎi* (Cortex Phellodendri Chinensis), *chì sháo* (Radix Paeoniae Rubra), *bái sháo* (Radix Paeoniae Alba) and *shēng gān cǎo* (Radix et Rhizoma Glycyrrhizae).

With kidney essence deficiency, the formula was modified with the addition of *Wǔ Zǐ Yǎn Zōng Wán* (五子衍宗丸) [45].

Dr. Ou treated 182 cases of necrospermia with *yín yáng huò* (Herba Epimedii) 15g, *dāng guī* (Radix Angelicae Sinensis) 12g, *tù sī zǐ* (Semen Cuscutae) 12g, *shú dì huáng* (Radix Rehmanniae Praeparata) 30g, *táo rén* (Semen Persicae) 9g, *hóng huā* (Flos Carthami) 12g and *chuān xiōng* (Rhizoma Chuanxiong) 12g.

➤ With kidney deficiency, *suǒ yáng* (Herba Cynomorii) and *hé shǒu wū* (Radix Polygoni Multiflori) were added.

➤ With qi deficiency, *dǎng shēn* (Radix Codonopsis) and *shān yào* (Rhizoma Dioscoreae) were added.

➤ With blood stasis, *sān léng* (Rhizoma Sparganii) and *é zhú* (Rhizoma Curcumae) were added.

Administered once daily, with 30 days constituting one treatment course.

Results showed 67 subjects recovered, 57 with excellent effect, 36 effective and 22 ineffective [48].

Dr. Yang treated 76 cases of necrospermia with modified *Táo Hóng Sì Wù Tāng* (桃红四物汤) consisting of *táo rén* (Semen Persicae) 10g, *hóng huā* (Flos Carthami) 10g, *chuān xiōng* (Rhizoma Chuanxiong) 10g, *bái sháo* (Radix Paeoniae Alba) 10g, *yín yáng huò* (Herba Epimedii) 10g, *lù lù tōng* (Fructus Liquidambaris) 10g, *xù duàn* (Radix Dipsaci) 10g, *shú dì huáng* (Radix Rehmanniae Praeparata) 20g, *huáng qí* (Radix Astragali) 20g and *kūn cǎo* (Herba Leonuri) 15g.

➤ With inflammation, *zǐ huā dì dīng* (Herba Violae) and *yě jú huā* (Flos Chrysanthemi Indici) were added.

➤ With yang deficiency, *lù róng* (Cornu Cervi Pantotrichum), *ròu guì* (Cortex Cinnamomi) and *tù sī zǐ* (Semen Cuscutae) were added.

Administered once daily, with 30 days constituting one treatment course. After three courses, results showed 46 cases recovered, 24 effective and 6 cases ineffective [49].

Dr. Zhang treated 18 cases of necrospermia with the empirical formula *Yì Shèn Shēng Jīng Tāng* (益肾生精汤) consisting of *yín yáng huò* (Herba Epimedii) 15g, *shú dì huáng* (Radix Rehmanniae Praeparata) 15g, *ròu cōng róng* (Herba Cistanches) 15g, *tù sī zǐ* (Semen Cuscutae) 20g, *gǒu qǐ zǐ* (Fructus Lycii) 20g, *huáng qí* (Radix Astragali) 30g and *dāng guī* (Radix Angelicae Sinensis) 10g.

➢ With hyperactivity of fire due to yin deficiency, *shú dì huáng* was replaced with *shēng dì huáng* (Radix Rehmanniae Recens) and *zhī mǔ* (Rhizoma Anemarrhenae) 15g, with *chì sháo* (Radix Paeoniae Rubra) 15g and *pú gōng yīng* (Herba Taraxaci) 30g added.

➢ With downpouring of damp-heat, *bì xiè* (Rhizoma Dioscoreae Hypoglaucae) 15g, *chē qián zǐ* (Semen Plantaginis) 15g and *tǔ fú líng* (Rhizoma Smilacis Glabrae) 30g were added.

➢ With liver constraint and blood stasis, *chái hú* (Radix Bupleuri) 10g, *chì sháo* (Radix Paeoniae Rubra) 10g, *bái sháo* (Radix Paeoniae Alba) 10g and *yù jīn* (Radix Curcumae) 15g were added.

➢ With kidney qi deficiency, *bā jǐ tiān* (Radix Morindae Officinalis) 15g and *shān yào* (Rhizoma Dioscoreae) 30g were added.

Results showed 7 cases recovered, 8 cases effective and 3 cases ineffective [50].

Dr. Zhou treated 68 cases of male infertility due to necrospermia with *Yì Shèn Shēng Jīng Tāng* (益肾生精汤). The medicinals included *shú dì huáng* (Radix Rehmanniae Praeparata) 15g, *shān zhū yú* (Fructus Corni) 10g, *gǒu qǐ zǐ* (Fructus Lycii) 15g, *tù sī zǐ* (Semen Cuscutae) 15g, *shān yào* (Rhizoma Dioscoreae) 20g, *bā jǐ tiān* (Radix Morindae Officinalis)10g, *yín yáng huò* (Herba Epimedii)10g, *lù jiǎo jiāo* (Colla Cornus Cervi) 10g, *zhì fù zǐ* (Radix Aconiti Lateralis Praeparata)(stir-fried) 10g, *ròu guì* (Cortex Cinnamomi) 6g, *zǐ shí yīng* (Fluoritum) 10g, *wǔ wèi zǐ* (Fructus Schisandrae Chinensis) 6g, *fù pén zǐ* (Fructus Rubi) 15g, *dǎng shēn* (Radix

Codonopsis) 15g and *huáng qí* (Radix Astragali) 20g.

➢ With internal heat due to yin deficiency, *fù zǐ* (Radix Aconiti Lateralis Praeparata) and *ròu guì* (Cortex Cinnamomi) were removed, with *zhī mǔ* (Rhizoma Anemarrhenae) 10g and *huáng bǎi* (Cortex Phellodendri Chinensis) 10g added.

➢ With damp-heat brewing internally, *fù zǐ* (Radix Aconiti Lateralis Praeparata) and *ròu guì* (Cortex Cinnamomi) were removed. *Lóng dǎn cǎo* (Gentianae Radix) 6g, *zhī zǐ* (Fructus Gardeniae) 10g, *huáng qín* (Radix Scutellariae) 10g, *tǔ fú líng* (Rhizoma Smilacis Glabrae) 15g and *chē qián cǎo* (Herba Plantaginis) 15g were added.

Results showed 22 cases with excellent effect and 8 cases effective, (with 30 women achieving pregnancy), and 8 cases ineffective. The total effective rate reached 88.3% [51].

(3) Non-liquefaction of Semen

In Chinese medicine, non-liquefaction of semen is associated with patterns of seminal cold, seminal heat, or seminal turbidity. Causes may involve hyperactivity of fire due to yin deficiency, downpouring of damp-heat, phlegm and static blood binding together, essence and blood deficiency, or seminal cold due to yang deficiency. The treatment principles include enriching yin, downbearing fire, clearing heat, disinhibiting dampness, quickening the blood, transforming stasis, warming the palace of essence, and dissipating congealing cold.

Dr. Guo treated 65 cases of non-liquefaction of semen with *Yè Huà Tāng* (液 化 汤) consisting of *yín yáng huò* (Herba Epimedii) 15g, *shú dì huáng* (Radix Rehmanniae Praeparata) 15g, *bì xiè* (Rhizoma Dioscoreae Hypoglaucae) 15g, *tù sī zǐ* (Semen Cuscutae) 12g, *jiǔ xiāng chóng* (Aspongopus) 12g, *gǒu qǐ zǐ* (Fructus Lycii) 12g, *chē qián zǐ* (Semen Plantaginis) 9g, *huáng bǎi* (Cortex Phellodendri Chinensis) 6g, *chuān shān jiǎ* (Squama Manis) 6g and *guì zhī* (Ramulus Cinnamomi) 3g.

With blood stasis, *dān shēn* (Radix et Rhizoma Salviae Miltiorrhizae Miltiorrhizae) *zhè chóng* (Eupolyphaga seu Opisthoplatia) and *niú xī* (Radix Achyranthis Bidentatae) were added.

Taken once daily, with 30 days as one treatment course. Results showed 35 cases recovered, 21 cases effective and 9 cases ineffective [52].

Dr. San treated 32 cases of non-liquefaction of semen with *Zī Yīn Huà Tán Tāng* (滋阴化痰汤) consisting of *shēng dì huáng* (Radix Rehmanniae Recens) 20g, *quán guā lóu* (Fructus Trichosanthis) 20g, *zhī mǔ* (Rhizoma Anemarrhenae) 20g, *mài mén dōng* (Radix Ophiopogonis) 20g, *zhè bèi mǔ* (Bulbus Fritillariae Thunbergii) 20g, *xuán shēn* (Radix Scrophulariae) 20g, *zhú huáng* (Concretio Silicea Bambusae) 15g, *hǎi fú shí* (Pumice) 15g and *gān cǎo* (Radix et Rhizoma Glycyrrhizae) 6g.

➤ With qi stagnation, *zhǐ qiào* (Fructus Aurantii) 10g and *chuān liàn zǐ* (Fructus Toosendan) 10g were added.

➤ With qi deficiency, *dǎng shēn* (Radix Codonopsis) 10g and *shān yào* (Rhizoma Dioscoreae) 10g were added.

➤ With hyperactivity of fire, *huáng bǎi* (Cortex Phellodendri Chinensis) 10g and *huáng lián* (Rhizoma Coptidis) 10g were added.

Results showed 26 cases recovered and 6 cases ineffective [53].

Dr. Yi treated 90 cases of non-liquefaction of semen with *Lù Zhú Gān Cǎo Tāng* (鹿竹甘草汤). The formula contains *zhú yè* (Folium bambusae) 10g, *bì xiè* (Rhizoma Dioscoreae Hypoglaucae) 10g, *huáng bǎi* (Cortex Phellodendri Chinensis) 30g, *gān cǎo* (Radix et Rhizoma Glycyrrhizae) 30g, *fú líng* (Poria) 15g, *gǒu qǐ zǐ* (Fructus Lycii) 15g, *bái sháo* (Radix Paeoniae Alba) 15g, *mài mén dōng* (Radix Ophiopogonis) 15g, *lù lù tōng* (Fructus Liquidambaris) 15g and *zhī mǔ* (Rhizoma Anemarrhenae) 20g.

Results showed 68 subjects recovered, 14 effective, and 8 ineffective [54].

Dr. Cai treated 84 cases of non-liquefaction semen with Modified *Gù Zhēn Tāng* (加味固真汤) consisting of *chái hú* (Radix Bupleuri), *shēng má* (Rhizoma Cimicifugae), *qiāng huó* (Rhizoma et Radix Notopterygii), *dāng guī* (Radix Angelicae Sinensis), *zhī mŭ* (Rhizoma Anemarrhenae), *huáng bǎi* (Cortex Phellodendri Chinensis), *lóng dăn căo* (Gentianae Radix), *jīn yín huā* (Flos Lonicerae Japonicae), *cāng zhú* (Rhizoma Atractylodis), *zé xiè* (Rhizoma Alismatis), *dān shēn* (Radix et Rhizoma Salviae Miltiorrhizae Miltiorrhizae), *chē qián zĭ* (Semen Plantaginis), *sāng gēn* (Cortex Mori) and *gān căo* (Radix et Rhizoma Glycyrrhizae).

Results showed 44 cases recovered, 27 cases with excellent effect, 8 cases effective, and 5 cases ineffective [55].

Dr. Dai treated 65 cases of non-liquefaction sperm with the empirical formula *Miăn Bù No. 2* (免不Ⅱ号) to enrich yin, downbear fire, resolve toxin and resolve stasis. The medicinals include *zhī mŭ* (Rhizoma Anemarrhenae) 10g, *huáng bǎi* (Cortex Phellodendri Chinensis) 10g, *shēng dì huáng* (Radix Rehmanniae Recens) 10g, *shān zhū yú* (Fructus Corni) 10g, *shān yào* (Rhizoma Dioscoreae) 10g, *dān pí* (Cortex Moutan) 10g, *dān shēn* (Radix et Rhizoma Salviae Miltiorrhizae Miltiorrhizae) 10g, *fú líng* (Poria) 10g, *chì sháo* (Radix Paeoniae Rubra) 10g, *pú gōng yīng* (Herba Taraxaci) 20g, *jīn yín huā* (Flos Lonicerae Japonicae) 20g, *mŭ lì* (Concha Ostreae) 20g, *shēng dà huáng* (Radix et Rhizoma Rhei) 5g and *chái hú* (Radix Bupleuri) 5g.

The total effective rate was 92.3%. The liquefaction period, seminal viscosity, and tartrate-resistant acidic phosphatase levels significantly improved after treatment ($p<0.01$) [56].

Dr. Zhang treated 15 cases of non-liquefaction of sperm with *Yè Jīng Tāng* (液精汤). The medicinals included *zhī mŭ* (Rhizoma Anemarrhenae) 15g, *dāng guī* (Radix Angelicae Sinensis) 15g, *shēng dì huáng* (Radix Rehmanniae Recens) 15g, *dān shēn* (Radix et Rhizoma Salviae Miltiorrhizae Miltiorrhizae)15g, *xuán shēn* (Radix Scrophulariae) 12g, *bái máo gēn* (Rhizoma Imperatae) 12g, *huáng bǎi* (Cortex Phellodendri Chinensis) 10g, *chì sháo* (Radix Paeoniae Rubra) 10g, *bái sháo* (Radix Paeoniae Alba) 10g and *zhú yè* (Folium bambusae) 6g.

➤ With severe damp-heat, *bái sháo* (Radix Paeoniae Alba) was eliminated, the dosages of *dāng guī* (Radix Angelicae Sinensis) and *xuán shēn* (Radix Scrophulariae) were reduced, and *bì xiè* (Rhizoma Dioscoreae Hypoglaucae), *qú mài* (Herba Dianthi) and *chē qián zǐ* (Semen Plantaginis) were added.

➤ With kidney deficiency, *bái máo gēn* (Rhizoma Imperatae) was eliminated, the dosages of *zhī mǔ* (Rhizoma Anemarrhenae), *huáng bǎi* (Cortex Phellodendri Chinensis) and *zhú yè* (Folium bambusae) were reduced, and *huáng qí* (Radix Astragali), *gǒu qǐ zǐ* (Fructus Lycii), *xiān máo* (Rhizoma Curculiginis) and *yín yáng huò* (Herba Epimedii) were added.

➤ With liver constraint, *chái hú* (Radix Bupleuri), *xiāng fù* (Rhizoma Cyperi) and *yù jīn* (Radix Curcumae) were added.

➤ With asthenospermia, *huáng qí* (Radix Astragali), *dù zhòng* (Cortex Eucommiae) and *bā jǐ tiān* (Radix Morindae Officinalis) were added.

➤ With spermacrasia, modified *Wǔ Zǐ Yǎn Zōng Wán* (五子衍宗丸) was added.

Decocted in water and taken once daily. One month constituted one treatment course. After 1 to 5 treatment courses, results showed 10 cases recovered (women became pregnant), 3 cases clinically cured and 2 cases ineffective [57].

Dr. Zhu treated 128 cases of non-liquefaction of semen with the empirical formula *Huà Jīng Tāng* (化精汤) consisting of *yì zhì rén* (Fructus Alpiniae Oxyphyllae) 15g, *yì yǐ rén* (Semen Coicis) 12g, *shēng dì huáng* (Radix Rehmanniae Recens) 15g, *xiān líng pí* (Herba Epimedii) 12g, *chē qián zǐ* (Semen Plantaginis) 12g, *shān zhā* (Fructus Crataegi) 15g and *mài yá* (Fructus Hordei Germinatus) 12g.

The formula was decocted and one divided dose was taken twice daily. 30 days constituted one treatment course.

After 1 to 3 courses, results showed 70 cases recovered with a rate of 54.7%, 40 cases effective with a rate of 31.2% and 18 cases ineffective with a rate of 14.1%. The total effective rate reached 85.9% [58].

Dr. Shen Jian-hua treated 31 cases of non-liquefaction of semen with *Jiā Wèi Liǎng Dì Tāng* (加味两地汤). The medicinals included *shēng dì huáng* (Radix Rehmanniae Recens) 30g, *dì gǔ pí* (Cortex Lycii) 30g, *mài dōng* (Radix Ophiopogonis) 15g, *bái sháo* (Radix Paeoniae Alba) 15g, *xuán shēn* (Radix Scrophulariae) 15g, *bái wéi* (Radix et Rhizoma Cynanchi Atrati) 15g, *nǚ zhēn zǐ* (Fructus Ligustri Lucidi) 15g, *hàn lián cǎo* (Ecliptae Prostratae) 15g, *shí hú* (Caulis Dendrobii) 12g and *ē jiāo* (Asini Gelatium Corii) 10g.

30 cases in the control group were treated with *Zhī Bǎi Dì Huáng Tāng* (知柏地黄汤) consisting of *shú dì huáng* (Radix Rehmanniae Praeparata) 24g, *shān zhū yú* (Fructus Corni) 12g, *shān yào* (Rhizoma Dioscoreae) 12g, *zé xiè* (Rhizoma Alismatis) 9g, *fú líng* (Poria) 9g, *mǔ dān pí* (Cortex Moutan) 9g, *zhī mǔ* (Rhizoma Anemarrhenae) 10g and *huáng bǎi* (Cortex Phellodendri Chinensis) 10g.

The recovery and total effective rates in the treatment group were 90.30% and 93.55% respectively, with 66.70% and 73.33% in the control group ($p<0.01$)[59].

Dr. Fan Chang-qing treated 120 cases of non-liquefaction of semen with *Yè Huà Tāng* (液化汤) consisting of *zhī mǔ* (Rhizoma Anemarrhenae) 10g, *huáng bǎi* (Cortex Phellodendri Chinensis) 10g, *chì sháo* (Radix Paeoniae Rubra) 10g, *bái sháo* (Radix Paeoniae Alba) 10g, *mǔ dān pí* (Cortex Moutan) 10g, *tiān dōng* (Radix Asparagi) 10g, *tiān huā fěn* (Radix Trichosanthis) 10g, *fú líng* (Poria) 10g, *chē qián zǐ* (Semen Plantaginis) 10g, *shēng dì huáng* (Radix Rehmanniae Recens) 20g, *shú dì huáng* (Radix Rehmanniae Praeparata) 20g, *lián qiào* (Fructus Forsythiae) 12g, *dān shēn* (Radix et Rhizoma Salviae Miltiorrhizae Miltiorrhizae) 30g, *yín yáng huò* (Herba Epimedii) 15g, *gǒu qǐ zǐ* (Fructus Lycii) 15g, *shēng gān cǎo* (Radix et Rhizoma Glycyrrhizae) 6g and *wú gōng* (Scolopendra) 1/3 piece (powdered).

Results showed 76 cases recovered (63.3%), 18 cases improved

(15%), 11 cases effective (9.1%) and 15 cases ineffective (12.6%). The total effective rate reached 87.4% [60].

Dr. Tan Qing-lan treated 42 cases of non-liquefaction of semen by dividing them into three treatment groups.

➤ For hyperactivity of fire due to yin deficiency, the treatment principle was to enrich yin and downbear fire. Modified *Zhī Bǎi Dì Huáng Tāng* (知柏地黄汤) was used. Medicinals included *zhī mǔ* (Rhizoma Anemarrhenae) 12g, *huáng bǎi* (Cortex Phellodendri Chinensis) 15g, *shēng dì huáng* (Radix Rehmanniae Recens) 15g, *shú dì huáng* (Radix Rehmanniae Praeparata) 15g, *tiān dōng* (Radix Asparagi) 15g, *shí hú* (Caulis Dendrobii) 15g, *gǒu qǐ zǐ* (Fructus Lycii) 15g, *shān zhū yú* (Fructus Corni) 15g, *tù sī zǐ* (Semen Cuscutae)15g, *shān zhā* (Fructus Crataegi) 30g, *mài yá* (Fructus Hordei Germinatus) 30g and *wǔ wèi zǐ* (Fructus Schisandrae Chinensis) 10g.

➤ For downpouring of damp-heat, the treatment principles were to clear heat and dissipate dampness. A modified combination of *Lóng Dǎn Xiè Gān Tāng* (龙胆泻肝汤) and *Bì Xiè Shèn Shī Tāng* (萆薢渗湿汤) was used. The medicinals included *lóng dǎn cǎo* (Gentianae Radix) 10g, *huáng bǎi* (Cortex Phellodendri Chinensis) 15g, *huáng qín* (Radix Scutellariae) 12g, *zé xiè* (Rhizoma Alismatis) 15g, *bì xiè* (Rhizoma Dioscoreae Hypoglaucae) 20g, *chē qián zǐ* (Semen Plantaginis) 20g, *yì yǐ rén* (Semen Coicis) 30g, *zhī zǐ* (Fructus Gardeniae) 15g, *mǔ dān pí* (Cortex Moutan) 12g, *tǔ fú líng* (Rhizoma Smilacis Glabrae) 30g, *hǔ zhàng* (Rhizoma et Radix Polygoni Cuspidati) 15g, *shān zhā* (Fructus Crataegi) 30g and *mài yá* (Fructus Hordei Germinatus 30g).

➤ For stasis-phlegm obstruction, the treatment principle was to transform phlegm and resolve stasis. A modified combination of *Dǎo Tán Tāng* (导痰汤) and *Shào Fǔ Zhú Yū Tāng* (少腹逐瘀汤) was used. The medicinals included *dǎn nán xīng* (Arisaema cum Bile) 10g, *bàn xià* (Rhizoma Pinelliae) 10g, *dān shēn* (Radix et Rhizoma Salviae Miltiorrhizae

Miltiorrhizae) 20g, *chì sháo* (Radix Paeoniae Rubra) 15g, *xiǎo huí xiāng* (Fructus Foeniculi) 3g, *niú xī* (Radix Achyranthis Bidentatae) 15g, *pú huáng* (Pollen Typhae) 10g, *dāng guī* (Radix Angelicae Sinensis)10g, *lù lù tōng* (Fructus Liquidambaris) 20g, *chuān xiōng* (Rhizoma Chuanxiong) 6g, *wǔ líng zhī* (Faeces Togopteri) 10g, *shān zhā* (Fructus Crataegi) 30g and *mài yá* (Fructus Hordei Germinatus) 30g.

36 cases in the control group were treated with α-chymontrypsin, vitamin E, trimethoprim-sulfamethoxazole, and zinc gluconate.

The recovery and total effective rates in the treatment group were 54.8% and 85.7% respectively, with 33.3% and 61.1% in the control group ($p<0.001$)[61].

(4) Male Infertility due to Varicocele

The biomedical approach to the treatment of male infertility due to varicocele generally involves early surgical intervention. However, current research shows that Chinese medicine can also effectively treat this condition, especially when combined with surgery.

Dr. Qi treated 70 subjects with male infertility due to varicocele with the empirical formula *Lǐ Jīng Jiān* (理 精 煎) to quicken the blood, transform stasis, and supplement the kidney and liver. The medicinals included *dān shēn* (Radix et Rhizoma Salviae Miltiorrhizae Miltiorrhizae), *é zhú* (Rhizoma Curcumae), *niú xī* (Radix Achyranthis Bidentatae), *zhè chóng* (Eupolyphaga seu opisthoplatia), *dāng guī wěi* (Radix Angelicae Sinensis), *shú dì huáng* (Radix Rehmanniae Praeparata), *gǒu jǐ* (Rhizoma Cibotii), *yín yáng huò* (Herba Epimedii), *ròu cōng róng* (Herba Cistanches), *lù jiǎo shuāng* (Cornu Cervi Degelatinatum) and *hóng zǎo* (Fructus Jujubae).

Within 3-6 months, 25 women became pregnant. Results also showed normal or improved seminal fluid in 29 cases, and 16 cases ineffective.

Dr. Qi also treated 102 cases of male infertility due to varicocele with

Tōng Jīng Jiān (通精煎) consisting of *shēng huáng qí* (Radix Astragali), *shēng mǔ lì* (Concha Ostreae), *é zhú* (Rhizoma Curcumae), *chuān niú xī* (Radix Cyathulae), *dān shēn* (Radix et Rhizoma Salviae Miltiorrhizae Miltiorrhizae) and *chái hú* (Radix Bupleuri).

In this study, 39 women became pregnant. Results showed 38 cases improved and 25 cases ineffective, with a total effective rate of 75.49% [62].

Dr. Jia holds that the pathogenesis of male infertility most often involves kidney and essence deficiency with stasis and toxin brewing and binding.

39 male infertility patients with varicocele were administered *Yì Tōng No. 3* (益通 III 号) to transform stasis, resolve toxin, supplement the kidney, and replenish essence. The medicinals included *dāng guī* (Radix Angelicae Sinensis), *chuān xiōng* (Rhizoma Chuanxiong), *dān shēn* (Radix et Rhizoma Salviae Miltiorrhizae Miltiorrhizae), *jī xuè téng* (Caulis Spatholobi), *zé lán* (Herba Lycopi), *yì mǔ cǎo* (Herba Leonuri), *mǔ dān pí* (Cortex Moutan), *niú xī* (Radix Achyranthis Bidentatae), *dù zhòng* (Cortex Eucommiae), *shēng dì huáng* (Radix Rehmanniae Recens), *shú dì huáng* (Radix Rehmanniae Praeparata), *lù jiǎo shuāng* (Cornu Cervi Degelatinatum), *ròu cōng róng* (Herba Cistanches) and *shēng gān cǎo* (Radix et Rhizoma Glycyrrhizae).

Results showed 15 cases recovered, 24 improved and 3 ineffective. The total effective rate reached 92.9% [63].

Dr. Wang treated 64 subjects with male infertility due to varicocele with *Fù Shén Tōng Zàn Yù Tāng* (附神通赞育汤) consisting of *dāng guī* (Radix Angelicae Sinensis) 15g, *shēng dì huáng* (Radix Rehmanniae Recens) 15g, *chuān xiōng* (Rhizoma Chuanxiong) 15g, *dān shēn* (Radix et Rhizoma Salviae Miltiorrhizae Miltiorrhizae) 15g, *tōng cǎo* (Medulla Tetrapanacis) 15g, *wáng bù liú xíng* (Semen Vaccariae) 15g, *lù lù tōng* (Fructus Liquidambaris) 15g, *gǒu qǐ zǐ* (Fructus Lycii) 30g and *yín yáng huò* (Herba Epimedii) 30g.

➢ With cold congealing and blood stasis, *xiǎo huí xiāng* (Fructus Foeniculi), *ròu guì* (Cortex Cinnamomi) and *wú zhū yú* (Fructus Evodiae) were added.

➢ With qi stagnation, *zhǐ shí* (Fructus Aurantii Immaturus), *bái sháo* (Radix Paeoniae Alba) and *yù jīn* (Radix Curcumae) were added.

➢ With yin deficiency, *nǚ zhēn zǐ* (Fructus Ligustri Lucidi), *yán huáng bǎi* (Cortex Phellodendri Chinensis)(stir-fried with brine) and *mài mén dōng* (Radix Ophiopogonis) were added.

➢ With qi deficiency, *huáng qí* (Radix Astragali), *shān zhū yú* (Fructus Corni) and *shé chuáng zǐ* (Fructus Cnidii) were added.

➢ With damp-heat, *lóng dǎn cǎo* (Gentianae Radix), *yì yǐ rén* (Semen Coicis) and *chē qián zǐ* (Semen Plantaginis) were added.

One daily dose was decocted in water for oral use. The dregs of the decoction were also soaked in warm water (T<30℃) as an external wash. Three months constituted one treatment course. Alcohol and spicy foods were also prohibited.

Following 1-3 courses of treatment, results showed 35 cases recovered, 15 cases effective and 14 cases ineffective, with a total effective rate of 82.5%. The seminal fluid volume, sperm counts, and sperm survival and motility rates were significantly improved ($p<0.001$ or $p<0.05$) [65].

Dr. Qi Guang-cong divided 75 male infertility patients with grade II or grade Ⅲ varicole accompanied by dysspermia into two groups. 44 subjects in a Chinese medicinal group were treated with *Tōng Jīng Chōng Jì* (通精冲剂) consisting of *zǐ dān shēn* (Radix et Rhizoma Salviae Miltiorrhizae Miltiorrhizae), *é zhú* (Rhizoma Curcumae), *chuān niú xī* (Radix Cyathulae), *dāng guī wěi* (Radix Angelicae Sinensis), *táo rén* (Semen Persicae), *chái hú* (Radix Bupleuri), *shēng mǔ lì* (Concha Ostreae) and *shēng huáng qí* (Radix Astragali). 31 subjects in a surgery group were treated with high ligation of the spermatic vein or shunting of the inferior epigastric vein.

In the Chinese medicinal and surgery groups, 11 and 7 women became pregnant, respectively. (25.0% and 22.58%) No significant difference in the pregnancy rate was observed between the two groups (*p*>0.05). However, the Chinese medicinal group displayed improved seminal fluid density with higher active counts and motility, speed, and forward movement rates (*p*<0.01)[66].

Dr. Sun Zhong–ming randomly divided 278 cases of male infertility due to varicocele into three treatment groups.

96 subjects in group A were treated with Chinese medicinals including *zhì hé shǒu wū* (Radix Polygoni Multiflori) 10g, *chǎo dāng guī* (Radix Angelicae Sinensis) (stir-fried) 15g, *táo rén* (Semen Persicae) 10g, *dān shēn* (Radix et Rhizoma Salviae Miltiorrhizae Miltiorrhizae) 9g, *chǎo chuān xù duàn* (Radix Dipsaci) (stir-fried) 10g, *bǔ gǔ zhī* (Fructus Psoraleae) 10g, *yín yáng huò* (Herba Epimedii) 12g, *shēng huáng qí* (Radix Astragali) 20g, *xiān máo* (Rhizoma Curculiginis) 10g, *chǎo zhǐ qiào* (Fructus Aurantii) (stir-fried) 9g, *gān cǎo* (Radix et Rhizoma Glycyrrhizae) 9g, *chóng cǎo jùn* (Cordyceps) 6g and *wú gōng* (Scolopendra) 2 pieces. Modifications were also applied according to pattern identification.

94 subjects in group B were treated with high ligation of the spermatic vein.

88 subjects in group C were treated with both surgery and Chinese medicinals.

The recovery and total effective rates reached 39. 6%, 83.3%; 28.7%, 57.4% and 51.1%, 86.4% in groups A, B and C respectively, with significant differences observed among the three groups (*p*<0.01)[67].

Dr. Xu Ji-xiang treated 269 patients with male infertility due to varicocele with *Jiā Wèi Guì Zhī Fú Líng Wán* (加味桂枝茯苓丸). The medicinals included *guì zhī* (Ramulus Cinnamomi) 10g, *fú líng* (Poria) 10g, *mǔ dān pí* (Cortex Moutan) 10g, *sháo yào* (Radix Paeoniae Alba) 10g, *táo rén* (Semen Persicae) 10g, *dāng guī* (Radix Angelicae Sinensis) 12g, *huáng qí* (Radix Astragali) 15g, *hé shǒu wū* (Radix Polygoni Multiflori) 15g, *gǒu qǐ zǐ* (Fructus Lycii) 20g, *niú xī* (Radix Achyranthis Bidentatae) 20g and *gān cǎo* (Radix et Rhizoma Glycyrrhizae) 6g.

➢ With liver depression, *jú hé* (Semen Citri Reticulatae) 10g and *wū yào* (Radix Linderae) 10g were added.

➢ With downpouring of damp-heat, *chē qián zǐ* (Semen Plantaginis) 10g and *huáng bǎi* (Cortex Phellodendri Chinensis) 10g were added.

➢ With qi deficiency, *dǎng shēn* (Radix Codonopsis) 10g and *bái zhú* (Rhizoma Atractylodis Macrocephalae) 10g were added.

➢ With yang deficiency, *wú zhū yú* (Fructus Evodiae) 3g and *fù zǐ* (Radix Aconiti Lateralis Praeparata) 6g were added.

➢ With yin deficiency, *zhī mǔ* (Rhizoma Anemarrhenae) 10g and *biē jiǎ* (Carapax Trionycis) 10g were added.

Results showed 97 cases recovered, 101 cases with excellent effect, 34 cases effective and 37 cases ineffective. The total effective rate reached 86.25% [68].

Dr. Zhang Jian treated 52 patients with male infertility due to varicocele with *Jiā Wèi Táo Hóng Sì Wù Tāng* (加味桃红四物汤) consisting of *shēng dì huáng* (Radix Rehmanniae Recens), *chì sháo* (Radix Paeoniae Rubra), *dāng guī* (Radix Angelicae Sinensis), *chuān xiōng* (Rhizoma Chuanxiong), *táo rén* (Semen Persicae), *hóng huā* (Flos Carthami), *lì zhī hé* (Semen Litchi), *huáng qí* (Radix Astragali), *guì zhī* (Ramulus Cinnamomi), *dǎng shēn* (Radix Codonopsis) and *chái hú* (Radix Bupleuri). Three months constituted one treatment course and semen analysis routine was performed monthly.

After 2-3 treatment courses, results showed 19 cases recovered (12 pregnancies), 12 cases with excellent effect, 8 cases effective, and 13 cases ineffective. This study suggests that the formula *Jiā Wèi Táo Hóng Sì Wù Tāng* is effective for the treatment of male infertility due to varicocele [69].

Dr. Liu treated 72 patients with male infertility due to varicocele with the empirical formula *Shēn Qū Zhù Yù Tāng* (伸曲助育汤) to course the liver, resolve constraint, rectify qi and alleviate pain. The medicinals included *zhì xiāng fù* (Rhizoma Cyperi), *lì zhī hé* (Semen Litchi), *dāng guī* (Radix Angelicae Sinensis), *chì sháo yào* (Radix Paeoniae Rubra), *bái sháo yào* (Radix Paeoniae Alba), *zhǐ shí* (Fructus Aurantii Immaturus), *qīng pí* (Pericarpium Citri Reticulatae Viride), *chén pí* (Pericarpium Citri Reticulatae) and *zhì gān cǎo* (Radix et Rhizoma Glycyrrhizae Praeparata cum Melle). 15 days constituted one treatment course.

After 2-4 courses, results showed 28 cases recovered, 35 cases effective and 9 cases ineffective, with an overall effective rate of 87.5% [70].

3. ACUPUNCTURE AND MOXIBUSTION

The selection of acupuncture and moxibustion points must also be applied according to accurate pattern differentiation. In most cases, the simultaneous application of Chinese medicinal treatment yields a superior therapeutic effect. Many of the protocols described in the following acupuncture and moxibustion studies also include the application of several treatment modalities.

Dr. Pei treated 23 cases of oligospermatism and azoospermia with *Dāng Guī Zhù Shè Yè* (当归注射液) and biostimulin point injection.

【Point selection】

(1) ST 36 (*zú sān lǐ*) (left), BL 23 (*shèn shù*) (left), SP 6 (*sān yīn jiāo*) (right) and RN 4 (*guān yuán*).

(2) ST 36 (right), BL 23 (right), SP 6 (left) and DU 4 (*mìng mén*).

Both groups of points were used alternately. After three months of treatment, the average density of sperm increased from 11 million/ml to 33 million/ml in 19 cases, or 83% [71].

Dr. Zheng treated 297 cases of male infertility with a combination of acupuncture, point injection and Chinese medicinals. BL 23, BL 20 (*pí shù*), BL 26 (*guān yuán shù*), BL 32 (*cì liáo*), SP 6 and RN 4 were selected for acupuncture. *Lù Róng Zhù Shè Yè* (鹿茸注射液) was injected into bilateral BL 25 (*dà cháng shù*) and BL 23. One pair of points was selected per day, and 1 ml was injected into each point.

Tù sī zǐ (Semen Cuscutae), *ròu cōng róng* (Herba Cistanches), *lù jiǎo jiāo* (Colla Cornus Cervi), *shān zhū yú* (Fructus Corni), *nǚ zhēn zǐ* (Fructus Ligustri Lucidi), *bái zhú* (Rhizoma Atractylodis Macrocephalae), *jīn yīng zǐ* (Fructus Rosae Laevigatae) and *shú dì huáng* (Radix Rehmanniae Praeparata) were used as the formula.

After 2 to 4 months of treatment, 142 cases recovered, a proportion of 47.8%, and the total effective rate was 92.9%. This study suggests that the combination of the above three methods is effective for the treatment of male infertility [72].

Dr. Bai treated 66 cases of male infertility with catgut embedding therapy at RN 4 threaded through to RN 3 (*zhōng jí*), SP 6 and DU 4.

28 cases recovered with a proportion of 42.42%, and the total effective rate was 87.87% [73].

Dr. Chen treated 189 cases of male infertility by dividing them into three types based on pattern differentiation.

➤ For kidney yang deficiency, the treatment was boosting the kidney and warming yang. BL 52 (*zhì shì*), BL 23, DU 4 and RN 6 (*qì hǎi*) were selected.

➤ For cold congealing and blood stasis, the treatment was to quicken the blood, transform stasis and warm and free the channels. BL 52, BL 23, BL 24 (*qì hǎi shù*), DU 4, RN 6 and RN 4 were selected.

➤ For kidney yin deficiency, the treatment was to enrich kidney yin. BL 52, BL 23, KI 6 (*zhào hǎi*), SP 6 and RN 4 were selected.

Bilateral BL 52, BL 23 and BL 24 were punctured and then stimulated using lifting and thrusting methods. Needle sensation was propogated to the genital region. Moxabustion was also applied to points RN 6 and RN 4 for 10 minutes.

169 cases experienced a clinical recovery, among which 128 spouses became pregnant with a proportion of 67.72%. The total effective rate was 98.42% [74].

Dr. Lian treated 83 cases of male infertility with acupuncture and moxibustion according to pattern differentiation. The patients were divided into four types.

➢ For kidney yang deficiency, the treatment was warming the kidney and invigorating yang. DU 4, RN 4, KI 12 (*dà hè*), BL 33 (*zhōng liáo*), ST 36 and KI 3 (*tài xī*) were needled with supplementation. 10 cones of moxa on ginger were applied to DU 4, RN 4 and ST 36. Some patients received pole moxibustion for 20 to 30 minutes.

➢ For kidney yin deficiency, the treatment was to enrich yin and replenish essence. BL 23, RN 4, RN 6 and SP 6 were needled and supplemented with rotation.

➢ For qi stagnation and blood stasis, the treatment was to rectify qi and quicken the blood. RN 3, LV 11 (*yīn lián*), LV 3 (*tài chōng*), LV 2 (*xíng jiān*) and SP 6 were needled with drainage.

➢ For phlegm-damp brewing internally, the treatment was to dissipate damp and dispel phlegm. RN 3, KI 13 (*qì xué*), SP 3 (*tài bái*) and SP 9 (*yīn líng quán*) were needled with drainage.

56 cases recovered, 19 cases improved and the treatment was ineffective in 8 cases. Among the effective cases, the treatment courses were from 2 to 14 months, with an average of 4.5 months [75].

Dr. Ban treated 260 male patients with fertility problems due to dysspermia with a combination of acupuncture and Chinese medicinals.

【Point selection】

(1) DU 4, BL 23, BL 18 (*gān shù*), BL 20 (*pí shù*), DU 3 (*yāo yáng guān*), BL 52, BL 31-34 (*bā liáo*) and KI 3.

(2) RN 4, RN 6, RN 3, RN 2, SP 6, ST 36 and LV 3.

Six points were selected in each group, and each group of points was used alternately. Each point was needled with neutral lifting, thrusting and twirling supplementation and drainage with moderate stimulation for 30 seconds. The needling sensation on RN 4 and BL 31-34 radiated downward, but on SP 6 upward, both to the genitalia. Needles were retained for 30 minutes. Treatment was applied once a day during the first 15 days of each month.

Meanwhile, *xióng cán é* (male silk moth) 120g, *lù jiǎo piàn* (Cornu Cervi) 10g, *shú dì huáng* (Radix Rehmanniae Praeparata) 10g, *huáng jīng* (Rhizoma Polygonati) 10g, *yín yáng huò* (Herba Epimedii) 180g, *hǎi gǒu shèn* (Callorhini Testes et Penis) 30g, *jí xìng zǐ* (Semen Impatientis) 30g, *tù sī zǐ* (Semen Cuscutae) 110g, *gǒu qǐ zǐ* (Fructus Lycii) 90g, *chì sháo* (Radix Paeoniae Rubra) 60g, *fēng fáng* (Nidus Vespae) 50g, *chǎo chuān shān jiǎ* (Squama Manis stir-fried) 20g and *chái hú* (Radix Bupleuri) 10g were also used, modified according to pattern differentiation. The medicinals were ground into powder and divided into 90 portions; taken twice daily. Three months constituted one treatment course. Cigarettes, alcohol and spicy foods were prohibited during treatment.

165 cases were recovered, 71 cases with excellent effect, 8 cases improved and in 16 cases treatment was ineffective. The total effective rate was 93.8% [76].

Dr. Yu treated 34 males with infertility by regulating the kidney and freeing the collaterals.

【Point selection】

(1) Cervical points: DU 17 (*nǎo hù*), DU 16 (*fēng fǔ*), DU 15 (*yǎ mén*) and 6 points between DU 17 and the root of mastoid process, 15 stimulation points in all.

(2) Sacral points: BL 31-34. Each point was needled three times, 24 times in all.

(3) Body points: RN 3, ST 36, SP 6, KI 3, and RN 3 were needled using the burning mountain fire method in addition to moxibustion.

The cervical points were needled in the morning every day, and the sacral or body points were needled alternately in the afternoon every other day. Ten sessions constituted one treatment course.

25 cases were recovered (22 spouses became pregnant), 6 cases improved and in 3 cases treatment was ineffective. The total effective rate was 91.18% [77].

Dr. Wang selected BL 23, BL 31-34, RN 4, RN 2, SP 12, SP 6, RN 1 (huì yīn) and RN 6 to treat 13 males with infertility. Methods of lifting, thrusting and twirling manipulations were applied. For yang qi deficiency, warming needles were applied. Ten sessions constituted one treatment course, with an interval of 5 days between courses. Sexual intercourse, cigarettes and alcoholic beverages were prohibited during treatment.

➤ For debilitation of life gate fire, DU 4 was needled with supplementation.

➤ For heart-spleen deficiency, HT 5 was needled with neutral supplementation and drainage and ST 36 with supplementation.

➤ For liver constraint, LV 3 (tài chōng) was needled with drainage.

➤ For emotional depression, psychological counseling was applied.

8 cases recovered, 3 cases improved and in 2 cases treatment was ineffective. The total effective rate was 84.6%. The number of treatments given ranged from 5 to 50 sessions [78].

Dr. Zhao treated 87 cases of male infertility and sexual disorders with acupuncture and moxibustion.

Selection of main points: (1) BL 23, KI 3, BL 32 and DU 4. (2) RN 2, RN 4, SP 6 and ST 36. Points in both groups were needled using filiform needles with moxibustion alternately once a day. Acupuncture was applied after 10 minutes of moxibustion and the needles were retained for 30 minutes. 25 sessions constituted one treatment course with an interval of 5 to 7 days between courses. Supporting points were needled according to pattern differentiation. The content of zinc, copper and iron in the hair was measured before and after treatment to observe the therapeutic effect.

After 3 treatment courses, the content of zinc, copper and iron in the hair increased to various degrees [79].

Dr. Pang treated 128 males with infertility due to oligospermatism with acupuncture. BL 23, RN 4, BL 20 and ST 36 were needled with neutral supplementation and drainage once a day. 25 days constituted one treatment course. There was an interval of 7 days between courses.

After 4 treatment courses, 42 cases recovered, treatment was effective in 76 cases and in 10 cases treatment was ineffective, with a total effective rate of 92.19%. This study suggests that acupuncture therapy can improve sperm production.[80]

Dr. Fu randomly and equally divided 100 males with infertility with positive AsAb into two groups. For the group treated with acupuncture and Chinese medicinals, BL 18, BL 23, LV 3, KI 3, BL 15 (xīn shù), BL 17 (gé shù), HT 7 (shēn mén) and SP 10 were needled and they were also given Liù Wèi Dì Huáng Wán (六味地黄丸). For the prednisone group, prednisone was given orally. The therapeutic effect and change of AsAb were observed.

A total effective rate of 90% was observed in the acupuncture and Chinese medicinals group, which was superior to 64% in the prednisone group ($p<0.05$). The positive rate of AsAb in blood serum and sperm was reduced in both groups, especially in the acupuncture and Chinese medicinals group ($p<0.05$). This study suggests that the combination of acupuncture and Chinese medicinals is effective for the treatment of male immune infertility through regulation of AsAb and improvement of the immune condition [81].

Dr. Lun equally randomly divided 40 males with infertility with positive AsAb into an electroacupuncture group and a biomedicine group. The method of combining transport and source points was used in the electroacupuncture group, while prednisone was used in the biomedicine group. After two treatment courses, the changes of nitrogen monoxide (NO) and other microelements were observed.

For the electroacupuncture group, the content of NO in the blood serum obviously decreased and the content of zinc, copper and iron in the hair had increased to various degrees, more than in the biomedicine group ($p<0.05$). This suggests that electroacupuncture, applied to transport and source points is effective for male infertility, and may also regulate the content of NO and other microelements [82].

Dr. Luo treated 110 male immune infertility cases. 40 cases were treated by the combination of acupuncture and *Guī Shèn Wán* (归肾丸), 40 cases only by *Guī Shèn Wán* (归肾丸) and 30 cases by prednisone.

Method: BL 32 and BL 26 were needled bilaterally. The needling sensation should reach the genitalia. Neutral supplementation and drainage stimulation was given every 5 minutes; the needles were retained for 15 to 20 minutes. Treatment was given once every other day.

The total effective rates were 92.50%, 87.50% and 66.67% in the acupuncture and *Guī Shèn Wán*, *Guī Shèn Wán* and prednisone groups respectively. This suggests that the combination of acupuncture and *Guī Shèn Wán* is effective for immune male infertility by supplementing kidney qi, enriching kidney yin and improving immune function [83].

Experimental Studies

1. RESEARCH ON SINGLE MEDICINALS

Tù sī zǐ (Semen Cuscutae), *xiān máo* (Rhizoma Curculiginis) and *bā jǐ tiān* (Radix Morindae Officinalis) can markedly improve the motility and membrane function of sperm in vitro, especially *tù sī zǐ* (Semen Cuscutae) [84].

Lycium barbarum polysaccharides can obviously improve the sexual function of partially castrated mice such as shortening the incubation period of penis erection and mounting action, reducing the level of E2 and raising the rate of mounting action, level of testosterone, organic quotient of the accessory sex glands, sperm counts and the motility of sperm. The mechanism is not as a substitution of androgen, but might be relevant to the regulation of the hypothalamus-pituitary-sexual gland axis [85].

A solution of *tù sī zǐ* (Semen Cuscutae) at proper concentration displays a significant intervening effect on the membrane, anterior head cap and mitochondrial function of sperm damaged by active oxygen, which surpasses Vitamin C. [86]

Yě shān zhā gēn (Radix Crataegi) has a certain effect on asthenospermia as it can improve sperm motility in vitro. [87]

The effective constituents of *bǔ gǔ zhī* (Fructus Psoraleae), *shé chuáng zǐ* (Fructus Cnidii), *tù sī zǐ* (Semen Cuscutae) and *yín yáng huò* (Herba Epimedii) can increase the serum level of testosterone of Sprague-Dawley rats, especially *yín yáng huò* (Herba Epimedii).[88]

The effective constituents of *yín yáng huò* (Herba Epimedii) can increase the weight of the testicles and serum level of testosterone and improve the sexual ability of Wistar rats [89].

2. Research on the Efficacy of Herbal Prescriptions

Shēng Jīng Zhòng Zǐ Tāng (生精种子汤) consisting of *huáng qí* (Radix Astragali), *yín yáng huò* (Herba Epimedii), *xù duàn* (Radix Dipsaci), *hé shǒu wū* (Radix Polygoni Multiflori), *dāng guī* (Radix Angelicae Sinensis), *sāng shèn* (Fructus Mori), *gǒu qǐ zǐ* (Fructus Lycii), *tù sī zǐ* (Semen Cuscutae), *wǔ wèi zǐ* (Fructus Schisandrae Chinensis), *fù pén zǐ* (Fructus Rubi) and *chē qián zǐ* (Semen Plantaginis) can increase the amount of wheat germ agglutinin receptor and improve the fluorescence intensity of 1, 8-ANS on the sperm membrane surface of males with infertility [90].

Nán Xìng Bù Yù Fāng II (男性不育 II 号方) consisting of *zhī mǔ* (Rhizoma Anemarrhenae), *huáng bǎi* (Cortex Phellodendri Chinensis), *shēng dì huáng* (Radix Rehmanniae Recens), *shú dì huáng* (Radix Rehmanniae Praeparata), *dān shēn* (Radix et Rhizoma Salviae Miltiorrhizae Miltiorrhizae), *gǒu qǐ zǐ* (Fructus Lycii), *xuán shēn* (Radix Scrophulariae), *bái sháo* (Radix Paeoniae Alba) and *yín yáng huò* (Herba Epimedii) can increase the testicular tissue weight of mice [91].

Yù Jīng Hé Jì (育精合剂) consisting of *ròu guì* (Cortex Cinnamomi), *jiǔ cài zǐ* (Semen Allii Tuberosi), *yín yáng huò* (Herba Epimedii) and *bā jǐ tiān* (Radix Morindae Officinalis) and *Yù Yīn Jīng Hé Jì* (育阴精合剂) consisting of *dāng guī* (Radix Angelicae Sinensis), *shú dì huáng* (Radix Rehmanniae Praeparata), *nǚ zhēn zǐ* (Fructus Ligustri Lucidi) and *tù sī zǐ* (Semen Cuscutae) can promote sperm generation in the testicles [92].

Èr Xiān Tāng (二仙汤) consisting of *yín yáng huò* (Herba Epimedii), *xiān máo* (Rhizoma Curculiginis), *bā jǐ tiān* (Radix Morindae Officinalis), *dāng guī* (Radix Angelicae Sinensis), *zhī mǔ* (Rhizoma Anemarrhenae) and *huáng bǎi* (Cortex Phellodendri Chinensis) can improve the spermatid and spermatic microstructure and increase the amount of SDH reactive granules in aged rats [93].

Zhī Bǎi Dì Huáng Wán (知柏地黄丸) is effective for immune male infertility, which might be relevant to its action of inhibiting the content of antigen-antibody in the testicles, seminal vesicles, spermatic duct and prostate directly or indirectly [94].

Yōu Shēng Bǎo (优生宝) has a similar function to androgen on immature rats in raising the weight of the prostate, seminal vesicles and levator ani muscle and increasing the serum level of testosterone. Meanwhile it can inhibit gossypol and protect the seminiferous epithelium cells of the testicles to increase the amount and motility of sperm and promote fertility [95].

Self-designed *Yè Huà Líng* (液化灵) is superior to biomedicine in improving the pH level, liquefaction time, 1 hour liquefaction rate, viscosity, motility and vitality of sperm ($p<0.05$ or $p<0.01$) [96].

Bǔ Shèn Shēng Jīng Tāng (补肾生精汤) can restore the pathological spermatogenic processes of the testicles to normal, increase the count, motility rates and activity of sperm, improve fertility, decrease the level of luteotrophic hormone and testosterone, increase the level of cortisol [97].

Yù Jīng Kē Lì (愈精颗粒) can increase the weight of the testicles and epididymis, the level of testosterone (T), the count, motility rate and activity of sperm and the pregnancy rate of female rats, decrease the level of estradiol (E2) and the ratio of E2/T and restore the seminiferous epithelium and mesenchyme cells.

Yù Jīng Kē Lì (愈 精 颗 粒) is effective for male infertility in rats due to its ability to improve the testicular function and quality of sperm and regulate the level of gonad hormones, and its effect is superior to that of clomiphene [98].

Yù Jīng Yīn (育 精 阴) consisting of *huáng qí* (Radix Astragali), *shān yú ròu* (Fructus Corni), *gǒu qǐ zǐ* (Fructus Lycii), *dāng guī* (Radix Angelicae Sinensis), *shú dì* (Radix Rehmanniae Praeparata), *xiān máo* (Rhizoma Curculiginis), *tù sī zǐ* (Semen Cuscutae), *nǚ zhēn zǐ* (Fructus Ligustri Lucidi) and *wǔ wèi zǐ* (Fructus Schisandrae Chinensis) can reduce and repair damage to the testicles and epididymis caused by experimental allergy and improve the quality of sperm in the epididymis [99].

Yì Kàng Líng (抑抗灵) consisting of *táo rén* (Semen Persicae), *shé chuáng zǐ* (Fructus Cnidii), *dāng guī* (Radix Angelicae Sinensis), *nǚ zhēn zǐ* (Fructus Ligustri Lucidi), *ròu cōng róng* (Herba Cistanches), *yì zhì rén* (Fructus Alpiniae Oxyphyllae), *yín yáng huò* (Herba Epimedii), *shān yú ròu* (Fructus Corni), *wǔ wèi zǐ* (Fructus Schisandrae Chinensis), *gǒu qǐ zǐ* (Fructus Lycii) and *gān cǎo* (Radix et Rhizoma Glycyrrhizae) can make AsAb in the serum and seminal plasma negative, increase the motility rate and velocity of sperm, and improve overall sperm quality, especially with low doses applied over 45 days of treatment [100].

Bǔ Shèn Shēng Jīng Wán (补肾生精丸) can improve the fertility of rats with kidney yang deficiency[101].

Dr. Zhou An-fang's empirical formula *Bǔ Shèn Yù Lín Tāng* (补肾毓麟 汤) can improve the fertility of male rats, and is superior to the effect of clomiphene. It has been shown to improve the quality of the testicles and epididymis, and also increase sperm count as well as the weight, density, and motility rates of sperm [102].

3. Research on New Forms of Medicinals

Gù Zhēn Soluble Granules (固真冲剂) are mainly composed of *fù pén zǐ* (Fructus Rubi) and *ròu cōng róng* (Herba Cistanches). *Bǎo Zhēn Soluble Granules* (葆真冲剂) are mainly composed of *hé shǒu wū* (Radix Polygoni Multiflori) and *nǔ zhēn zǐ* (Fructus Ligustri Lucidi). Both have been shown to improve the proportion of A and B cells in the supraoptic nucleus of the hypothalamus and paraventricular nucleus, increase the cell population of prehypophyseal somatotroph, luteotropic, and follicle-stimulating hormone and also to improve the structure of reproductive organs and the activity of related enzymes [103].

Wǔ Zǐ Yǎn Zōng Oral Liquid (五子衍宗液) can decrease the content of 5-hydroxytryptamine and the ratio of estradiol and testosterone and increase the plasmic level of testosterone in rats 18 to 24 months old. It possibly improves the level of sexual hormones and fertility by regulating monoamine transmitters in the hypothalamus [104].

Kāng Níng Oral Liquid (康宁口服液) consisting of *rén shēn* (Radix et Rhizoma Ginseng), *lù róng* (Cornu Cervi Pantotrichum), *shú dì huáng* (Radix Rehmanniae Praeparata), *xiān líng pí* (Herba Epimedii), *xiān máo* (Rhizoma Curculiginis), *ròu cōng róng* (Herba Cistanches), *gǒu qǐ zǐ* (Fructus Lycii) and *tù sī zǐ* (Semen Cuscutae) is effective for male infertility due to kidney deficiency. It can restore damage to spermatogenic cells in rats due to tripterygium wilfordii glycosides by promoting the repair of the mitochondrion and membranous structure in spermatocytes and spermatids [105].

Jīng Tài Lái Granules (精 泰 来 颗 粒 剂) can accelerate the delayed type hypersensitivity of mice due to cyclophosphamide. This suggests that *Jīng Tài Lái Granules* may effect the regulation of cell immunity. *Jīng Tài Lái Granules* can obviously decrease the phagocytic quotient α, and 40.0g/kg can decrease phagocytic quotient K as well. This suggests that *Jīng Tài Lái Granules* have a certain depressant effect on non-specific immunity function. 20.0g/kg and 40.0g/kg of *Jīng Tài Lái Granules* can obviously inhibit the production of serum hemolysin in mice. It suggests that *Jīng Tài Lái Granules* can inhibit the humoral immunity of mice. Results show that *Jīng Tài Lái Granules* can directly and indirectly balance immunity by regulating hormones, neural transmitters and through the reticuloendothelial system, promoting the recovery of T-cell function, inhibiting autoantibody production and antibody degradation of B-cells [106].

Jīng Zhī Zhù Capsule (精 之 助 胶 囊) consisting of *dǎng shēn* (Radix Codonopsis), *huáng qí* (Radix Astragali), *bái zhú* (Rhizoma Atractylodis Macrocephalae), *shú dì* (Radix Rehmanniae Praeparata), *dāng guī* (Radix Angelicae Sinensis), *sháo yào* (Radix Paeoniae Alba), *tù sī zǐ* (Semen Cuscutae) and *wǔ wèi zǐ* (Fructus Schisandrae Chinensis) can obviously improve the sperm indexes in oligospermatism and asthenospermia patients and reverse the pathological changes of ultrastructure in mice testicles and epididymis [107].

Shǒu Wū Huán Jīng Capsule (首乌还精胶囊) can obviously increase sperm velocity (VAP, VCL, VSL), ALH, BCF, density of forward moving sperm, acrosome reaction rate of sperm and fertility rate and index of ovum with a certain dose-effect relationship. This suggests that *Shǒu Wū Huán Jīng Capsule* can improve both sperm motility and fertility rates [108].

Zēng Jīng Granules (增 精 颗 粒) are effective for male infertility by regulating epididymal function such as decreasing the content of glycerol-3-phosphocholine in the spermatic membrane, increasing the content of sialic acid in the epididymal fluid and improving the density, motility and deformity rates of sperm [109].

The main medicinals of *Zhuàng Jīng Hé Jì Oral Liquid* (壮精合剂口服 液) were *huáng bǎi* (Cortex Phellodendri Chinensis) 10g, *zhī mǔ* (Rhizoma Anemarrhenae) 10g, *shēng dì* (Radix Rehmanniae Recens) 10g, *shú dì* (Radix Rehmanniae Praeparata) 10g, *gǒu qǐ* (Fructus Lycii) 10g, *chē qián zǐ* (Semen Plantaginis) 10g, *tù sī zǐ* (Semen Cuscutae) 10g, *bā jǐ tiān* (Radix Morindae Officinalis) 10g, *yín yáng huò* (Herba Epimedii) 10g, *shān zhū yú* (Fructus Corni) 10g, *ròu cōng róng* (Herba Cistanches) 10g, *suǒ yáng* (Herba Cynomorii) 10g and *lù jiǎo piàn* (Cornu Cervi) 6g. It can obviously improve sperm quality and significantly increase sperm quantity [110].

Shēng Jīng Granules (生精冲剂) consisting of *gǒu qǐ zǐ* (Fructus Lycii), *tù sī zǐ* (Semen Cuscutae), *sāng shèn zǐ* (Fructus Mori), *wǔ wèi zǐ* (Fructus Schisandrae Chinensis), *fù pén zǐ* (Fructus Rubi), *huáng qí* (Radix Astragali), *dān shēn* (Radix et Rhizoma Salviae Miltiorrhizae Miltiorrhizae), *dāng guī* (Radix Angelicae Sinensis), *táo rén* (Semen Persicae) and *hóng huā* (Flos Carthami) can obviously increase the activity of SOD, CAT and ACE, and decrease the content of LPO and NO in rat varicocele[111].

(Chen Zhi-qiang, Dai Rui-xin, Wang Shu-sheng, Bai Zun-guang)

REFERENCES

[1] Zhen Chang-qin. Clinical Observation on the Treatment of 180 Oligospermatism Patients Based on Syndrome Differentiation (辨证分型治疗少精症180例临床观察). *Clinical Journal of Anhui Traditional Chinese Medicine* (安徽中医临床杂志), 1996, 8 (1): 14.

[2] Lu Shao-guang. Explore the Curative Effects of Different Methods in Treating 208 Male Infertility Patients Due to Abnormal Sperm (精液异常不育症208例不同疗法的治疗效果探讨). *Fujian Medical Journal* (福建医学杂志), 1996, 18(5): 1.

[3] Qiu De-ze. Analysis and Clinical Observation on Methods of Supplementing the Kidney and Replenishing Essence in Improving Sperm Quality of 66 Cases (补肾填精法改善精子质量66例临床观察分析). *Jiangxi Journal of Traditional Chinese Medicine* (江西中医药), 1997, 28 (5): 12.

[4] Bai Yu-zheng. 49 Male Infertility Patients Treated by the Self-designed Formula *Shēng Yù Tāng* (自拟生育汤治疗男性不育症49例). *Beijing Journal of Traditional Chinese Medicine* (北京中医), 1997, (5): 57.

[5] Chen Xiao-yuan. Treatment Methods of Warming the Spleen and Kidney, Nourishing the Heart, and Replenishing Essence in 25 Male Infertility Patients (温补脾肾养心填精法治疗男性不育25例). *New Journal of Traditional Chinese Medicine* (新中医), 1998, 30 (5): 38.

[6] Zhang Qi-hua. Treatment Based on Syndrome Differentiation in 400 Male Infertility Patients (辨证分型论治男性不育症400例). *Journal of Shanxi College of Traditional Chinese Medicine* (陕西中医), 1998, 19 (10): 449-450.

[7] Jin Xin. Clinical Observation of Chinese Medicinals in the Treatment of 57 Immune Male Infertility Patients (中医药治疗免疫性不育57例临床观察). *Gansu Journal of Traditional Chinese Medicine* (甘肃中医), 12 (2): 22.

[8] Yan Zheng-jun. Treatment with *Chūn Fù Lín* Capsules in 109 Male Infertility Patients (春复灵胶囊治疗男性不育症109例). *Journal of Shanxi College of Traditional Chinese Medicine* (陕西中医), 2002, 23 (4): 319-319.

[9] Yang De-fang, Yin Yong. Methods of Tonifying the Spleen and Replenishing Qi used to Treat 66 Male Infertility Patients (健脾益气法治疗男性不育症68例). *Journal of Shanxi College of Traditional Chinese Medicine* (陕西中医), 2003, 24 (4): 330.

[10] Cai Xin, Wang Li-wen, He Ying. Beginning Explorations on the Relationship among the Types of Male Infertility According to Syndrome Differentiation, Seminal Fluid Indexes and Serum Sexual Hormones (男性不育症中医证型与精液参数及血清性激素关系的初步探讨). *National Journal of Andrology* (中华男科学), 2003, 9(5): 396-398.

[11] Wang Tong, Chen Sheng. Clinical Observation of 100 Male Infertility Patients due to Non-liquefaction Sperm Treated by Syndrome Differentiation (辨证治疗精液不液化男性不育症100例临床观察). *Chinese Journal for Clinicians* (中国临床医生), 2005, 33 (12): 29-31.

[12] Mi Yang. Treatment with *Yi Qì Bǔ Shèn Jiě Dú Tāng* in 64 Immune Male Sterility Patients (益气补肾解毒汤治疗免疫性不育症64例). *Chinese Journal of Information on Traditional Chinese Medicine* (中国中医药信息杂志), 1997, 10 (13): 45.

[13] Huang Bai-lin. Treatment with *Zhuǎn Yīn Tāng* in 35 Male Infertility Patients with Positive AsAb (转阴汤治疗男性不育血清抗精子抗体阳性35例). *Journal of Practical Traditional Chinese Internal Medicine* (实用中医内科杂志), 1997, 11 (1): 46.

[14] Wang Li-qun. Treatment using Combinations of Chinese Medicine and Biomedicine in 31 Cases of Immune Male Infertility (中西医结合治疗免疫性不育31例). *Shaxxi Journal of Traditional Chinese Medicine* (山西中医), 1997, 13 (5): 24.

[15] Dai Ning. Clinical Observation of the Empirical Formula *Miǎn Yì* II in the Treatment of 48 Immune Male Infertility Patients withf Hyperactive Fire Due to Yin Deficiency (免疫 II 号治疗男性阴

虚火旺型免疫性不育48例临床观察). *Chinese Journal of Integrated Traditional and Western Medicine* (中国中西医结合杂志), 1998, 18 (4): 239-240.

[16] Xu Fu-song, Shi Yun-hua, Liu Cheng-yong. The Clinical Efficacy and Safety of *Jīng Tài Lái* in the Treatment of Male Infertility (精泰来治疗男性免疫性不育的疗效和安全性). *National Journal of Andrology* (中华男科学), 2001, 7 (1): 67-70.

[17] He Yan-ping, Tang Chun-zhi, Liang Guo-zheng. Clinical Observation of *Guī Shèn Wán* in the Treatment of 46 Cases of Immune Male Infertility (归肾丸治疗男性免疫性不育症46例疗效观察). *New Journal of Traditional Chinese Medicine* (新中医), 2002, 34 (12): 25-26.

[18] Yue Chen, Zhang Pei-yong, Yan Zhao-song. Clinical Observation of *Kàng Miǎn Cù Yù Wán* in the Treatment of Immune Male Infertility (抗免促育丸治疗男性免疫性不育疗效观察). *Hubei Journal of Traditional Chinese Medicine* (湖北中医杂志), 2004, 26 (8): 15-17.

[19] He Yan-ping, Tang Chun-zhi, Li Gong-ying. A Clinical Study on the Effects of *Guī Shèn Wán* on Seminal Fluid IL-6 in Male Immune Sterility (归肾丸对男性免疫性不育症患者精浆IL-6影响的临床研究). *New Journal of Traditional Chinese Medicine* (新中医), 2004, 36 (8): 15-18.

[20] Chen Qi-hua. Treatment with *Yì Qì Chú Shī Tāng* in 40 Immune Male Sterility Patients (益气除湿汤为主治疗免疫性不育症40例). *The Chinese Journal of Human Sexuality* (中国性科学), 2004, 13 (11): 24.

[21] Zhou Qiang, Ou-yang Hong-gen, Jin Guan-yu. Clinical Observation of *Hǔ Zhàng Dān shēn Yǐn* in the Treatment of 50 Male Sterility Patients with Positive AsAb (虎杖丹参饮治疗男性抗精子抗体阳性不育50例疗效观察). *New Journal of Traditional Chinese Medicine* (新中医), 2005, 37 (3): 43-44.

[22] Jiang Rui-feng. The Progression of Chinese Medicine in Diagnosing and Treating Impotence (阳痿的中医诊治进展). *New Journal of Traditional Chinese Medicine* (新中医), 1986, 18(10): 50.

[23] Ye Guang-yu, Wen Xue-fen. Treatment of No-sperm Syndrome with *Shēng Jīng Tōng Guān Tāng* (生精通关汤治疗无精子症). *Hebei Journal of Traditional Chinese Medicine* (河北中医), 1994, 16(4): 22–23.

[24] Wang Guan-jian, Chen Yu-chuan, Hu Fang-yan. Treatment of No-sperm Syndrome with Warming Methods for Reinforcing Kidney Yin (从"强肾之阴，热之尤可"谈无精子症的治疗). *New Journal of Traditional Chinese Medicine* (新中医), 1994, 26(7): 44–45.

[25] Zhao Guang-an, Zhang Zong-sheng. Treatment with *Huà Yū Tián Jīng Tāng* in 46 Inflammatory and Obstructive Azoospermia Patients (化瘀填精汤治疗炎症性梗阻性无精子症46例). *Beijing Journal of Traditional Chinese Medicine* (北京中医), 1998, (1): 44-45.

[26] Ji Hong-xia. Zhu Qing-guo. Liu Xian-yun. Understanding Differentiation and Treatment Methods of Azoospermia (无精症的辨证论治体会). *Inner Mongol Journal of Traditional Chinese Medicine* (内蒙古中医药), 2004, 19(6): 6-7.

[27] Hu Bing-de. Treatment of 36 Azoospermia Cases with the Self–designed Formula *Shēng Jīng Tāng* (自拟生精汤治疗无精症36例). *Jilin Journal of Traditional Chinese Medicine* (吉林中医药), 2004, 24(9): 35.

[28] Han Xiao-feng. Clinical Observation of the Self–designed Formula *Sì Jūn Shēng Jīng Tāng* in the Treatment of Azoospermia (自拟四君生精汤治疗无精子症疗效观察). *Health Vocational Education* (卫

生职业教育), 2005, 23(8): 57.

[29] Guang Chuan Shi Lang (光川史郎). The Experience of *Bǔ Zhōng Yì Qì Tāng* in the Treatment of Male Sterility Patients (男子不妊症患者补中益气汤使用经验). *Japan Sterility Association Journal* (日本不妊学会杂志), 1984, (4): 50.

[30] Qi Wang. Research Report on Chinese Herbs for Improving Human Spermatic Quality (关于中药提高人类精子质量的研究报告). The Collection of Theses of 2nd National Chinese Andriatry Research and Discussion Conference (第二届全国中医男科学研讨会论文集), 1988.

[31] Zheng Jin. The Effects of Self–designed Formula *Yùn Yù Dān* Capsules on Male Fertility Patients, with Attached Clinical Evaluation (自制孕育丹胶囊对男性生殖功能的影响：附 "例疗效评价"). *Clinical Journal of Anhui Traditional Chinese Medicine* (安徽中医临床杂志), 1997, 9(5): 236–237.

[32] Zhang Rong-kun, Li Ya-ping. The Clinical Analysis of *Shēng Jīng Tāng* in the Treatment of 86 Spermacrasia Patients (生精汤治疗少精症85例临床分析). *Journal of Journal of Zhejiang University of Traditional Chinese Medicine* (浙江中医学院学报), 1998, 22(4): 22.

[33] Wang An-pu. Clinical Observation of the Self–designed Formula *Yú Biào Shēng Jīng Tāng* in the Treatment of Spermacrasia and Asthenospermia (自拟鱼鳔生精汤治疗少精症和精子活力低的临床观察). *Xinjiang Journal of Traditional Chinese Medicine* (新疆中医药), 1999, 17(1): 20-22.

[34] Liu Bao-guang. Clinical Observation of *Sàn Yù Tāng* in the Treatment of Male Sterility (散郁汤治疗男性不育临床观察). *Shandong Journal of Traditional Chinese Medicine* (山东中医杂志), 1999, 18(5): 203-204.

[35] Zeng Jin-xiong, Dai Xi-hu, Yang Jia-hui. Clinical and Experimental Study of *Shǒu Wū Huán Jīng* Capsule in the Treatment of 180 Male Sterility Patients (首乌还精胶囊治疗男性不育症180例临床及实验研究). *Journal of Traditional Chinese Medicine* (中医杂志), 2000, 41(1): 33–35.

[36] Li Jin-kun, Shen Ming, Xu Shao-lin. Clinical Observation of *Shēng Jīng Zhù Yù Tāng* in the Treatment of 120 Male Sterility Patients (生精助育汤治疗男性不育症120例临床观察). *Journal of Traditional Chinese Medicine* (中医杂志), 2000, 41(12): 728–729.

[37] Zhu Yu-fen. Treatment of 158 Spermacrasia Male Patients According to Syndrome Differentiation in Chinese Medicine (中医辨证分型治疗男性不育少精子症158例). *Forum of Traditional Chinese Medicine* (国医论坛), 2002, 17(4): 20–21.

[38] Chen Lei, Xia Wei-ping, Zhou Zhi-heng. Treatment with the Self–designed Formula *Èr Xiān Tāng* in 46 Teratospermia Patients (自拟二仙汤治疗畸形精子过多不育症46例). *Shanghai Journal of Traditional Chinese Medicine* (上海中医药杂志), 2002, (5): 29.

[39] Zhuang Tian-zai. Clinical Observation of Methods for Tonifying the Kidney and Soothing the Liver in the Treatment of 40 Weak Sperm Patients (补肾疏肝法治疗弱精子症40例临床观察). *Hunan Guiding Journal of Traditional Chinese Medicine and Pharmacology* (湖南中医药导报), 2002, 8 (12): 763.

[40] He Yi-xin. Clinical Observation of *Huó Jīng Zhòng Zǐ Tāng* in the Treatment of 168 Asthenospermia Sterility Patients (活精种子汤治疗精子活力低下不育症168例临床观察). *Jiangxi Journal of Traditional Chinese Medicine* (江西中医药), 2003, 34(9): 28.

[41] Qu Xi-chai. Clinical Observation of 82 Mycoplasmal Infection Teratospermia Patients Treated with Combinations of Chinese Medicine and Biomedicine (中西医结合治疗解脲支原体感

染性畸形精子症82例疗效观察). *Hebei Journal of Traditional Chinese Medicine* (河北中医), 2004, 26(10): 791-792.

[42] Ou-yang Hong-gen, Jin Guan-yu. Clinical Study of *Shēng Jīng Fāng* in the Treatment of 50 Asthenospermia Sterility Patients (生精方治疗少精子症50例临床研究). *Journal of Practical Traditional Chinese Internal Medicine* (实用中医内科杂志), 2005, 19(1): 79-80.

[43] Li Bo, Jiang Li-jun, Bi Jian-cheng. Clinical Study on the Improvement of Spermatic Ability and Epididymis Function after Treatment with *Bǔ Fèi Zhuàng Jīng Tāng* (补肺壮精汤提高精子活力及附睾功能的临床研究). *New Journal of Traditional Chinese Medicine* (新中医), 2005, 37(2): 26-27.

[44] Zhu Tong, Ding Pei-chun. Treatment with *Shēng Jīng* Capsules in 30 Idiopathic Spermacrasia Patients (生精胶囊治疗特发性少精子症30例). *Journal of Sichuan Traditional Chinese Medicine* (四川中医), 2005, 23(5): 45-46.

[45] Li Guang-wen. Chinese Medicine Treatment of Male Sterility (男性不育症的中医治疗). *Journal of Shandong University of Traditional Chinese Medicine* (山东中医学院学报), 1979, (2): 29.

[46] Zeng Chao-wen. Treatment of Male Sterility with *Shēng Jīng Sǎn* with Attached Analysis of 500 Cases (生精散治疗男性不育症一附500例分析). *Journal of Guiyang College of Traditional Chinese Medicine* (贵阳中医学院学报), 1986, (4): 43.

[47] Li Liong-zhong. Clinical Summary of 700 Male Sterility Cases (700例男性不育临床小结). *Yunnan Journal of Traditional Chinese Medicine and Materia Medica* (云南中医杂志), 1988, 5 (5): 2.

[48] Ou Chun, Chen Zi-sheng. Clinical Observation of 182 Excessive Dead Sperm Syndrome Cases (182例死精过多症临床观察). *Shanghai Journal of Traditional Chinese Medicine* (上海中医药杂志), 1990, (5): 28-29.

[49] Yang Cong-bing. Clinical Observation of 76 Dead Sperm Patients Treated with Combinations of Chinese Medicine and Biomedicine (中西医结合治疗死精子症76例疗效观察). *Beijing Journal of Traditional Chinese Medicine* (北京中医), 1994, (6): 31.

[50] Zhang Luo. Treatment of Dead Sperm Syndrome with *Yì Shèn Shēng Jīng Tāng* (益肾生精汤治疗死精症), *Hubei Journal of Traditional Chinese Medicine* (湖北中医杂志), 2002, 24(8) :46

[51] Zhou Lei-zhi. Treatment of Excessive Dead Sperm Syndrome with *Yì Shèn Shēng Jīng Tāng* ("益肾生精汤"治疗死精子过多症). *The Journal of Medical Theory and Practice* (医学理论与实践), 2002, 15(9): 1049.

[52] Guo Zhi-rong. Clinical Observation of *Yè Huà Shēng Jīng Tāng* in the Treatment of 65 Male Sterility Patients (液化生精汤治男性不育65例疗效观察). *Jiangxi Journal of Traditional Chinese Medicine* (江西中医药), 1991, 22(3): 21-23.

[53] San Jing-chun, Liu Hong-sheng. Treatment with *Zī Yīn Huà Tán Tāng* of 32 Non-liquefaction Sperm Patients (滋阴化痰汤治疗精液不液化32例). *Jiangxi Journal of Traditional Chinese Medicine* (江西中医药), 1992, 33(1): 15.

[54] Yi Guo-xin. Treatment with *Lù Zhú Gān cǎo Tāng* on 90 Non-liquefaction of Sperm Patients (鹿竹甘草汤治疗精液不液化90例). *Liaoning Journal of Traditional Chinese Medicine* (辽宁中医杂志), 1992, 19(2): 265.

[55] Cai Qing-tong, Cai Kai. Clinical Observation of Modified *Gù Zhēn Tāng* in the Treatment of

88 Non-liquefaction of Sperm Patients (加减固真汤治疗精液不液化88例临床观察). *Beijing Journal of Traditional Chinese Medicine* (北京中医), 1993, (4): 27.

[56] Dai Ning. Clinical Research on 66 Non-liquefaction of Sperm Patients treated with *Miǎn Bù No. 2* (免不 II 号治疗精液不液化症65例临床研究). *Journal of Anhui Traditional Chinese Medical College* (安徽中医学院学报), 1998, 17(2): 25-26.

[57] Zhang Hong. Treatment with *Yè Huà Tāng* on 15 Patients with Abnormal Liquefaction of Sperm (液化汤治精液液化异常15例). *Jiangxi Journal of Traditional Chinese Medicine* (江西中医药), 1998, 29(5): 8.

[58] Zhu Qing-sheng. Treatment with *Huà Jīng Tāng* on 128 Non-liquefaction of Sperm Patients ("化精汤"治疗精液不液化症128例). *Jiangsu Journal of Traditional Chinese Medicine* (江苏中医), 2000, 21(12): 29.

[59] Sheng Jian-hua, Li Shu-ping, Qiu Yun-qiao. Clinical Observation of *Jiā Wèi Liǎng Dì Tāng* in the Treatment of Non-liquefaction of Sperm (加味两地汤治疗精液不液化症31例疗效观察). *New Journal of Traditional Chinese Medicine* (新中医), 2001, 33(6): 23-24.

[60] Huan Ming-qing. Treatment with *Yè Huà Tāng* on 120 Non-liquefaction of Sperm Patients (液化汤治疗精液不液化120例). *Journal of Sichuan Traditional Chinese Medicine* (四川中医), 2002, 20(10): 38.

[61] Tan Qing-lan. Clinical Observation of 42 Non-liquefaction of Sperm Cases Treated with Syndrome Differentiation of Chinese Medicine (中医辨证分型治疗精液不液化症42例疗效观察). *The Journal of Practical Medicine* (实用医学杂志), 2005, 21(5): 540–541.

[62] Qi Guang-cong, et al. Clinical Observation of *Tōng Jīng Jiān* in the Treatment of 102 Male Sterility Combined with Varicocele Patients (通精煎治疗精索静脉曲张合并不育症102例临床观察). *Chinese Journal of Integrated Traditional and Western Medicine* (中西医结合杂志), 1987, 7(10): 626.

[63] Jia Yan-bo. Clinical Observation of 42 Male Infertility Due to Varicocele Patients Treated with Chinese Medicine (精索静脉曲张所致男性不育症的中医治疗—附42例临床观察). *Hebei Journal of Traditional Chinese Medicine* (河北中医), 1990, 12(2): 31.

[64] Cui Yun, Zheng Wu, Wan Zhou. Clinical Observation of 37 Male Sterility Patients Treated with Combinations of *Tōng Jīng Líng* and High Level Disconnection of Vena Spermatica Interna (通精灵结合精索内静脉高位断流术治疗不育症37例的临床观察). *Journal of Zhejiang University of Traditional Chinese Medicine* (浙江中医学院学报), 1998, 22(6): 30-31.

[65] Wang Jun-gui. Treatment using the Dredging Method on Male Sterility Due to Varicocele Patients with the Freeing Method, and Attached Clinical Observation of *Fù Shén Tōng Zàn Yù Tāng* on 80 Cases (通法为主治疗精索静脉曲张合并不育：附神通赞育汤治疗80例疗效观察). *Beijing Journal of Traditional Chinese Medicine* (北京中医), 1999, 18(1): 46-47.

[66] Qi Guan-cong, Lu Hu-kun, Jue Qin-ling. Clinical Research on Male Sterility Due to Varicocele when Treated with *Tōng Jīng Chōng Jì* and Surgery (通精冲剂与手术治疗精索静脉曲张不育症的临床研究). *Chinese Journal of Integrated Traditional and Western Medicine* (中国中西医结合杂志), 2001, 21(6): 412–415.

[67] Sun Zhong-ming, Bao Yan-zhong. Clinical Observation of the Treatment of Male Sterility

Due to Varicocele (精索静脉曲张所致不育症临床治疗观察). *Chinese Journal of Andrology* (中国男科学杂志), 2003, 17(2): 123-124.

[68] Xu Ji-xiang. Treatment using *Jiā Wèi Guì zhī Fú líng Wán* on 269 cases of Male Sterility Due to Varicocele (加味桂枝茯苓丸治疗精索静脉曲张型不育症269例). *Journal of Shanxi College of Traditional Chinese Medicine* (陕西中医), 2003, 24(9):783-785.

[69] Zhang Jian. Treatment with *Jiā Wèi Táo Hóng Sì Wù Tāng* on 52 Male Sterility Due to Varicocele Patients (加味桃红四物汤治疗精索静脉曲张不育症52例), *Journal of Sichuan Traditional Chinese Medicine* (四川中医), 2004, 22(12): 49-50.

[70] Liu Jian-rong, Wang Huai-xiu. Clinical Research on *Shēn Qū Zhù Yù Tāng* in the Treatment of Male Sterility Due to Varicocele (伸曲助育汤治疗精索静脉曲张及其不育的临床研究), *Shanghai Journal of Traditional Chinese Medicine* (上海中医药杂志), 2005, 39(3): 33-34.

[71] Pei Ye-ming. Clinical Observation of 23 Spermacrasia and Asthenospermia Patients when Treated with Point Injection (药物穴位注射治疗少精、弱精症23例临床观察). *Jiangxi Journal of Traditional Chinese Medicine* (江西中医药), 1994, 25(2): 24.

[72] Zheng Zong-chang. Analysis of the Clinical Effects on 29 Male Sterility Patients when Treated with Combinations of Acupuncture and Chinese Herbs (针药并用治疗男性不育297例疗效分析). *Journal of Traditional Chinese Medicine* (中医杂志), 1995, 36(6): 349.

[73] Bai Dong. Clinical Observation of Catgut Embedding Therapy in the Treatment of 66 Male Sterility Patients (穴位埋线治疗男性不育66例疗效观察). *Chinese Acupuncture and Moxibustion* (中国针灸), 1996, 16(11): 41.

[74] Chen Peng. Clinical Explorations on Combinations of Acupuncture and Moxibustion in the Treatment of 189 Male Sterility Patients (针灸并举治疗男性不育症189例临床探讨). *Modern Diagnosis & Treatment* (现代诊断与治疗), 1997, 8(2): 115.

[75] Lian Yu-ling. Clinical Observation of 83 Male Sterility Patients Treated with Acupuncture and Moxibustion According to Syndrome Differentiation (针灸辨证治疗男性不育症83例疗效观察). *Journal of Clinical Acupuncture and Moxibustion* (针灸临床杂志), 1998, 14(3): 19-21.

[76] Ban Xu-sheng, Guan Jian-mei, Zhang Yong-mei. Treatment with Combinations of Acupuncture and Chinese Medicinals in 260 Male Sterility Patients Due to Abnormal Seminal Fluid (针刺配中药冲剂治疗精液异常性不育症260例). *Chinese Acupuncture and Moxibustion* (中国针灸), 1998, 18(4): 213-214.

[77] Yu Zheng-bei. Treatment of 34 Male Sterility Patients with Acupuncture and Moxibustion (针灸治疗男性不育症34例). *Shanghai Acupuncture and Moxibustion Journal* (上海针灸杂志), 2000, 19(6): 31.

[78] Wang Sui-zhu, Si Ji-chun. Clinical Observation of 13 Male Sterility Patients Treated with Acupuncture and Moxibustion (针灸治疗男性不育症13例临床观察). *Gansu Journal of Traditional Chinese Medicine* (甘肃中医), 2001, 14(5): 54.

[79] Zhao Xing-yu. The Curative Effects of Acupuncture and Moxibustion in the Treatment of Male Infertility and Microelement Analysis (针灸治疗男性不育及性功能障碍疗效及微量元素分析). *Journal of Clinical Acupuncture and Moxibustion* (针灸临床杂志), 2003, 19(2): 6–7.

[80] Peng Bao-zheng, Zhao Huan-yun. Treatment of 128 Male Sterility Due to Spermacrasia Cases with Acupuncture (针刺治疗少精不育128例). *Heilongjiang Journal of Traditional Chinese Medicine* (黑龙江中医药杂志), 2004(1): 42–43.

[81] Fu Bing, Lun Xin, Gong Yu-zhuo. Clinical Observation of 50 Immune Male Sterility Patients with Combinations of Acupuncture and Chinese Medicinals (针药结合治疗男性免疫性不育症50例疗效观察). *New Journal of Traditional Chinese Medicine* (新中医), 2004, 36(8): 48–49.

[82] Lun Xin. The Influence of Electric Stimulation on NO and Micro–elements when Treating Immune Male Sterility (电针治疗对男性免疫性不育症一氧化氮及微量元素的影响). *Chinese Acupuncture and Moxibustion* (中国针灸), 2004, 24(12): 854–856.

[83] Luo Qi-wei, Tang Chun-zhi, Yang Jun-jun. Clinical Observation of Immune Male Sterility Treated with Combinations of Acupuncture and *Guī Shèn Wán* (针刺结合归肾丸治疗男性免疫性不育症疗效观察). *Journal of Traditional Chinese Medicine University of Hunan* (湖南中医学院学报), 2005, 25(3): 50–52.

[84] Peng Shou-qing. Research on the Influence of Semen Cuscutae, Rhizoma Curculiginis and Radix Morindae Officinalis on the Movement and Membrance Function of Human Sperm in Vitro (菟丝子、仙茅、巴戟天对人精子体外运动和膜的功能影响的研究). *Chinese Journal of Integrated Traditional and Western Medicine* (中国中西医结合杂志), 1997, 17(3): 145.

[85] Luo Qiong, Huang Xiao-lan, Li Zhuo-neng. The Influence of Polysaccharose of Lycium Barbarum Polysaccharide on Sexual Function and Fertility of Male Mice (枸杞多糖对雄性大鼠性功能及生殖功能的影响). *Acta Nutrimenta Sinica* (营养学报), 2006, 28(1): 62-70.

[86] Yan Zhi-zhong, Yang Xin, Ding Cai-fei. The Interference Action of Semen Cuscutae on the Oxidizing Damaged Anterior Head Cap and Ultrastructure of Sperm (菟丝子对人精子顶体和超微结构氧化损伤的干预作用). *Chinese Archives of Traditonal Chinese Medicine* (中医药学刊), 2006, 24(2): 266-268.

[87] Hu Lian, Xiong Cheng-liang. The External Research on the Influence of Blood Serum Containing Crataegus cuneata Sieb.et Zucc. Root on Sperm Motility Parameters of Asthenospermia Patients (野山楂根含药血清对弱精子症患者精子运动参数影响的体外研究). *China Journal of Chinese Materia Medica* (中国中药杂志), 2006, (31)4 : 333–335.

[88] Wang Xing-sheng, Jie Guang-yan, Shi Xue-li. The Influence of Four Chinese Medicinals including Herba Epimedii on the Reproductive Hormones of Male SD Mice (淫羊藿等四味中药对SD雄性大鼠生殖内分泌的影响). *Chinese Journal of Traditional Medical Science and Technology* (中国中医药科技), 2005, 12(6): 380–381.

[89] Zhang Zhong-quan, Yang Bao-hua. The Effects of Herba Epimedii on Immunity and Reproductive Function of Experimental Animals (淫羊藿对实验动物免疫、生殖功能的影响). *Journal of Medical Forum* (医药论坛杂志), 2003, 24(24): 14–15.

[90] Liu Xiu-de, Li Guang-wen, Sui Yi-zhuang. The Influence of Chinese Medicinals on the Spermatic Plasma Membrane of Male Sterility Patients (中药对男性不育患者精子质膜的影响). *Chinese Journal of Integrated Traditional and Western Medicine* (中西医结合杂志), 1990, 10(9): 519.

[91] Wang Shu-rong, Sun Zhi-guang, Li Guang-wen. Experimental Study of *Nán Xìng Bù Yù*

Fāng II when Applied to Animals (男性不育 II 号方的动物实验研究). *Shanghai Journal of Traditional Chinese Medicine* (上海中医药杂志), 1991, (2): 17.

[92] Zhou Zhi-han, Xia Wei-ping, Jiang Xue-shi. Experimental Study on the Principle of Reinforcing the Kidney Method in Promoting Sperm Generation of the Testicle (补肾法促进睾丸生精原理的实验研究). *Shanghai Journal of Traditional Chinese Medicine* (上海中医杂志), 1992, (7): 24.

[93] Fang Zhao-qing. The Effects of *Èr Xiān Tāng* and its Modifications on Spermatic Cells and the Ultrastructure and the SDH of Mature Mice (中药二仙汤及其拆方对老年大鼠精子细胞和精子的亚微结构和SDH的作用). *Reproduction and Contraception* (生殖与避孕), 1993, (1): 62.

[94] Chen Xiao-ping. *Zhī Bǎi Dì Huáng Wán* in the Treatment of Male Immune Sterility and its Influence on Humoral Immunity (知柏地黄丸治疗男子免疫不育及其对体液免疫的影响). *Journal of Traditional Chinese Medicine* (中医杂志), 1994, (10): 610.

[95] Yi Jing, Yi Ping. Experiment Research on the Mechanism of *Yōu Shēng Bǎo* in the Treatment of Male Sterility with the Principles of Reinforcing the Liver and Kidney (优生宝补益肝肾治疗男性不育机理的实验研究). *Chinese Journal of Basic Medicine in Traditional Chinese Medicine* (中国中医基础医学杂志), 1996, 2(5): 33-34.

[96] Yang Xin．Clinical Study of *Yè Huà Líng* in the Treatment of Non-liquefaction of Sperm (液化灵治疗精液不液化症的临床研究). *Journal of Traditional Chinese Medicine* (中医杂志), 1996, 37(11): 682.

[97] Yue Guang-ping. Experimental Research on *Bǔ Shèn Shēng Jīng Tāng* and the Influence on Mice Models with Damaged Testicular Function and Kidney-yang Deficiency (补肾生精汤对肾阳虚睾丸功能损害大鼠模型作用的实验研究). *Chinese Journal of Integrated Traditional and Western Medicine* (中国中西医结合杂志), 1997, 17(5): 289.

[98] Zhong Bai-ling, Lv Wei. Pharmacodynamic Research on *Yù Jīng Kē Lì* in the Treatment of Male Sterility (愈精颗粒治疗男性不育症药效学研究). *Shandong Journal of Traditional Chinese Medicine* (山东中医杂志), 2002, 21(3): 177-179.

[99] Chen Lei, Xia Wei-ping, Xu Xin-jian. Experimental Research on *Yù Jīng Yīn* in the Treatment of Male Guinea Pigs with Immune Sterility (育精阴对雄性豚鼠免疫性不育的实验研究). *Chinese Journal of Andrology* (中国男科学杂志), 2002, 16(2): 92-94.

[100] Cui Ying-xia, Huang Yu-feng, Wang Yong-mei. Experimental Research on *Yì Kàng Líng* in the Treatment of Immune Sterility with Positive AsAb (中药抑抗灵治疗抗精子抗体介导的免疫性不育的实验研究). *National Journal of Andrology* (中华男科学), 2003, 9(8): 628–631.

[101] Li Hai-song, Li Ri-qing. Experimental Research on *Bǔ Shèn Shēng Jīng Wán* in the Treatment of Male Sterility (补肾生精丸治疗男性不育症的实验研究). *The Chinese Journal of Human Sexuality* (中国性科学), 2003, l2(1): 16–17.

[102] Huang Qiong-xia, Cao Ji-gang. Experimental Research on *Bǔ Shèn Yù Lín Tāng* in the Fertility of Mice with Damaged Reproduction Function and Kidney Deficiency (补肾毓麟汤对肾虚性生殖功能障碍大鼠生育力影响的实验研究). *Hubei Journal of Traditional Chinese Medicine* (湖北中医学院学报), 2005, 7(3): 7–9.

[103] Ma Zheng-li, Shi Yu-hua, Wang Li-ya. Morphological Research on the Hypothalmus-pituitary-sexual gland-thymus axis of Mature Mice after Treatment with Chinese Medicinals that

Tonify Essence and Kidney Function (填精补肾中药对老年大鼠下丘脑—垂体—性腺—胸腺轴的形态学研究). *Journal of Traditional Chinese Medicine* (中医杂志), 1989, (8): 45.

[104] Wang Xue-mei, Xie Zhu-fan, Liu Gen-xing. The Influence of *Wǔ Zǐ Yǎn Zōng* Oral Liquid on Hypothalamus Monoamine Transmitters, Sexual Hormones and Spermatogenic Functions of Male Mice (五子衍宗液对雄性大鼠下丘脑单胺类递质、性激素和生精能力的影响). *Chinese Journal of Integrated Traditional and Western Medicine* (中国中西医结合杂志), 1993, 13(6): 349.

[105] Fang Quan, Jiang Xue-zhou, Xia Wei-ping. Morphological Research on the Testicles of Sterile Mice with Kidney Deficiency caused by Tripterygium Glycosides after Treatment with *Kāng Níng* Oral Liquid (康宁口服液治疗雷公藤多甙所致肾虚不育症大鼠的睾丸形态学研究). *Acta Universitatis Traditionis Medicalis Sinensis Pharmacologiaeque Shanghai* (上海中医药大学学报), 2000, 14(4): 50-53.

[106] Zhu Xuan-xuan, Xu Fu-song, Shi Rong-shan. The Influence of *Jīng Tài Lái* Powder on Immune Function and AsAb (精泰来颗粒剂对免疫功能及抗精子抗体的影响). *Drug Standards of China* (中国药品标准), 2002, 3(2): 62–64.

[107] Wang Huai-xiu, Li Hong. Research on the Influence of *Jīng Zhì Zhù* Capsule on Reproductive Function ("精之助"胶囊对生殖功能影响的研究). *Chinese Journal of Andrology* (中国男科学杂志), 2002, 16(3): 201–204.

[108] Zeng Jin-xiong, Dai Xi-hu, Liu Jian-hua. The Influence of *Shǒu wū Huán Jīng* Capsules on Movement Ability and Fertilization of Human Sperm in Vitro (首乌还精胶囊体外对人精子运动能力和受精能力的影响). *National Journal of Andrology* (中华男科学杂志), 2003, 9(6): 476–479.

[109] Du Wei-liang, Chang De-gui, Ding Zhi-de. The Influence of *Zēng Jīng* Granules on the Sexual Indexes of Mice Epididymal Function --- GPC and SA (增精颗粒对大鼠附睾功能性指标GPC及SA的影响). *Chinese Journal of Andrology* (中国男科学杂志), 2004, 18(1): 22–25.

[110] Jie Ri-bo, Zhang Bao-guo. Clinical Observation of *Zhuàng Jīng Hé Jì* in the Treatment of Male Sterility (壮精合剂治疗男性不育症疗效观察). *Liaoning Journal of Traditional Chinese Medicine* (辽宁中医杂志), 2004, 31(10): 857.

[111] An Li-wen, Shui Yong, Hou Gao-feng. Experimental Research on *Shēng Jīng* Granules in Resisting Oxidation Damage on Mice Testicular Tissue with Varicocele (生精冲剂对精索静脉曲张大鼠睾丸组织抗过氧化损伤的实验研究). *Heilongjiang Medical Journal* (黑龙江医学), 2005, 29(3): 184-185.

Female Infertility

by **Li Li-yun**

Professor of Chinese Medicine Gynecology

Xu Min,

Ph.D. TCM, Associate Chief Physician of Chinese Medicine Gynecology

OVERVIEW

Infertility is defined as the inability for a couple to concieve following one year of unprotected sexual intercourse. The condition may be divided into two types, primary and secondary infertility. It is estimated that 80% of couples will conceive after one year of attempting to become pregnant, while 90% should conceive after two years. Women over 30 years of age should seek medical help when unable to achieve pregnancy after one year of regular sexual intercourse. After the age of 30, the chances of achieving a natural pregnancy are reduced as the quality of the ovum begins to decline.

Female infertility can also be categorized into absolute and relative infertility. Absolute infertility is the term used to describe an inability to conceive due to anatomical or functional defects, whereas relative infertility describes a less serious condition that will often respond favorably to treatment.

A variety of associated signs and symptoms may be observed, depending on the associated medical condition.

Obesity, weight gain, excessive bodyhair growth, and enlarged or distended ovaries may indicate polycystic ovarian syndrome (PCOS). Hyperlactation may appear due to amenorrhea galactorrhea syndrome. When infertility is secondary to endometriosis, a distended uterus with referred pain or ovarian cystic masses with fixed indurations may be palpated. With uterine fibroids or endometrioma, palpation may also reveal an enlarged uterus with an uneven surface or hypogastric masses. When pelvic or fallopian tube inflammation is involved, hypogastric tenderness and a fixed uterus may be found. Thyroid disorders often present with goiter or eye problems, where Cushing's disease manifests with obesity and acne. At the same time, many infertility patients will display asymptomatic presentations.

Gonadotropic hormone evaluations associated with ovarian function include FSH, LH, PRL, T and E2. These are generally tested during the follicular or ovulation phase, where progesterone should be tested in the middle of the beta phase. Thyroid exams include T3, T4, 17-hydroxycorticosteroids or PGI tests. Blood testing may be performed on the 2nd or 3rd day of the menstrual cycle to evaluate ovarian storage.

Laparoscopy and X-ray exams are used to identify fallopian tube obstruction, uterine fibroids and endometrial tuberculosis. Ultrasound exams and endometrial biopsy may also be used evaluate ovulatory function. BBT, hormone level, cervical mucus, and vaginal cell testing may also be performed. A postcoital test (PCT) can also be used to identify possible immune reactions that cause female infertility.

Treatment should be determined according to the specific cause of infertility. Active treatment is required for organic conditions involving tumors or inflammation, and also structural abnormalities such as transverse vaginal septum or other congenital conditions. When infertility is associated with anovulation, biomedicines may be prescribed to induce ovulation. Surgical procedures may be required to treat obstruction of the fallopian tube, and artificial insemination may be applied for narrowing of the cervix or in cases of male dysfunction. In vitro fertilization (IVF) and embryo transfer methods are currently used to treat tubal infertility, as well as conditions associated with endometriosis, PCOS, or aging.

Methods of prevention and health maintainence include physical exercise, stress management, reproductive health education, and routine screening for STD and other associated medical conditions.

Disorders associated with female infertility were first recorded in the Chinese medical literature as early as 2000 years ago.

The *Treatise on Bone Hollow* in the *Plain Questions* (素问·骨空论 , *Sù Wèn. Gǔ Kōng Lùn*) states: "When the penetrating vessel is in dysfunction, women may present with infertility." [1]

In *Compendium of Mountains and Rivers* (山海经 , *Shān Hǎi Jīng*), the condition was refered to as *childlessness*.

A Thousand Gold Pieces Emergency Formulary (千金要方 , *Qiān Jīn Yào Fāng*) uses the terms *complete childlessness* or *absence of progeny*.

Other historical references appear with such names as *attempting pregnancy*, *bearing children*, *offspring*, or *conception*.

CHINESE MEDICAL ETIOLOGY AND PATHOMECHANISM

The causes of female infertility are often complex. The *Treatise on Offspring* from *Rare Book of the Stone House* (石室秘录 · 子嗣论 , *Shí Shì Mì Lù. Zǐ Sì Lùn*) states, "There are ten kinds of disorders that lead to female infertility." [2]

These ten categories of disease include: uterine cold, spleen-stomach cold, urgent girdling vessel, depressed liver qi, exuberant phlegm-qi, effulgent ministerial fire, debilitated kidney water, governing vessel disease, inhibited bladder qi transformation, and qi and blood deficiency.

The *Treatise on Heavenly Truth from Remote Antiquity* from *Plain Questions* (素问 · 上古天真论 , *Sù Wèn. Shàng Gǔ Tiān Zhēn Lùn*) states, "In the female, kidney qi is exuberant by the age of 7. At the age of 14, *tian gui* arrives, the conception vessel flows and the great penetrating vessel fills, the menses arrive periodically, and [she] can bear children."[3]

The *Thousand Gold Pieces Emergency Formulary* (备急千金要方 , *Bèi Jí Qiān Jīn Yào Fāng*) states, "Couples remain childless when afflicted by the five taxations, seven damages, or weakness and deficiency."[4] This statement also points out that infertility is associated with both male and

---

[1] 见 《素问 · 骨空论》: "督脉者……此生病……其女子不孕。"

[2] 见 《石室秘录 · 子嗣论》: "女子不能生子, 有十病。"

[3] 见 《素问 · 上古天真论》: "女子七岁, 肾气盛……二七而天癸至, 任脉通, 太冲脉盛, 月事以时下, 故有子……"

[4] 见 《备急千金要方》: "凡人无子, 当为夫妇具有五劳七伤, 虚羸百病所致, 故有绝嗣之殃。"

female factors.

The *Sages' Salvation Records* (圣济总录 , *Shèng Jì Zǒng Lù*) states, "Female infertility results from insufficiency of the penetrating and conception vessels, or kidney qi deficiency cold." [5]

The *Treatise on Attempting to Become Pregnant* from *A Standard of Gynecology* (妇科玉尺·求嗣 , *Fù Kē Yù Chǐ. Qiú Sì*) quotes physician Wan Quan's commentary as follows. "The male is controlled by essence, whereas the female is governed by blood. Yang essence spills out and drains without exhaustion, while yin blood descends periodically and with regularity. The embryo settles and generation increases when yin and yang interact and essence and blood interconnect." [6] This statement shows that the material basis of generation involves both kidney qi, *tian gui*, male essence, and female blood.

Furthermore, "The uterine collaterals are connected with the kidney", "The kidney governs hibernation, is the root of storage, and the place of essence", and "The kidney governs the penetrating and conception vessels. The penetrating vessel is the sea of blood; the conception vessel governs the fetus". Deficiency of the kidney is therefore viewed as the fundamental cause in most cases of infertility.

Many conditions involve pathological interactions of the bowels, viscera, channels, and vessels, as well as transformations of cold, dampness, phlegm, heat, and stasis. Complex patterns of disharmony often lead to pathological changes of the kidney, and also the penetrating and conception vessels.

The most common patterns associated with female infertility are kidney deficiency, blood deficiency, liver constraint, phlegm-damp, damp-heat, and blood stasis.

---

[5] 见《圣济总录》："女子所以无子者，冲任不足，肾气虚寒也。"
[6] 见《妇科玉尺·求嗣》引万全语："男子以精为主，女子以血为主，阳精溢泻而不竭，阴血时下而不愆，阴阳交畅，精血合凝，胚胎结而生育滋矣。"

(1) Kidney Deficiency

A. Kidney yang deficiency

Kidney yang deficiency may result from congenital deficiency, kidney qi deficiency, and delayed or insufficient *tian gui*. This pattern also appears as a result of intemperate sexuality, chronic disease, or yin depletion involving yang. These factors lead not only to to kidney yang deficiency, but also debilitation of life gate fire, insufficiency of the penetrating and conception vessels, and uterine cold infertility.

B. Kidney yin deficiency

Kidney yin deficiency is caused by excessive sexual activity and taxation, essence damage from blood loss, and dual depletion of essence and blood. Yin depletion can also result from the overconsumption of hot and spicy foods as well as emotional factors, including impatience. As kidney yin and essence become deficient, the penetrating and conception vessels are also deprived of nourishment, leading to dryness of the uterus and infertility. Effulgent yin deficiency fire and excessive heat entering the sea of blood can also result in failure to retain essence.

C. Dual deficiency of kidney yin and yang

Patterns of kidney yin or kidney yang deficiency can develop simultaneously, or they may give way to one another in succession. Manifestations include combinations of the signs and symptoms listed above.

(2) Blood Deficiency

Blood is the material basis of menstruation and fertility; and patterns of blood deficiency often manifest in those with a weak physical constitution. The source of its transformation may become insufficient as a result of spleen-stomach deficiency, and fluids may become damaged by blood loss or chronic disease. These factors often lead to deficiency of the penetrating and conception vessels, and the uterus being deprived of nourishment. When the material basis is lacking due to blood deficiency, infertility may result.

(3) Liver Constraint

The female is said to be governed by blood, and the liver stores blood. The liver is also associated with orderly reaching and the free flow of qi and blood. The proper regulation of qi and blood also depends on the penetrating vessel since it governs the sea of blood. Emotional disturbances and unfufilled desires lead to dysfunction of orderly reaching, depression of the qi dynamic, constraint of liver qi, and eventually patterns of qi stagnation and blood stasis. Qi is the commander of blood, where the smooth movement of blood depends on the proper functioning of qi. Therefore, qi and blood disharmony patterns often manifest with irregular menstruation. When the penetrating and conception vessels are not adequately supplied with qi and blood, conception becomes difficult.

Infertility can also result when liver stagnation transforms into fire. Constrained heat can enter the penetrating and conception vessels, leading to disharmonies of the sea of blood and uterus.

(4) Phlegm-damp

The accumulation of phlegm-damp is most often associated with the spleen and kidney. When spleen and kidney yang become deficient, phlegm will form and fluids will gather. When the function of transportation and transformation is disturbed, the circulation of water and essence becomes inhibited. Phlegm-damp is a very sticky and persistent yin pathogen that can easily obstruct qi circulation, or even damage yang qi in some cases. When phlegm-damp inhibits the qi dynamic and obstructs the penetrating and conception vessels, irregular menstruation and infertility may result.

The excess consumption of fatty meats, refined grains, and strong flavors will damage the spleen and stomach. When the functions of transportation and transformation become affected, phlegm-damp accumulates internally. External cold-damp invading the spleen and stomach can also result in the formation of phlegm-damp. When phlegm-damp flows downward to the lower burner causing congestion of the uterus and stagnation of the penetrating and conception vessels, infertility may result.

(5) Damp-heat

Damp-heat patterns appear when spleen deficiency engenders dampness which later transforms into heat. The excess consumption of fatty and sweet foods often leads to this condition. Liver-spleen disharmony may also be involved. Environmental factors such as exposure to rain, heat, and humidity can also contribute to this pattern. Internal damp-heat may flow to the lower burner and affect the uterus and its vessels, or external dampness may invade the penetrating, conception, and girdling vessels directly. The penetrating and girdling vessels may fail to control blood, and the penetrating and conception vessels can become obstructed. Under these conditions, conception also becomes difficult.

(6) Blood Stasis

Patterns of blood stasis may result from inhibition of the qi dynamic or other internal factors. Blood also becomes static when not properly eliminated during menstruation or the postpartum period. Congealing cold or heat depression may also result in stasis obstruction. Blood stasis and qi stagnation can lead to concretions, conglomerations, accumulations, and gatherings. When the free flow of qi and blood becomes affected, menstruation becomes irregular and conception becomes difficult. Furthermore, when qi becomes deficient, the movement of blood is also inhibited. This may lead to static blood or other pathogens lodging in the uterine gate.

The etiology and pathomechanism of female infertility can be considered from the perspective of six individual mechanisms. Although a single cause may be identified, clinical presentations often involve more complex presentations.

CHINESE MEDICAL TREATMENT

The general principles for treatment include supplementing kidney qi, increasing essence-blood, nourishing the penetrating and conception vessels, and regulating menstruation. The proper treatment method must be selected in accordance with the specific clinical presentation. A number of approaches are possible, depending on the predominance of deficiency or excess, deficiencies of yin and yang, or patterns of phlegm-damp, blood stasis, or liver constraint. Complex patterns manifesting with signs and symptoms of both excess and deficiency are also quite common. In many cases, surgical intervention or other biomedical approaches may be required. Psychological and lifestyle counseling is also quite helpful in most cases.

Pattern Differentiation and Treatment

Infertility can result from a number of causative factors. However, the accurate differentiation of deficiency and excess patterns remains primary, regardless of the cause. Deficiency presentations generally include patterns involving the kidney, spleen, and blood. Typical excess patterns include liver constraint, damp-heat, phlegm-damp and blood stasis.

To distinguish more complex patterns of deficiency and excess, all symptoms and signs associated with menstruation must be carefully considered, along with the patient's congenital constitution and age of menarche.

Patterns of kidney deficiency are often associated with constitutional insufficiency. Manifestations include delayed menarche, thin clear vaginal discharge, aching lumbus, cold in the lower abdomen, and delayed menstruation with scant thin and dark menses.

Patterns of blood deficiency can manifest with emaciation and delayed menstruation with scant thin and pale menses.

Patterns of spleen deficiency with phlegm-damp often manifest with a thick sticky and profuse vaginal discharge, obesity, and a bright white facial complexion.

Patterns of blood stasis can manifest with severe lesser abdominal or lumbosacral pain that refuses pressure, appearing before or during menstruation. The pain is generally relieved after the passing of clotted menses. Menstruation is usually delayed, with menses appearing scant or profuse and dark purple with clots.

Patterns of liver constraint often manifest with dysmenorrhea, vexation, irascibility, and mental depression. Menstruation may be delayed, with menses appearing profuse or scant.

Patterns of damp-heat can manifest with lower abdominal discomfort and profuse, thick or yellow leukorrhea with a foul odor.

(1) Kidney Deficiency

A. Kidney yang deficiency

【Syndrome Characteristics】

Infertility with amenorrhea or delayed menstruation with scant or pale menses. Other signs and symptoms include frigidity, cold sagging in the lower abdomen, soreness of lumbar region, a lusterless complexion, cold limbs, and long voidings of clear urine or nocturia. The tongue appears pale. Pulses are deep and slow.

【Treatment Principle】

Warm the kidney and uterus and tonify the penetrating vessel.

【Commonly Used Medicinals】

To tonify the kidney and replenish essence and marrow, select *shú dì huáng* (Radix Rehmanniae Praeparata), *lù jiǎo shuāng* (Cornu Cervi Degelatinatum), and *zǐ hé chē* (Placenta Hominis).

To warm and tonify kidney yang, select *tù sī zǐ* (Semen Cuscutae), *xiān líng pí* (Herba Epimedii), *ròu cōng róng* (Herba Cistanches), and *bā jǐ tiān* (Radix Morindae Officinalis).

【Representative Formula】

Combine *Yòu Guī Wán* (Right-Restoring Pill) with *Èr Xiān Tāng* (Two Immortals Decoction).

【Ingredients】

熟附子	*shú fù zǐ*	6g	Radix Aconiti Lateralis Praeparata
肉桂	*ròu guì*	0.5g	Cortex Cinnamomi
熟地黄	*shú dì huáng*	15g	Radix Rehmanniae Praeparata
当归	*dāng guī*	9g	Radix Angelicae Sinensis
枸杞子	*gǒu qǐ zǐ*	15g	Fructus Lycii
鹿角霜	*lù jiǎo shuāng*	15g	Cornu Cervi Degelatinatum
巴戟天	*bā jǐ tiān*	9g	Radix Morindae Officinalis
补骨脂	*bǔ gǔ zhī*	12g	Fructus Psoraleae
肉苁蓉	*ròu cōng róng*	15g	Herba Cistanches
山药	*shān yào*	15g	Rhizoma Dioscoreae
益智仁	*yì zhì rén*	9g	Fructus Alpiniae Oxyphyllae
仙茅	*xiān máo*	15g	Rhizoma Curculiginis
仙灵脾	*xiān líng pí*	15g	Herba Epimedii

Decoct in 500 ml water until 100 ml remains. Take 50 ml warm, twice daily.

【Formula Analysis】

Shú fù zǐ (Radix Aconiti Lateralis Praeparata) and *ròu guì* (Cortex Cinnamomi) warm the kidney and uterus. *Shú dì huáng* (Radix Rehmanniae Praeparata), *dāng guī* (Radix Angelicae Sinensis) and *gǒu qǐ zǐ* (Fructus Lycii) nourish the kidney and blood.

Lù jiǎo shuāng (Cornu Cervi Degelatinatum), *bǔ gǔ zhī* (Fructus Psoraleae), *ròu cōng róng* (Herba Cistanches), *xiān máo* (Rhizoma Curculiginis), *xiān líng pí* (Herba Epimedii) and *bā jǐ tiān* (Radix Morindae Officinalis) warm the kidney and invigorate yang.

Shān yào (Rhizoma Dioscoreae) and *yì zhì rén* (Fructus Alpiniae Oxyphyllae) fortify the spleen and obtain the essence.

These two formulas combined act to warm the kidney and uterus, assist yang, and benefit the penetrating and conception vessels.

【Modifications】

➢ With spleen deficiency, add *dǎng shēn* (Radix Codonopsis), *bái zhú* (Rhizoma Atractylodis Macrocephalae), *zhì gān cǎo* (Radix et Rhizoma Glycyrrhizae Praeparata cum Melle), and *huáng qí* (Radix Astragali) to fortify the spleen and supplement qi.

➢ With kidney deficiency with phlegm-damp, add *dǎn nán xīng* (Arisaema cum Bile), *cāng zhú* (Rhizoma Atractylodis), and *chén pí* (Pericarpium Citri Reticulatae) to dry dampness and transform phlegm.

B. Kidney yin deficiency

【Syndrome Characteristics】

Infertility with early menstruation, delayed menstruation, or amenorrhea. Menses appear scant and red without clots. Other signs include dizziness, blurred vision, and vexing heat in the five hearts. The tongue appears red with scant coating. Pulses are thready.

【Treatment Principle】

Enrich the kidney, nourish essence, and benefit the penetrating vessel.

【Commonly Used Medicinals】

To nourish the liver and kidney, select *nǚ zhēn zǐ* (Fructus Ligustri Lucidi), *hàn lián cǎo* (Herba Ecliptae), and *gǒu qǐ zǐ* (Fructus Lycii).

To nourish yin and moisten dryness, select *shí hú* (Caulis Dendrobii) and *yù zhú* (Rhizoma Polygonati Odorati).

To enrich the kidney, replenish essence, tonify qi and strengthen the spleen, select *huáng jīng* (Rhizoma Polygonati).

To nourish yin and subdue yang, select *guī jiǎ* (Carapax et Plastrum Testudinis) and *biē jiǎ* (Carapax Trionycis).

【Representative Formula】

Zuǒ Guī Wán (左归丸) modified with *Èr Zhì Wán* (二至丸).

【Ingredients】

熟地黄	*shú dì huáng*	30g	Radix Rehmanniae Praeparata
枸杞	*gǒu qǐ*	15g	Fructus Lycii
山茱萸	*shān zhū yú*	15g	Fructus Corni
鹿胶	*lù jiāo*	15g	Colla Cornus Cervi
龟胶	*guī jiāo*	15g	Colla Carapax et Plastrum Testudinis
菟丝子	*tù sī zǐ*	15g	Semen Cuscutae
紫河车	*zǐ hé chē*	15g	Placenta Hominis
山药	*shān yào*	15g	Rhizoma Dioscoreae
女贞子	*nǚ zhēn zǐ*	20g	Fructus Ligustri Lucidi
旱莲草	*hàn lián cǎo*	15g	Herba Ecliptae

Decoct in 500 ml water until 100 ml remains. Take 50 ml warm, twice daily.

【Formula Analysis】

Shú dì huáng (Radix Rehmanniae Praeparata) enriches the kidney and nourishes yin. *Gǒu qǐ zǐ* (Fructus Lycii) benefits the essence. *shān zhū yú* (Fructus Corni) obtains the essence. *Lù jiāo* (Colla Cornus Cervi) and *guī jiāo* (Colla Carapax et Plastrum Testudinis) are medicinals with an affinity to flesh and blood. *Lù jiāo* (Colla Cornus Cervi) more strongly tonifies yang, while *guī jiāo* (Colla Carapax et Plastrum Testudinis) is superior for nourishing yin. Their combining can replenish essence and marrow while also interacting with the conception and governing vessels. This approach acts to tonify yin by "seeking yin within yang". *Tù sī zǐ* (Semen Cuscutae) tonifies both yin and yang. *Zǐ hé chē* (Placenta Hominis) tonifies both essence and blood. *Shān yào* (Rhizoma Dioscoreae) nourishes the spleen and stomach.

Èr Zhì Wán (Double Supreme Pill) tonifies the liver and kidney and nourishes yin blood. These two formulas combined act to regulate menstruation and promote conception by nourishing the kidney, fostering yin, and subduing yang.

【Modifications】

➢ With kidney yin deficiency with heat, add *zhī mǔ* (Rhizoma Anemarrhenae), *huáng bǎi* (Cortex Phellodendri Chinensis) and *guī jiǎ* (Carapax et Plastrum Testudinis) to enrich yin and clear heat.

➢ With liver-kidney yin depletion, add *yú zhú* (Rhizoma Polygonati Odorati), *shā shēn* (Radix Adenophorae) and *sāng shèn zǐ* (Fructus Mori) to enrich the liver and kidney.

➢ With kidney yin and kidney yang dual deficiency, add *shú fù zǐ* (Radix Aconiti Lateralis Praeparata), *bā jǐ tiān* (Radix Morindae Officinalis), *bǔ gǔ zhī* (Fructus Psoraleae), and *yì zhì rén* (Fructus Alpiniae Oxyphyllae) to tonify both yin and yang.

(2) Qi and Blood Deficiency

【Syndrome Characteristics】

Infertility with amenorrhea or delayed menstruation with scant clear menses. Other signs include dizziness, blurred vision, palpitations, fearful throbbing, and lusterless skin with a bright white or withered-yellow complexion. The tongue appears pale with thin coating. Pulses are thready and weak.

【Treatment Principle】

Supplement qi, nourish blood, and regulate menstruation.

【Commonly Used Medicinals】

Select *dǎng shēn* (Radix Codonopsis), *huáng qí* (Radix Astragali), *dà zǎo* (Fructus Jujubae), *tài zǐ shēn* (Radix Pseudostellariae), *shān yào* (Rhizoma

Dioscoreae), *bái zhú* (Rhizoma Atractylodis Macrocephalae) and *huáng jīng* (Rhizoma Polygonati).

To tonify blood, select *shú dì huáng* (Radix Rehmanniae Praeparata), *dāng guī* (Radix Angelicae Sinensis), *shǒu wū* (Radix Polygoni Multiflori), and *bái sháo* (Radix Paeoniae Alba).

To tonify and invigorate blood, select *chuān xiōng* (Rhizoma Chuanxiong) and *jī xuè téng* (Caulis Spatholobi).

【Representative Formula】

Modified *Yù Lín Zhū* (毓麟珠).

【Ingredients】

当归	*dāng guī*	9g	Radix Angelicae Sinensis
川芎	*chuān xiōng*	6g	Rhizoma Chuanxiong
熟地黄	*shú dì huáng*	30g	Radix Rehmanniae Praeparata
白芍	*bái sháo*	12g	Radix Paeoniae Alba
党参	*dǎng shēn*	20g	Radix Codonopsis
白术	*bái zhú*	12g	Rhizoma Atractylodis Macrocephalae
茯苓	*fú líng*	15g	Poria
炙甘草	*zhì gān cǎo*	6g	Radix et Rhizoma Glycyrrhizae Praeparata cum Melle
鹿角霜	*lù jiǎo shuāng*	15g	Cornu Cervi Degelatinatum
菟丝子	*tù sī zǐ*	15g	Semen Cuscutae
杜仲	*dù zhòng*	12g	Cortex Eucommiae
何首乌	*hé shǒu wū*	20g	Radix Polygoni Multiflori
鸡血藤	*jī xuè téng*	30g	Caulis Spatholobi
黄精	*huáng jīng*	15g	Rhizoma Polygonati

Decoct in 500 ml water until 100 ml remains. Take 50 ml warm, twice daily.

【Formula Analysis】

Tù sī zǐ (Semen Cuscutae), *lù jiǎo shuāng* (Cornu Cervi Degelatinatum) and *dù zhòng* (Cortex Eucommiae) tonify the kidney, strengthen the lumbus and knees, and replenish essence and marrow.

Sì Jūn Zǐ Tāng (四君子汤) tonifies qi, where *Sì Wù Tāng* (四物汤) is added to nourish blood. *Huáng jīng* (Rhizoma Polygonati) nourishes the kidney and spleen. *Jī xuè téng* (Caulis Spatholobi) invigorates blood and tonifies without cloying.

These medicinals act in combination to nourish the kidney qi and engender marrow, while also tonifying the spleen qi to transform blood. Medicinals that regulate and harmonize the blood and vessels are also added here. When essence and blood are made sufficient and the penetrating and conception vessels are well-nourished, the chance of conception is also greatly increased.

【Modifications】

➤ With poor sleep, add *yè jiāo téng* (Caulis Polygoni Multiflori) and *suān zǎo rén* (Semen Ziziphi Spinosae) to nourish the heart and quiet the spirit.

➤ With poor stomach intake, remove *shú dì huáng* (Radix Rehmanniae Praeparata). Add *chūn shā rén* (Fructus Amomi) and *shān yào* (Rhizoma Dioscoreae) to harmonize the stomach and fortify the spleen.

(3) Binding Constraint of Liver Qi

【Syndrome Characteristics】

Infertility and irregular menstruation with dark clotted menses, premenstrual breast distention, depression, vexation, and irascibility. The tongue appears dusky pale with a thin white coating. Pulses are wiry.

【Treatment Principle】

Course the liver, resolve constraint, and regulate the penetrating vessel.

【Commonly Used Medicinals】

To course the liver and regulate qi, select *chái hú* (Radix Bupleuri), *yù jīn* (Radix Curcumae), *qīng pí* (Pericarpium Citri Reticulatae Viride), *zhǐ qiào* (Fructus Aurantii), *sù xīn huā* (Flos Jasmini Officinalis), and *fó shǒu piàn* (Fructus Citri Sarcodactylis).

To nourish yin and emolliate the liver, select *bái sháo* (Radix Paeoniae Alba).

To tonify liver and kidney yin, select *shān zhū yú* (Fructus Corni), *nǚ zhēn zǐ* (Fructus Ligustri Lucidi), *hàn lián cǎo* (Herba Ecliptae), *sāng shèn zǐ* (Fructus Mori), *gǒu qǐ zǐ* (Fructus Lycii), and *sāng jì shēng* (Herba Taxilli).

【Representative Formula】

Modified *Kāi Yù Zhòng Yù Tāng* (开郁种玉汤).

【Ingredients】

当归	*dāng guī*	12g	Radix Angelicae Sinensis
白芍	*bái sháo*	15g	Radix Paeoniae Alba
香附	*xiāng fù*	9g	Rhizoma Cyperi
牡丹皮	*mǔ dān pí*	12g	Cortex Moutan
白术	*bái zhú*	9g	Rhizoma Atractylodis Macrocephalae
茯苓	*fú líng*	9g	Poria
花粉	*huā fěn*	15g	Radix Trichosanthis

Decoct in 500 ml of water until 100 ml remains. Take warm, twice daily.

【Formula Analysis】

Dāng guī (Radix Angelicae Sinensis) and *bái sháo* (Radix Paeoniae Alba) nourish blood and emolliate the liver. *Xiāng fù* (Rhizoma Cyperi) regulates qi and moves stagnation to resolve liver constraint. *Mǔ dān pí* (Cortex Moutan) cools and invigorates blood. *Bái zhú* (Rhizoma Atractylodis Macrocephalae) and *fú líng* (Poria) fortify the spleen and harmonize the stomach to enrich the source of transformation. *Huā fěn* (Radix Trichosanthis) benefits the stomach and engenders fluids. This main action of this formula is to course the liver, regulate the spleen, and nourish blood.

【Modifications】

➢ With liver constraint transforming into fire, add *zhī zǐ* (Fructus

Gardeniae) and *huáng bǎi* (Cortex Phellodendri Chinensis) to clear heat.

➤ For severe premenstrual breast distention and pain or with galactorrhea, add *chǎo mài yá* (dry-fried Fructus Hordei Germinatus), *zhǐ qiào* (Fructus Aurantii), *māo zhuǎ cǎo* (Radix Ranunculi Ternati), and *quán guā lóu* (Fructus Trichosanthis) to move qi and free the collaterals.

➤ For breast distention with lumps, add *wáng bù liú xíng* (Semen Vaccariae), *lù lù tōng* (Fructus Liquidambaris), and *jú hé* (Semen Citri Reticulatae) to break qi and move stagnation.

➤ For distending breast pain with severe heat, add *chǎo huáng lián* (fried Rhizoma Coptidis) and *pú gōng yīng* (Herba Taraxaci) to clear heat and drain fire.

➤ For profuse dreaming and poor sleep, add *chǎo zǎo rén* (dry-fried Semen Ziziphi Spinosae Frictum) and *yè jiāo téng* (Caulis Polygoni Multiflori) to quiet the heart and spirit.

(4) Blood Stasis

A. Qi stagnation and blood stasis

【Syndrome Characteristics】

Infertility with irregular menstruation and breast distention, or dysmenorrhea with abdominal pain that is relieved after the passing of dark clotted menses, or longstanding concretions and conglomerations. The tongue appears dusky with purple macules at the margins. Pulses are wiry.

【Treatment Principle】

Regulate qi, invigorate blood, and dispel stasis.

【Commonly Used Medicinals】

To course the liver and regulate qi, select *mù xiāng* (Radix Aucklandiae), *xiāng fù* (Rhizoma Cyperi), and *yù jīn* (Radix Curcumae). To course the liver and drain heat, select *chuān liàn zǐ* (Fructus Toosendan). To move qi and disperse accumulation, select *chuān pò* (Cortex Magnoliae Officinalis) and *zhǐ shí* (Fructus Aurantii Immaturus). To invigorate blood and dispel stasis, select *dāng guī* (Radix Angelicae Sinensis), *chuān xiōng* (Rhizoma Chuanxiong), *hóng huā* (Flos Carthami), and *dān shēn* (Radix et Rhizoma Salviae Miltiorrhizae).

【Representative Formula】

Modified *Gé Xià Zhú Yū Tāng* (膈下逐瘀汤).

【Ingredients】

当归	*dāng guī*	9g	Radix Angelicae Sinensis
川芎	*chuān xiōng*	6g	Rhizoma Chuanxiong
赤芍	*chì sháo*	9g	Radix Paeoniae Rubra
桃仁	*táo rén*	6g	Semen Persicae
红花	*hóng huā*	6g	Flos Carthami
丹参	*dān shēn*	15g	Radix et Rhizoma Salviae Miltiorrhizae
牡丹皮	*mǔ dān pí*	9g	Cortex Moutan
香附	*xiāng fù*	9g	Rhizoma Cyperi
枳壳	*zhǐ qiào*	12g	Fructus Aurantii
郁金	*yù jīn*	9g	Radix Curcumae

Decoct in 500 ml water until 100 ml remains. Take 50 ml warm, twice daily.

【Formula Analysis】

Dāng guī (Radix Angelicae Sinensis) acts to invigorate blood. *Chuān xiōng* (Rhizoma Chuanxiong) treats the qi within the blood. *Hóng huā* (Flos Carthami), *táo rén* (Semen Persicae), *chì sháo* (Radix Paeoniae Rubra), *mǔ dān pí* (Cortex Moutan) and *dān shēn* (Radix et Rhizoma Salviae Miltiorrhizae) invigorate blood and dispel stasis. *Xiāng fù* (Rhizoma Cyperi), *zhǐ qiào* (Fructus Aurantii) and *yù jīn* (Radix Curcumae) act to course the liver and regulate qi. This main action of this formula is to invigorate blood and dispel stasis.

【Modifications】

For severe qi stagnation, add *sù xīn huā* (Flos Jasmini Officinalis), *shā rén* (Fructus Amomi) and *hòu pò* (Cortex Magnoliae Officinalis) to promote the movement of qi.

B. Congealing cold and blood stasis

【Syndrome Characteristics】

Infertility with painful menstruation, light or dark menses with clots, lower abdominal cold, cold limbs, and a bright white complexion. The tongue appears dusky and pale. Pulses are sunken and rough.

【Treatment Principle】

Warm the channels, dissipate cold, and dispel stasis.

【Commonly Used Medicinals】

To tonify kidney fire and assist yang, select *fù zǐ* (Radix Aconiti Lateralis Praeparata) and *ròu guì* (Cortex Cinnamomi). To warm the middle and dissipate cold, select *gān jiāng* (Rhizoma Zingiberis) and *xiǎo huí xiāng* (Fructus Foeniculi). To invigorate blood and dispel stasis, select *dāng guī* (Radix Angelicae Sinensis), *chuān xiōng* (Rhizoma Chuanxiong), *táo rén* (Semen Persicae), and *hóng huā* (Flos Carthami).

【Representative Formula】

Modified *Shào Fù Zhú Yū Tāng* (少腹逐瘀汤).

【Ingredients】

小茴香	xiǎo huí xiāng	3g	Fructus Foeniculi
干姜	gān jiāng	3g	Rhizoma Zingiberis
延胡索	yán hú suǒ	6g	Rhizoma Corydalis
当归	dāng guī	9g	Radix Angelicae Sinensis
川芎	chuān xiōng	3g	Rhizoma Chuanxiong
肉桂	ròu guì	1g	Cortex Cinnamomi
赤芍	chì sháo	9g	Radix Paeoniae Rubra
蒲黄	pú huáng	6g	Pollen Typhae
五灵脂	wǔ líng zhī	6g	Faeces Togopteri
吴茱萸	wú zhū yú	3g	Fructus Evodiae
艾叶	ài yè	6g	Folium Artemisiae Argyi

Decoct in 500 ml water until 100 ml remains. Take 50 ml warm, twice daily.

【**Formula Analysis**】

Ròu guì (Cortex Cinnamomi), *gān jiāng* (Rhizoma Zingiberis) and *xiǎo huí xiāng* (Fructus Foeniculi) warm the channels and dissipate cold. *Yán hú suǒ* (Rhizoma Corydalis), *wǔ líng zhī* (Faeces Togopteri) and *pú huáng* (Pollen Typhae) dispel stasis and relieve pain. *Dāng guī* (Radix Angelicae Sinensis), *chuān xiōng* (Rhizoma Chuanxiong) and *chì sháo* (Radix Paeoniae Rubra) invigorate blood. *Wú zhū yú* (Fructus Evodiae) and *ài yè* (Folium Artemisiae Argyi) warm the uterus and dissipate cold. The main action of this formula is to warm the channels, dissipate cold, dispel stasis, and invigorate blood.

【**Modifications**】

➢ With severe abdominal pain, add *shuǐ zhì* (Hirudo) and *é zhú* (Rhizoma Curcumae) to dispel stasis and relieve pain.

➢ With painful menstruation, add *guǎng mù xiāng* (Radix Aucklandiae) 9g and *tái wū* (Radix Linderae) 9g to move qi and relieve pain.

C. Binding of stasis and heat

【**Syndrome Characteristics**】

Infertility and fixed lower abdominal pain, profuse yellow leukorrhea, intermittent low-grade fever, dry mouth with a bitter taste, and bound stool. The tongue appears dusky red with a yellow coating. Pulses are slightly rapid and wiry.

【**Treatment Principle**】

Invigorate blood, dispel stasis, and clear the penetrating vessel.

【**Commonly Used Medicinals**】

To clear heat, resolve toxin and disinhibit dampness, select *pú gōng yīng* (Herba Taraxaci), *yú xīng cǎo* (Herba Houttuyniae), *shé shé cǎo* (Herba Hedyotis), *yín huā* (Flos Lonicerae Japonicae), and *bài jiàng cǎo* (Herba Patriniae).

To clear heat and dry dampness, select *huáng qín* (Radix Scutellariae) and *huáng lián* (Rhizoma Coptidis). To clear heat and free the bowels, select *dà huáng* (Radix et Rhizoma Rhei). To clear the liver and drain fire, select *shān zhī zǐ* (Fructus Gardeniae) and *mǔ dān pí* (Cortex Moutan).

To move qi and invigorate blood, select *yù jīn* (Radix Curcumae). To dispel stasis and invigorate blood, select *dān shēn* (Radix et Rhizoma Salviae Miltiorrhizae), *táo rén* (Semen Persicae), *hóng huā* (Flos Carthami), *xuè jié* (Sanguis Draconis), *dāng guī* (Radix Angelicae Sinensis), and *jī xuè téng* (Caulis Spatholobi).

【Representative Formula】

Modified *Jiě Dú Huó Xuè Tāng* (解毒活血汤).

【Ingredients】

连翘	*lián qiào*	12g	Fructus Forsythiae
葛根	*gě gēn*	15g	Radix Puerariae Lobatae
忍冬藤	*rěn dōng téng*	20g	Caulis Lonicerae Japonicae
枳壳	*zhǐ qiào*	15g	Fructus Aurantii
柴胡	*chái hú*	9g	Radix Bupleuri
当归	*dāng guī*	9g	Radix Angelicae Sinensis
赤芍	*chì sháo*	9g	Radix Paeoniae Rubra
桃仁	*táo rén*	9g	Semen Persicae
红花	*hóng huā*	9g	Flos Carthami
牡丹皮	*mǔ dān pí*	12g	Cortex Moutan
地榆	*dì yú*	15g	Radix Sanguisorbae
大黄	*dà huáng*	9g	Radix et Rhizoma Rhei
蒲公英	*pú gōng yīng*	15g	Herba Taraxaci

Decoct in 500 ml water until 100 ml remains. Take 50 ml warm, twice daily.

【Formula Analysis】

Lián qiào (Fructus Forsythiae), *gě gēn* (Radix Puerariae Lobatae), *rěn dōng téng* (Caulis Lonicerae Japonicae) and *pú gōng yīng* (Herba Taraxaci) clear heat and course the collaterals. *Zhǐ qiào* (Fructus Aurantii) regulates qi and moves stagnation. *Chái hú* (Radix Bupleuri) courses the liver and resolves constraint. *Dāng guī* (Radix Angelicae Sinensis), *chì sháo* (Radix

Paeoniae Rubra), *táo rén* (Semen Persicae), and *hóng huā* (Flos Carthami) invigorate blood and dispel stasis. *Mǔ dān pí* (Cortex Moutan) and *dì yú* (Radix Sanguisorbae) cool the blood. *Dà huáng* (Radix et Rhizoma Rhei) frees the bowels and drains heat. This main action of this formula is to clear heat, cool and invigorate blood, and dispel stasis.

【Modifications】

With continuous low-grade fever, add *dì gǔ pí* (Cortex Lycii), *bái wēi* (Radix et Rhizoma Cynanchi Atrati), *shí hú* (Caulis Dendrobii) and *biē jiǎ* (Carapax Trionycis) to clear deficiency heat.

D. Qi deficiency with blood stasis

【Syndrome Characteristics】

Infertility with profuse menses and clots, sagging lower abdominal pain, lassitude of the spirit, weak limbs, and a bright white or lusterless complexion. The tongue appears dusky and pale with white coating. Pulses are thready and weak.

【Treatment Principle】

Tonify qi and blood and dispel stasis.

【Commonly Used Medicinals】

To tonify qi, select *dǎng shēn* (Radix Codonopsis), *běi qí* (Radix Astragali Septentrionalis), *bái zhú* (Rhizoma Atractylodis Macrocephalae), and *huái shān yào* (Rhizoma Dioscoreae). To invigorate blood, select *dāng guī* (Radix Angelicae Sinensis) and *chuān xiōng* (Rhizoma Chuanxiong).

【Representative Formula】

Modified *Dāng Guī Bǔ Xuè Tāng* (当归补血汤).

【Ingredients】

黄芪	*huáng qí*	30g	Radix Astragali
当归	*dāng guī*	9g	Radix Angelicae Sinensis
川芎	*chuān xiōng*	9g	Rhizoma Chuanxiong
党参	*dǎng shēn*	15g	Radix Codonopsis
熟地黄	*shú dì huáng*	20g	Radix Rehmanniae Praeparata

| 丹参 | dān shēn | 20g | Radix et Rhizoma Salviae Miltiorrhizae |
| 鸡血藤 | jī xuè téng | 20g | Caulis Spatholobi |

Decoct in 500 ml water until 100 ml remains. Take 50 ml warm, twice daily.

【Formula Analysis】

"Although blood is tangible, it cannot generate itself. The source of its engenderment is qi, which is intangible."

In this formula, large doses of *dǎng shēn* (Radix Codonopsis) and *huáng qí* (Radix Astragali) are selected to strongly tonify the qi of the spleen and lung. This approach aims to promote the source of qi and blood engendering and transformation.

Dāng guī (Radix Angelicae Sinensis) *chuān xiōng* (Rhizoma Chuanxiong) and *jī xuè téng* (Caulis Spatholobi) act together to nourish and invigorate blood and harmonize the nutrient aspect. *Dān shēn* (Radix et Rhizoma Salviae Miltiorrhizae) invigorates blood and dispels stasis. This main action of this formula is to benefit qi and invigorate blood.

【Modifications】

➢ With spleen deficiency, add *bái zhú* (Rhizoma Atractylodis Macrocephalae) 9g, *huái shān yào* (Rhizoma Dioscoreae) 15g, *zhì gān cǎo* (Radix et Rhizoma Glycyrrhizae Praeparata cum Melle) 6g and *dà zǎo* (Fructus Jujubae) 6g to fortify the spleen, boost qi, and engender blood.

➢ With kidney deficiency and lower burner deficiency cold, add *xiān máo* (Rhizoma Curculiginis) 12g, *xiān líng pí* (Herba Epimedii) 15g, *bǔ gǔ zhī* (Fructus Psoraleae) 9g, of *ròu guì* (Cortex Cinnamomi) 10g, *lù jiǎo jiāo* (Colla Cornus Cervi) 6g, and *zǐ hé chē* (Placenta Hominis) 9g to warm the kidney and assist yang.

➢ With severe blood deficiency, add 20g of *shǒu wū* (Radix Polygoni Multiflori) and *jī xuè téng* (Caulis Spatholobi) to tonify blood and boost essence.

(5) Damp-heat Brewing and Binding

【Syndrome Characteristics】

Infertility with profuse, sticky yellow putrid leukorrhea, and genital itching. The tongue appears red with a thick slimy yellow coating. Pulses are soggy.

【Treatment Principle】

Eliminate dampness, resolve toxin, and clear the penetrating vessel.

【Commonly Used Medicinals】

To clear heat and disinhibit dampness, select *pú gōng yīng* (Herba Taraxaci), *yú xīng cǎo* (Herba Houttuyniae), *shé shé cǎo* (Herba Hedyotis), *yín huā* (Flos Lonicerae Japonicae), and *bài jiàng cǎo* (Herba Patriniae).

To clear heat and dry dampness, select *huáng qín* (Radix Scutellariae) and *huáng lián* (Rhizoma Coptidis). To clear heat and free the bowels, select *dà huáng* (Radix et Rhizoma Rhei).

To clear the liver, cool the blood and resolve toxin, select *shān zhī zǐ* (Fructus Gardeniae).

【Representative Formula】

Modified *Wǔ Wèi Xiāo Dú Yǐn* (五味消毒饮).

【Ingredients】

蒲公英	*pú gōng yīng*	15g	Herba Taraxaci
金银花	*jīn yín huā*	15g	Flos Lonicerae Japonicae
野菊花	*yě jú huā*	12g	Flos Chrysanthemi Indici
紫花地丁	*zǐ huā dì dīng*	12g	Herba Violae
天葵	*tiān kuí*	9g	Radix Semiaquilegiae
土茯苓	*tǔ fú líng*	25g	Rhizoma Smilacis Glabrae
薏苡仁	*yì yǐ rén*	15g	Semen Coicis

Decoct in 500 ml water until 100 ml remains. Take 50 ml warm, twice daily.

【Formula Analysis】

Pú gōng yīng (Herba Taraxaci), *yín huā* (Flos Lonicerae Japonicae), *yě jú huā* (Flos Chrysanthemi Indici) and *zǐ huā dì dīng* (Herba Violae) clear heat and resolve toxin. *Tiān kuí* (Radix Semiaquilegiae), *tǔ fú líng* (Rhizoma Smilacis Glabrae) and *yì yǐ rén* (Semen Coicis) act together to disinhibit water and eliminate dampness while also clearing heat and resolving toxin.

【Modifications】

➤ With predominant damp, add *mián yīn chén* (Herba Artemisiae Scopariae) 15g and *pèi lán* (Herba Eupatorii) 9g to transform dampness.

➤ With severe heat, add *mǔ dān pí* (Cortex Moutan) 15g, *yú xīng cǎo* (Herba Houttuyniae) 20g, *huáng bǎi* (Cortex Phellodendri Chinensis) 10g, and *shé shé cǎo* (Herba Hedyotis) 20g.

(6) Phlegm-damp

【Syndrome Characteristics】

Infertility with irregular menstruation, profuse sticky white leukorhea, obesity, copious phlegm, chest oppression and abdominal distention, lassitude, and a bright white complexion. The tongue appears pale with slimy white coating. Pulses are slippery.

【Treatment Principle】

Fortify the spleen, dry dampness, and resolve phlegm.

【Commonly Used Medicinals】

To dry dampness and resolve phlegm, select *fǎ xià* (Rhizoma Pinelliae Praeparatum), *dǎn nán xīng* (Arisaema cum Bile) and *cāng zhú* (Rhizoma Atractylodis).

To fortify the spleen and eliminate dampness, select *fú líng* (Poria) and *bái zhú* (Rhizoma Atractylodis Macrocephalae).

To move qi, dry dampness and harmonize the stomach, select *hòu pò* (Cortex Magnoliae Officinalis), *chén pí* (Pericarpium Citri Reticulatae) and *shí chāng pú* (Rhizoma Acori Tatarinowii).

【Representative Formula】

Cāng Fù Dǎo Tán Wán (苍附导痰丸).

【Ingredients】

茯苓	fú líng	15g	Poria
半夏	bàn xià	10g	Rhizoma Pinelliae
陈皮	chén pí	10g	Pericarpium Citri Reticulatae
甘草	gān cǎo	6g	Radix et Rhizoma Glycyrrhizae
苍术	cāng zhú	12g	Rhizoma Atractylodis
制南星	zhì nán xīng	10g	Arisaema cum Bile
香附	xiāng fù	10g	Rhizoma Cyperi
枳壳	zhǐ qiào	15g	Fructus Aurantii
生姜	shēng jiāng	3 pieces	Rhizoma Zingiberis Recens
神曲	shén qū	15g	Massa Medicata Fermentata

Decoct in 500 ml water until 100 ml remains. Take 50 ml warm, twice daily.

【Formula Analysis】

Bàn xià (Rhizoma Pinelliae), *fú líng* (Poria), *chén pí* (Pericarpium Citri Reticulatae), *shēng jiāng* (Rhizoma Zingiberis Recens) and *gān cǎo* (Radix et Rhizoma Glycyrrhizae) are main ingredients in the formula *Èr Chén Tāng* (二陈汤), which acts to eliminate dampness and resolve phlegm. *Cāng zhú* (Rhizoma Atractylodis), *fú líng* (Poria) and *shí chāng pú* (Rhizoma Acori Tatarinowii) fortify the spleen, eliminate dampness, and disperse accumulation. *Xiāng fù* (Rhizoma Cyperi) and *zhǐ qiào* (Fructus Aurantii) act together to regulate qi and eliminate dampness.

【Modifications】

With severe nausea, vomiting, or fullness in the chest, add *hòu pò* (Cortex Magnoliae Officinalis) 10g, *zhǐ qiào* (Fructus Aurantii) 12g, and *zhú rú* (Caulis Bambusae in Taenia) 9g to loosen the center, downbear counterflow, and resolve phlegm.

With severe palpitation, add *yuǎn zhì* (Radix Polygalae) to resolve phlegm and quiet the heart and spirit.

With concretions of phlegm and static blood binding together, add *kūn bù* (Thallus Laminariae), *hǎi zǎo* (Sargassum), *sān léng* (Rhizoma

Sparganii) and *é zhú* (Rhizoma Curcumae) to soften hardness, resolve phlegm, and disperse concretions.

Additional Treatment Modalities

1. CHINESE PATENT MEDICINE

(1) *Nǚ Bǎo Jiāo Náng* (女宝胶囊)

Indicated for irregular menstruation, dysmenorrhea, and infertility due to kidney deficiency and blood stasis. This formula acts to regulate menstruation, stanch bleeding, warm the uterus, check vaginal discharge, expel stasis, and engender the new.

Take 4 pills, 3 times daily.

(2) *Zuǒ Guī Wán* (左归丸)

Indicated for infertility due to liver-kidney yin deficiency. This formula acts to enrich yin, tonify the kidney, and foster yin to nourish yang.

Take 1 pill, twice daily.

(3) *Hé Chē Dà Zào Wán* (河车大造丸)

Indicated for infertility due to insufficiency of the liver and kidney with depletion of essence and blood. This formula acts to tonify the kidney, enrich yin, clear heat, moisten the lung, replenish essence, and tonify blood.

Take 6 grams, twice daily.

(4) *Nǚ Jīn Wán* (女金丸)

Indicated for infertility and painful menstruation due to dual deficiency of qi and blood. This formula acts to regulate menstruation, nourish blood, regulate qi, and relieve pain.

Take 1 pill, twice daily.

(5) *Bā Bǎo Kūn Shun Wán* (八宝坤顺丸)

Indicated for infertility due to qi and blood depletion, especially when accompanied by liver constraint. This formula can nourish blood, regulate menstruation, tonify qi, and resolve constraint.

Take 1 pill, twice daily.

(6) *Xiāo Yáo Wán* (逍遥丸)

Indicated for infertility due to qi constraint. This formula acts to course the liver, resolve constraint, fortify the spleen, and nourish blood.

Take 6 to 9g, 3 times daily.

(7) *Qī Zhì Xiāng Fù Wán* (七制香附丸)

Indicated for infertility with painful menstruation due to liver constraint and qi stagnation. This formula acts to soothe constraint, harmonize the liver, regulate qi, nourish blood, and regulate menstruation.

Take 1 honey pill, twice daily. Water pills, 6g twice daily.

(8) *Ài Fù Nuǎn Gōng Wán* (艾附暖宫丸)

Indicated for infertility, painful menstruation, and leukorrhea due to uterine deficiency cold. This formula acts to regulate qi, nourish blood, warm the uterus, and regulate menstruation.

Take 1 pill, 2 to 3 times daily.

(9) *Shí Èr Wēn Jīng Wán* (十二温经丸)

Indicated for infertility due to penetrating vessel deficiency cold, congealing cold, and blood stasis. This formula acts to warm the channels, dissipate cold, nourish blood, dispel stasis, regulate menstruation, and free the vessels.

Take 6 to 9g, twice daily.

(10) *Shēn Guì Lù Róng Wán* (参桂鹿茸丸)

Indicated for infertility due to spleen-kidney yang deficiency, uterine deficiency cold, or congealing cold. This formula acts to nourish blood, boost essence, replenish marrow, and strengthen the body.

Take 1 pill, twice daily.

(11) Èr Chén Wán (二陈丸)

Indicated for infertility due to spleen deficiency with phlegm-damp. This formula acts to dry dampness, resolve phlegm, regulate qi, and harmonize the stomach.

Take 6 to 9g, twice daily.

(12) Yì Mǔ Wán (益母丸)

Indicated for infertility due to qi stagnation and blood stasis. This formula acts to nourish blood, regulate menstruation, dispel stasis, and engender the new.

Take 1 pill, twice daily.

2. ACUPUNCTURE AND MOXIBUSTION

Current research indicates that treatment with acupuncture and moxibustion shows a definite therapeutic effect when applied in cases of female infertility. The following section includes the most effective and commonly applied clinical methods.

(1) Ovulation Failure Infertility

A. Acupuncture

【Point Selection】

ST 29	*guī lái*	归来
RN 4	*guān yuán*	关元
EX-CA 1	*zǐ gōng*	子宫
RN 3	*zhōng jí*	中极
LI 4	*hé gǔ*	合谷
SP 6	*sān yīn jiāo*	三阴交

ST 36	*zú sān lǐ*	足三里

【Point Modifications】

With kidney deficiency, add BL 23 (*shèn shù*) and KI 3 (*tài xī*).

With liver constraint, add LV 3 (*tài chōng*).

With blood deficiency, add SP 10 (*xuè hǎi*).

With phlegm-damp, add SP 9 (*yīn líng quán*) and ST 40 (*fēng lóng*).

With blood stasis, add BL 17 (*gé shù*).

【Manipulation】

Needle EX-CA 1, LI 4 and ST 36 with supplementation.

Needle ST 36 with drainage, and RN 3 with neutral supplementation and drainage.

With kidney deficiency, needle BL 23 and KI 3 with supplementation.

With liver constraint, needle LV 3 with drainage.

With blood deficiency, needle SP 10 with supplementation.

With phlegm-damp, needle SP 9 and ST 40 with neutral supplementation and drainage.

With blood stasis, needle BL 17 with drainage.

B. Plum-blossom needle

【Point Selection】

Apply plum-blossom needling along the course of the channel from RN 2 to RN 13. Then stimulate the areas from DU 1 to DU 5, and also BL 22 to BL 30. Finally, apply stimulation along the girdling vessel at the inguinal region and near the genitalia.

C. Point injection therapy

【Point Selection】

Select several of the main points; alternate point selection with each treatment.

【Manipulation】

Placenta injection, Radix Angelica, HCG, and HMG may be applied.

D. Point embedding therapy

【Point Selection】

SP 6	sān yīn jiāo	三阴交

E. Auricular acupuncture

【Point Selection】

shenmen	TF4	shén mén	神门
subcortex	AT4	pí zhì xià	皮质下
endocrine	CO18	nèi fēn mì	内分泌
internal genitals	TF2	nèi shēng zhí qì	内生殖器
liver	CO12	gān	肝
kidney	CO10	shèn	肾

【Manipulation】

Embed ear tack needles or apply acupressure with ear seeds.

(2) Infertility due to Salpingemphraxis

A. Acupuncture

Method A:

【Point Selection】

SP 6	sān yīn jiāo	三阴交
EX-CA 1	zǐ gōng	子宫
RN 6	qì hǎi	气海
RN 3	zhōng jí	中极
LI 4	hé gǔ	合谷
KI 3	tài xī	太溪

【Point Modifications】

With qi stagnation and blood stasis, add BL 17, LV 3, and BL 18 (gān shù).

With damp-heat and stasis obstruction, needle RN 3 with drainage.

With cold-damp and stasis stagnation, apply moxabustion to BL 21 (wèi shù).

With binding of stasis and phlegm, needle ST 40 with even supplementation and drainage.

Method B:

【Point Selection】

Primarily apply abdominal cluster-needling.

The following acupoints may also be selected.

SP 6	*sān yīn jiāo*	三阴交
ST 36	*zú sān lǐ*	足三里

【Manipulation】

Point selecting method for abdominal cluster-needling: Locate two points two *cun* medial to the anterior superior iliac spine, lateral to RN 3. Divide the distance between these two points to locate a total of 8 points. Needle with even supplementation and drainage. Manipulate with caution to avoid damage to the peritoneum.

B. Plum-blossom needle

For patterns of liver constraint and qi stagnation:

【Point Selection】

SP 6	*sān yīn jiāo*	三阴交
RN 6	*qì hǎi*	气海
ST 25	*tiān shū*	天枢
LV 14	*qī mén*	期门

Also stimulate the bilateral areas of the 8th to the 12th vertebra. Then apply treatment to the lumbosacral area and lower abdomen. Finally, apply stimulation along the girdling vessel as well as to any obviously reactive points.

For patterns of damp-heat and blood stasis:

【Point Selection】

ST 36	*zú sān lǐ*	足三里
RN 12	*zhōng wǎn*	中脘
LI 11	*qū chí*	曲池

BL 17	*gé shù*	膈俞

Also stimulate the bilateral areas of the 8ᵗʰ to the 12ᵗʰ vertebra. Then apply treatment to the lumbosacral area and lower abdomen. Finally, apply stimulation along the medial aspect of the lower leg and groin, as well as to any obviously reactive points.

For deficiency with damage to the viscera and malnourishment of the penetrating and conception vessels:

【Point Selection】

Apply plum blossom needling to the bilateral areas of the 8ᵗʰ to the 12ᵗʰ vertebrae. Then apply treatment to the lumbosacral area. Finally, apply stimulation to the inguinal area along the course of the girdling vessel, as well as to any obviously reactive points.

The following acupoints may also be selected.

ST 36	*zú sān lǐ*	足三里
SP 6	*sān yīn jiāo*	三阴交
RN 12	*zhōng wǎn*	中脘
RN 4	*guān yuán*	关元
DU 14	*dà zhuī*	大椎

C. Point injection therapy

【Point Selection】

RN 4	*guān yuán*	关元
ST 29	*guī lái*	归来
EX-CA 1	*zǐ gōng*	子宫
RN 3	*zhōng jí*	中极
ST 28	*shuǐ dào*	水道
BL 31-34	*bā liáo*	八髎

Select several of the main points; alternate point selection with each treatment.

【Manipulation】

Placenta injection, *yú xīng cǎo* (Herba Houttuyniae), sodium benzylpenicillin, or cefazolin sodium injections may be applied, according to the specific condition.

D. Moxibustion during San fu

Note: "*San fu* " refers to the three periods of greatest heat during the summer season, according to the Chinese lunar calendar. *Geng* (庚) refers to the 7th Heavenly Stem, a specific calendar day within those periods.

【Point Selection】

Select points one *cun* lateral to the lumbar spinous processes.

【Method】

Materials: Grind *bái jiè zǐ* (Sinapis Semen), *gān jiāng* (Rhizoma Zingiberis) and *xì xīn* (Radix et Rhizoma Asari) into a fine powder, and mix with fresh ginger juice to make a paste. Treatments should be administered on each *geng* day, beginning at the first *fu* period. Continue treatment through all three *fu* periods.

E. Auricular acupuncture

internal genitals	TF2	*nèi shēng zhí qì*	内生殖器
endocrine	CO18	*nèi fēn mì*	内分泌
liver	CO12	*gān*	肝
sanjiao	CO17	*sān jiāo*	三焦
adrenal gland	TG2p	*shèn shàng xiàn*	肾上腺
cavitas pelvis	TF5	*pén qiāng*	盆腔

(3) Infertility due to Polycystic Ovarian Syndrome (PCOS)

A. Acupuncture

【Point Selection】

SP 6	*sān yīn jiāo*	三阴交
EX-CA 1	*zǐ gōng*	子宫
RN 3	*zhōng jí*	中极
RN 4	*guān yuán*	关元
BL 20	*pí shù*	脾俞

BL 23	*shèn shù*	肾俞
BL 18	*gān shù*	肝俞

【Manipulation】

Apply treatment once daily for 15 days, beginning on the 5th day of the menstrual period. Retain all needles for 30 minutes. Three menstrual cycles constitute one treatment course.

For obese patients, select the following points:

【Point Selection】

RN 4	*guān yuán*	关元
RN 6	*qì hǎi*	气海
RN 10	*xià wǎn*	下脘
RN 12	*zhōng wǎn*	中脘
SP 15	*dà héng*	大横
ST 24	*huá ròu mén*	滑肉门
ST 26	*wài líng*	外陵

【Manipulation】

In addition to standard acupuncture, embedding needles may be applied on SP 15, ST 24, ST 26, ST 21 (*liáng mén*), SP 10 and ST 25. Select 5–6 points per treatment, embedding needles once every two weeks. 7 treatments constitute one treatment course.

B. Plum-blossom needle

【Point Selection】

Apply plum blossom needling to the bilateral areas of the 1st to 5th lumbosacral vertebrae. Also stimulate the inner line of the bladder channel; the conception vessel below the umbilicus; and the spleen channel below the umbilicus.

C. Auricular acupuncture

【Point Selection】

kidney	CO10	*shèn*	肾
liver	CO12	*gān*	肝

endocrine	CO18	*nèi fēn mì*	内分泌
adrenal gland	TG2p	*shèn shàng xiàn*	肾上腺
ovary	luan chao	*luǎn cháo*	卵巢
brain point	nao dian	*nǎo diǎn*	脑点
uterus	zi gong	*zǐ gōng*	子宫

【Manipulation】

Apply treatment 2 to 3 times each week, selecting 4-5 points per session. Apply medium stimulation with filiform needles, or embed ear tack needles.

D. Point injection therapy

【Point Selection】

BL 20	*pí shù*	脾俞
BL 23	*shèn shù*	肾俞
BL 30	*bái huán shù*	白环俞
RN 4	*guān yuán*	关元
RN 6	*qì hǎi*	气海
SP 6	*sān yīn jiāo*	三阴交
KI 3	*tài xī*	太溪

【Manipulation】

Administer *dāng guī* (Radix Angelicae Sinensis) or vitamin B1 injection; 0.2-0.5 ml per point. Select 3 to 4 points per treatment, once every two days.

E. Moxibustion

【Point Selection】

RN 3	*zhōng jí*	中极
RN 4	*guān yuán*	关元
BL 20	*pí shù*	脾俞
BL 23	*shèn shù*	肾俞
SP 10	*xuè hǎi*	血海
SP 6	*sān yīn jiāo*	三阴交

DU 4	mìng mén	命门

(4) Infertility due to Endometriosis

A. Acupuncture

Combining front-*mu* and back-*shu* points:

【Point Selection】

BL 18	gān shù	肝俞
BL 20	pí shù	脾俞
BL 23	shèn shù	肾俞
LV 13	zhāng mén	章门
LV 14	qī mén	期门
GB 25	jīng mén	京门

【Manipulation】

Treat once daily, with 20 days constituting one course. Pause treatment for 10 days in between courses. Continue for 3 months.

Supplementary points:

【Point Selection】

RN 3	zhōng jí	中极
LI 4	hé gǔ	合谷
SP 6	sān yīn jiāo	三阴交
RN 4	guān yuán	关元
RN 6	qì hǎi	气海
RN 10	xià wǎn	下脘
RN 12	zhōng wǎn	中脘
LV 3	tài chōng	太冲
SP 10	xuè hǎi	血海

B. Auricular acupuncture

【Point Selection】

uterus	zi gong	zǐ gōng	子宫
endocrine	CO18	nèi fēn mì	内分泌
shenmen	TF4	shén mén	神门

subcortex	AT4	*pí zhì xià*	皮质下
liver	CO12	*gān*	肝
kidney	CO10	*shèn*	肾
sympathetic	AH6a	*jiāo gǎn*	交感
abdomen	AH8	*fù*	腹
lumbosacral vertebrae	AH9	*yāo dǐ zhuī*	腰骶椎

【Manipulation】

Select 4 to 5 points for needling or ear seed embedding for each treatment; 2 to 3 times per week.

C. Plum-blossom needle

【Point Selection】

Apply plum blossom needling along the course of the conception vessel in the area of the lower abdomen. Points on the stomach channel, kidney channel, spleen channel, the governing channel, bladder channel may also be selected. Also stimulate the *jia-ji* points of the lumbosacral region.

【Manipulation】

Use moderate to strong stimulation, according to the tolerance of the patient. Treat for 10 to 15 minutes per session.

D. Point injection therapy

【Point Selection】

ST 36	*zú sān lǐ*	足三里
SP 10	*xuè hǎi*	血海
SP 6	*sān yīn jiāo*	三阴交
BL 32	*cì liáo*	次髎

Points are grouped into pairs for treatment; ST 36 with SP 10, and SP 6 with BL 32. Treatment is applied 5 times per month, alternating between each pair of points.

【Manipulation】

Inject 2 ml *dān shēn* (Radix et Rhizoma Salviae Miltiorrhizae) compound into one pair of acupoints; begin 10 days before menstruation. 2 months constitute one treatment course. 3 to 5 courses are recommended.

E. Qī Hòu Sǎn (七厚散) umbilical compress

【Point Selection】

RN 8	shén què	神阙

【Method】

Mix 1g Qī Hòu Sǎn (七厚散) with a small amount of yellow rice wine and apply to RN 8. Moxa for 20 minutes, then apply a compress using Shè Xiāng Zhǐ Tòng Gāo (麝香止痛膏). For patients with sensitive skin, Fū Jī Níng (肤肌宁) may be selected. Change the compress every 48 hours. Begin treatment on the 10th day after menstruation and continue through the next menstrual period. 2 months constitute one treatment course; 2 to 4 courses are recommended.

(5) Immune Infertility

A. Acupuncture

【Point Selection】

BL 15	xīn shù	心俞
BL 17	gé shù	膈俞
BL 18	gān shù	肝俞
BL 23	shèn shù	肾俞
LV 3	tài chōng	太冲
SP 10	xuè hǎi	血海
KI 3	tài xī	太溪
SP 10	xuè hǎi	血海
HT 7	shén mén	神门

【Manipulation】

Needle all points with even supplementation and drainage; retain needles for 30 minutes. Apply treatment daily, with 2 months constituting one treatment course.

(6) Premature Ovarian Failure (POF)

A. Acupuncture

【Point Selection】

RN 3	*zhōng jí*	中极
RN 4	*guān yuán*	关元
RN 6	*qì hǎi*	气海
RN 10	*xià wǎn*	下脘
RN 12	*zhōng wǎn*	中脘
EX-CA 1	*zǐ gōng*	子宫
KI 12	*dà hè*	大赫
BL 23	*shèn shù*	肾俞

Also needle the *jia-ji* points from the 5th thoracic to the 4th lumbar vertebrae.

【Point Modifications】

With liver and kidney yin deficiency, add SP 6, SP 9, BL 18, HT 6 (*yīn xī*) and KI 7 (*fù liū*).

For spleen and kidney yang deficiency, add BL 20, DU 4, BL 32, and SP 8 (*dì jī*); warming needle moxabustion may also be applied.

【Manipulation】

Retain needles for 20 minutes. After their removal, apply cupping on the back-*shu* and *jia-ji* points for 5 to 10 minutes. 20 treatments constitute one course, with 5 to 7 days between courses. 6 treatment courses are recommended.

B. Plum-blossom needle

With liver and kidney yin deficiency:

【Point Selection】

Apply plum blossom needling along the back of the nape, and to the bilateral areas of the 8th to 10th thoracic vertebrae. Then stimulate the areas along the lumbosacral and iliac spine. Also treat the medial aspect of the calf, as well as any obviously reactive points.

The following acupoints may also be selected.

BL 18	gān shù	肝俞
BL 23	shèn shù	肾俞
LI 4	hé gǔ	合谷
SP 6	sān yīn jiāo	三阴交

With liver qi stagnation:
【Point Selection】

Apply plum blossom needling to the bilateral areas of the 7th to 10th thoracic vertebrae. Then stimulate areas on the sacrum, upper abdomen, and the medial aspect of the lower leg. Also treat the region along the course of the girdling vessel, and any other obviously reactive points.

The following acupoints may also be selected.

GB 20	fēng chí	风池
PC 6	nèi guān	内关

With non-interaction of heart and kidney:
【Point Selection】

Apply plum blossom needling along the back of the nape, the lumbar region, sacrum, inguinal area, and the medial aspect of the lower leg. Also treat the region along the course of the girdling vessel, and any other obviously reactive points.

The following acupoints may also be selected.

PC 6	nèi guān	内关
BL 15	xīn shù	心俞
BL 23	shèn shù	肾俞
RN 4	guān yuán	关元

With heart and spleen dual deficiency:
【Point Selection】

Apply plum blossom needling to the bilateral areas of the 5th to 12th thoracic vertebrae. Also stimulate the lumbus, lower abdomen, and along the course of girdling vessel. Also treat any other obviously reactive points.

The following acupoints may also be selected.

ST 36	*zú sān lǐ*	足三里
SP 6	*sān yīn jiāo*	三阴交
RN 12	*zhōng wǎn*	中脘
HT 7	*shén mén*	神门

【Manipulation】

Apply medium stimulation. For the most reactive areas, apply heavier stimulation whenever possible.

3. SIMPLE PRESCRIPTIONS AND EMPIRICAL FORMULAS

(1)

炒当归	*chǎo dāng guī*	10g	Radix Angelicae Sinensis
赤芍	*chì sháo*	10g	Radix Paeoniae Rubra
白芍	*bái sháo*	10g	Radix Paeoniae Alba
山药	*shān yào*	10g	Rhizoma Dioscoreae
山萸肉	*shān yú ròu*	9g	Fructus Corni
甘草	*gān cǎo*	6g	Radix et Rhizoma Glycyrrhizae
丹皮	*dān pí*	10g	Cortex Moutan
钩藤	*gōu téng*	15g	Ramulus Uncariae Cum Uncis
地黄	*dì huáng*	10g	Radix Rehmanniae

This formula acts to enrich yin and repress yang hyperactivity to treat infertility due to liver-kidney yin deficiency.

(2)

熟地	*shú dì*	30g	Radix Rehmanniae Praeparata
山药	*shān yào*	30g	Rhizoma Dioscoreae
白术	*bái zhú*	30g	Rhizoma Atractylodis Macrocephalae
茯苓	*fú líng*	30g	Poria
泽泻	*zé xiè*	20g	Rhizoma Alismatis

枸杞	gǒu qǐ	30g	Fructus Lycii
巴戟天	bā jǐ tiān	30g	Radix Morindae Officinalis
菟丝子	tù sī zǐ	30g	Semen Cuscutae
肉桂	ròu guì	20g	Cortex Cinnamomi
附子	fù zǐ	20g	Radix Aconiti Lateralis Praeparata
鹿胶	lù jiāo	30g	Colla Cornus Cervi
破故纸	pò gù zhǐ	30g	Fructus Psoraleae
陈皮	chén pí	10g	Pericarpium Citri Reticulatae
甘草	gān cǎo	20g	Radix et Rhizoma Glycyrrhizae

This formula acts to warm the kidney and assist yang to treat infertility due to kidney yang deficiency.

(3)

柴胡	chái hú	15g	Radix Bupleuri
香附	xiāng fù	15g	Rhizoma Cyperi
王不留行	wáng bù liú xíng	15g	Semen Vaccariae
红花	hóng huā	15g	Flos Carthami
桃仁	táo rén	20g	Semen Persicae
三棱	sān léng	20g	Rhizoma Sparganii
牛膝	niú xī	20g	Radix Achyranthis Bidentatae
莪术	é zhú	30g	Rhizoma Curcumae

This formula acts to warm yang and free the vessels to treat obstruction of the fallopian tube and infertility due to liver constraint, qi stagnation, and blood stasis.

(4)

官桂	guān guì	3g	Cortex Cinnamomi
鹿角片	lù jiǎo piàn	10g	Sectum Cervi Cornu
仙灵脾	xiān líng pí	12g	Herba Epimedii
仙茅	xiān máo	10g	Rhizoma Curculiginis
巴戟天	bā jǐ tiān	12g	Radix Morindae Officinalis
苍术	cāng zhú	10g	Rhizoma Atractylodis
白术	bái zhú	10g	Rhizoma Atractylodis Macrocephalae

姜半夏	*jiāng bàn xià*	10g	Rhizome Pinelliae Praeparata
胆星	*dǎn xīng*	6g	Arisaema cum Bile
椒目	*jiāo mù*	3g	Pericarpium Zanthoxyli
泽泻	*zé xiè*	9g	Rhizoma Alismatis
山楂	*shān zhā*	10g	Fructus Crataegi
石菖蒲	*shí chāng pú*	5g	Rhizoma Acori Tatarinowii
化橘红	*huà jú hóng*	9g	Exocarpium Citri Grandis

This formula acts to warm the channels and abduct phlegm to treat infertility due to phlegm-damp obstruction.

PROGNOSIS

There is no consensus regarding the prognosis of infertility because of the number of problems that may exist within an individual or couple trying to conceive. However, without any treatment intervention, 15% to 20% of couples previously diagnosed as infertile will eventually become pregnant, unless the woman is over 35 years of age. Generally speaking, the rates of conception are lower in those cases which require a longer course of treatment. Also, the prognosis for functional infertility is better than in those conditions associated with structural disease.

PREVENTIVE HEALTHCARE

Lifestyle Modification

(1) Lifestyle

Patients with infertility can take some control of their reproductive function by living healthy lifestyles. Heavy physical labor is to be avoided. Recommend that the patient create a reasonable schedule that balances both work and rest. To avoid essence damage and yin depletion, sexual activities should be limited to once or twice a week.

(2) Personal Hygiene

During menstruation, it is especially easy for pathogens to enter the blood chamber and uterine vessels. Therefore, good personal hygiene is essential. Sexual intercourse, swimming, bathing, and suppository medications should be avoided during the menstrual period.

(3) Monitoring BBT

Sexual intercourse at the proper time can increase the chances of conception. Monitoring of the basal body temperature should be performed by the patient in order to time sexual intercourse most effectively.

(4) Smoking and Alcohol

Tobacco use has been shown to affect the reproductive capacities of both men and women. In women, smoking can interfere with or damage ovarian functioning. As for men, smoking increases the rate of sperm abnormalities and also reduces the ability to produce an erection. Alcohol also has detrimental effects on fertility, so its consumption should be limited. Decreased conception rates have been found in women who drink between one and five alcoholic drinks a week.

(5) Family Planning

Couples who want to have children should first undergo a thorough medical examination to discover any possible congenital conditions or physiological defects that could lead to infertility. A number of conditions exist that may cause secondary infertility, or the inability to conceive after having given birth previously. Menstrual disorders, endometriosis, and pelvic inflammation can occur as a result of repeated or improper abortions. Furthermore, 40% of untreated chlamydia cervical infections cause PID (pelvic inflammatory disease). If a woman suffers with PID, she has a 20% chance of being infertile. These conditions should be addressed as soon as possible, regardless of their cause.

Dietary Recommendation

(1) Avoid Cold-natured Foods

Consuming an excessive amount of cold-natured foods may lead to cold evils settling internally. This can cause the blood to congeal and stagnate, and menstrual irregularities may occur as a result. Overindulging in these foods can eventually damage yang qi, and may lead to patterns of uterine deficient cold and infertility.

(2) Medicinal Diet

A. *Jī Zhǔ Yì Mǔ Cǎo* (鸡煮益母草)

| 乌鸡 | *wū jī* | 1 | Black chicken |
| 益母草 | *yì mǔ cǎo* | 500g | Herba Leonuri |

Divide the *yì mǔ cǎo* (Herba Leonuri) into 4 portions. First soak each portion in yellow rice wine, vinegar, ginger juice and *chuān xiōng* (Rhizoma Chuanxiong) juice respectively, then roast together until dry.

Put the processed *yì mǔ cǎo* (Herba Leonuri) into the chicken, and cook with water. The meat and soup should be eaten without spices, but it may be taken with medicinal wine.

Remove the bones and herbal dregs; bake to dry. Then add 120g *guī shēn* (Radix Angelicae Sinensis), 60g *xù duàn* (Radix Dipsaci) and 18g ginger; grind all ingredients into powder and make 9g honey pills. Take 1 pill, 3 times daily.

Indicated for chronic female infertility.

B. *Hóng Huā Yùn Yù Dàn* (红花孕育蛋)

| 鸡蛋 | *jī dàn* | 1 | Egg |
| 藏红花 | *zàng hóng huā* | 1.5g | Stigma Croci |

Poke a hole into the egg shell; place 1.5g *zàng hóng huā* (Stigma Croci) inside the egg and stir. Cook with steam and eat.

To be taken daily for 9 days; begin on the 2nd day of menstruation. Repeat for 3 to 4 cycles.

Indicated for infertility with patterns of qi deficiency and stasis.

C. Dāng Guī Yuǎn Zhì Jiǔ (当归远志酒)

全当归	quán dāng guī	150g	Radix Angelicae Sinensis
远志	yuǎn zhì	150g	Radix Polygalae
甜酒	tián jiǔ	1500g	Sweet wine

Mince the *quán dāng guī* (Radix Angelicae Sinensis); add *yuǎn zhì* (Radix Polygalae) and place into a cloth bag. Soak with wine in a clean and sealed container for 7 days. Discard the dregs and take warm each evening.

This preparation acts to invigorate blood, free the channels, and harmonize qi and blood.

Indicated for infertility, menstrual irregularities, and patterns of qi and blood insufficiency.

D. Zhà yù lán huā (炸玉兰花)

玉兰花	yù lán huā	10	Flos Magnoliae Denudatae (buds)

Decoct the flower buds in water. Alternately, they may be covered with flour, fried, and coated with sugar. They may also be eaten cold with sesame oil and salt.

Indicated for infertility and painful menstruation.

E. Shǒu Wū Gān Piàn (首乌肝片)

何首乌	hé shǒu wū	20g	Radix Polygoni Multiflori
鲜猪肝	xiān zhū gān	250g	Fresh pork liver
油菜	yóu cài	100g	Rape

Decoct *shǒu wū* (Radix Polygoni Multiflori) in 300 ml water for 20 minutes. Stir-fry the sliced pork liver with rape, and add to the decoction. May be taken once daily.

Indicated for infertility with patterns of blood deficiency.

F. *Táo Rén Mò Yú Tāng* (桃仁墨鱼汤)

桃仁	*táo rén*	6g	Semen Persicae
墨鱼	*mò yú*	15g	Cuttlefish

Remove the bones and skin, and decoct the cleaned cuttlefish with *táo rén* (Semen Persicae) in 500 ml of water until well-cooked. The soup and fish may be taken once daily.

Indicated for infertility with patterns of blood deficiency.

G. *Qī Yí Bǐng* (期颐饼)

生芡实米	*shēng qiàn shí mǐ*	180g	Semen Euryales (raw, ground)
生鸡内金	*shēng jī nèi jīn*	90g	Endothelium Corneum Gigeriae Galli (raw, ground)
白面	*bái miàn*	250g	White flour
白糖	*bái táng*	as needed	White sugar

Soak the powdered *jī nèi jīn* (Endothelium Corneum Gigeriae Galli) in 300 ml of boiled water for 4 hours. Then add *qiàn shí* (Semen Euryales), flour and sugar, and mix. Shape into thin pancakes and bake. 50 to 100 grams may be taken in between meals.

Indicated for infertility with patterns of phlegm-damp.

H. *Lái Fú Zǐ Zhōu* (莱菔子粥)

莱菔子	*lái fú zǐ*	20g	Semen Raphani
大米	*dà mǐ*	100g	Rice

Decoct both ingredients in 600 ml of water. To be taken once daily.

Indicated for infertility with patterns of liver constraint and qi stagnation.

I. *Lù Róng Jiǔ* (鹿茸酒)

鹿茸	*lù róng*	3g	Cornu Cervi Pantotrichum
山药	*shān yào*	30g	Rhizoma Dioscoreae
白酒	*bái jiǔ*	500ml	Distilled spirits

Place sliced *lù róng* (Cornu Cervi Pantotrichum) and *shān yào* (Rhizoma

Dioscoreae) into a gauze bag and soak with spirits in a clean and sealed container for 7 days. Take 10 ml, twice daily.

Indicated for infertility with patterns of uterine cold.

Regulation of Emotional and Mental Health

A balanced emotional state is very beneficial to a woman's reproductive health. The conscious cultivation of a positive mental attitude helps to regulate not only the emotions, but also the qi and blood of the penetrating and conception vessels. Agitation and vexation can damage the liver, causing stagnation which inhibits the free flow of qi and blood. Infertility may occur when the penetrating and conception vessels are affected. When a couple is infertile, they are generally anxious and worried, and this mental state can also lead to inhibition of the qi dynamic. It is therefore most important to regulate the emotions as much as possible to avoid this vicious cycle.

CLINICAL EXPERIENCE OF RENOWNED PHYSICIANS

Empirical Formulas

1. Yì Yáng Shèn Shī Tāng (益阳渗湿汤) for Infertility due to Kidney Yang Deficiency
(Han Bai-ling)

【Ingredients】

益阳渗湿汤 Yì Yáng Shèn Shī Tāng

熟地	shú dì	30g	Radix Rehmanniae Praeparata
山药	shān yào	30g	Rhizoma Dioscoreae
白术	bái zhú	30g	Rhizoma Atractylodis Macrocephalae
茯苓	fú líng	30g	Poria
泽泻	zé xiè	20g	Rhizoma Alismatis
枸杞	gǒu qǐ	30g	Fructus Lycii

巴戟天	bā jǐ tiān	30g	Radix Morindae Officinalis
菟丝子	tù sī zǐ	30g	Semen Cuscutae
肉桂	ròu guì	20g	Cortex Cinnamomi
附子	fù zǐ	20g	Radix Aconiti Lateralis Praeparata
鹿胶	lù jiāo	30g	Colla Cornus Cervi
破故纸	pò gù zhǐ	30g	Fructus Psoraleae
陈皮	chén pí	10g	Pericarpium Citri Reticulatae
甘草	gān cǎo	20g	Radix et Rhizoma Glycyrrhizae

【Indications】

Infertility with clear thin scant menses, persistent leukorrhea, aching lumbus and weak legs, cold limbs, thin loose stool, dizziness, poor memory, and a dull grayish complexion. The tongue appears pale and moist with white glossy coating. Pulses are deep and weak.

【Formula Analysis】

Shān yào (Rhizoma Dioscoreae) and *bái zhú* (Rhizoma Atractylodis Macrocephalae) fortify the spleen and boost the source of engendering and transformation. *Fú líng* (Poria) and *chén pí* (Pericarpium Citri Reticulatae) fortify the spleen and regulate qi. *Shú dì* (Radix Rehmanniae Praeparata) and *gǒu qǐ zǐ* (Fructus Lycii) nourish blood and regulate menstruation. *Lù jiāo* (Colla Cornus Cervi), *bā jǐ tiān* (Radix Morindae Officinalis), *ròu guì* (Cortex Cinnamomi), and *fù zǐ* (Radix Aconiti Lateralis Praeparata) warm the kidney and assist yang. *Tù sī zǐ* (Semen Cuscutae) and *pò gù zhǐ* (Fructus Psoraleae) tonify the kidney and invigorate yang. It is interesting to note that this empirical perscription contains a very high dosage of *ròu guì* (Cortex Cinnamomi), at 20g.

【Modifications】

➤ With clear thin and profuse vaginal discharge, add *lù jiǎo shuāng* (Cornu Cervi Degelatinatum) and *jīn yīng zǐ* (Fructus Rosae Laevigatae) to astringe and secure.

➤ With delayed menstruation and scant menses, add *dāng guī* (Radix

Angelicae Sinensis), *chuān xiōng* (Rhizoma Chuanxiong) and *huái niú xī* (Radix Achyranthis Bidentatae).

> With binding constraint of liver qi, add *yù jīn* (Radix Curcumae), *fó shǒu* (Fructus Citri Sarcodactylis) and *wū yào* (Radix Linderae).

(Han Bai-ling. *Bailing's Gynecology* 百灵妇科 . 1st edition. Heillongjiang: Heilongjiang People's Publishing House, 1980: 154)

2. *TIÁO CHŌNG CÙ YÙN TĀNG* (调冲促孕汤) FOR INFERTILITY DUE TO KIDNEY ESSENCE INSUFFICIENCY AND DEPLETION OF THE PENETRATING AND CONCEPTION VESSELS (ZHAO SONG-QUAN)

【Ingredients】

调冲促孕汤 *Tiáo Chōng Cù Yùn Tāng*

当归	*dāng guī*	10g	Radix Angelicae Sinensis
熟地	*shú dì*	10g	Radix Rehmanniae Praeparata
白芍	*bái sháo*	10g	Radix Paeoniae Alba
太子参	*tài zǐ shēn*	10g	Radix Pseudostellariae
巴戟天	*bā jǐ tiān*	10g	Radix Morindae Officinalis
菟丝子	*tù sī zǐ*	10g	Semen Cuscutae
枸杞子	*gǒu qǐ zǐ*	10g	Fructus Lycii
仙灵脾	*xiān líng pí*	10g	Herba Epimedii
山茱萸	*shān zhū yú*	10g	Fructus Corni
覆盆子	*fù pén zǐ*	10g	Fructus Rubi
制首乌	*zhì shǒu wū*	10g	Radix Polygoni Multiflori Praeparata cum Succo Glycines Sotae
山药	*shān yào*	15g	Rhizoma Dioscoreae
河车粉	*hé chē fěn*	3g	Placenta Hominis (powdered)
鹿角霜	*lù jiǎo shuāng*	10g	Cornu Cervi Degelatinatum

【Indications】

Infertility with uterine hypoplasia, ovarian hypofunction, and irregular menstruation with profuse or scant menses.

【Formula Analysis】

Dāng guī (Radix Angelicae Sinensis) nourishes blood and regulates menstruation. *Bái sháo* (Radix Paeoniae Alba) constrains yin, emolliates the liver, and frees the blood vessels. *Chuān xiōng* (Rhizoma Chuanxiong) acts to track liver qi and quicken the blood. *Shú dì* (Radix Rehmanniae Praeparata) enriches kidney yin. *Tài zǐ shēn* (Radix Pseudostellariae) and *huáng qí* (Radix Astragali) tonifies qi and nourishes the stomach to enrich the source of transformation. *Tù sī zǐ* (Semen Cuscutae), *gǒu qǐ zǐ* (Fructus Lycii), *fù pén zǐ* (Fructus Rubi) and *shǒu wū* (Radix Polygoni Multiflori) act together to replenish essence and boost marrow. *Cōng róng* (Herba Cistanches), *bā jǐ tiān* (Radix Morindae Officinalis) and *xiān líng pí* (Herba Epimedii) act together to strongly tonify the life gate while harmonizing yang with yin. *Zǐ hé chē* (Placenta Hominis) can strongly tonify the extraordinary vessels due to its affinity with flesh and blood. *Lù jiǎo* (Cornu Cervi) vitalizes yang qi in order to produce yin, while also freeing the governing vessel.

【Modifications】

➤ With predominant qi deficiency, add *dǎng shēn* (Radix Codonopsis) 12g, *huáng qí* (Radix Astragali) 15g, and remove *tài zǐ shēn* (Radix Pseudostellariae).

➤ With blood deficiency, add *ē jiāo* (Colla Corii Asini) 15g.

➤ With yang deficiency, add *fù zǐ* (Radix Aconiti Lateralis Praeparata) 9g, *ròu guì* (Cortex Cinnamomi) 1.5g, *bǔ gǔ zhī* (Fructus Psoraleae) 10g, and *xiān máo* (Rhizoma Curculiginis) 10g.

➤ With internal heat due to yin deficiency, add *guī bǎn* (Carapax et Plastrum Testudinis) 15g, *shēng dì* (Radix Rehmanniae Exsiccata seu Recens) 10g, *dān pí* (Cortex Moutan) 10g, and *nǚ zhēn zǐ* (Fructus Ligustri Lucidi) 10g.

➤ With scant menses, add *yì mǔ cǎo* (Herba Leonuri) 12g, *jī xuè téng* (Caulis Spatholobi) 10g, and *chuān xiōng* (Rhizoma Chuanxiong) 10g.

> ➢ With profuse menstruation, add *qiàn cǎo tàn* (Radix et Rhizoma Rubiae Carbonisatus) 6g, *wū zéi gǔ* (Endoconcha Sepiae) 15g, and *cè bǎi yè* (Cacumen Platycladi) 10g.

> ➢ With watery vaginal discharge, add *qiàn shí* (Semen Euryales) 15g, and *wū zéi gǔ* (Endoconcha Sepiae) 15g.

(Yang Si-shu, Yan Xiu-lan, Wang Xin-pei. *Collected Empirical Formulas of Renowned Physicians in Modern China* 中国现代名医验方荟海. 1ˢᵗ edition. Wuhan: Hubei Science and Technology Press, 1996: 1360-1361)

3. *Xiāo Yáo Zhù Yùn Tāng* (逍遥助孕汤) for Infertility due to Liver Qi Constraint

(Zhu Xiao-nan)

【Ingredients】

逍遥助孕汤 *Xiāo Yáo Zhù Yùn Tāng*

香附	*xiāng fù*	9g	Rhizoma Cyperi
郁金	*yù jīn*	9g	Radix Curcumae
当归	*dāng guī*	9g	Radix Angelicae Sinensis
茯苓	*fú líng*	9g	Poria
合欢皮	*hé huān pí*	9g	Cortex Albiziae
苏罗子	*sū luó zǐ*	9g	Semen Aesculi
路路通	*lù lù tōng*	9g	Fructus Liquidambaris
白术	*bái zhú*	6g	Rhizoma Atractylodis Macrocephalae
白芍	*bái sháo*	6g	Radix Paeoniae Alba
陈皮	*chén pí*	6g	Pericarpium Citri Reticulatae
柴胡	*chái hú*	4g	Radix Bupleuri

【Indications】

Infertility due to liver qi constraint.

【Formula Analysis】

Xiāng fù (Rhizoma Cyperi), *yù jīn* (Radix Curcumae) and *hé huān pí* (Cortex Albiziae) act to open constraint, move qi, and free liver-wood. *Dāng guī* (Radix Angelicae Sinensis) and *bái sháo* (Radix Paeoniae

Alba) nourish blood and constrain yin. *Bái zhú* (Rhizoma Atractylodis Macrocephalae), *chén pí* (Pericarpium Citri Reticulatae) and *fú líng* (Poria) fortify the spleen and harmonize the middle while tonifying deficiency to quiet the heart. *Sū luó zǐ* (Semen Aesculi) and *lù lù tōng* (Fructus Liquidambaris) act to free stagnation of the liver channel. *Chái hú* (Radix Bupleuri) clears depressed heat and eliminates vexation and agitation.

【Modifications】

➢ With menstrual swelling, add *guā lóu* (Fructus Trichosanthis), *jú yè* (Folium Citri Reticulatae) and *qīng pí* (Pericarpium Citri Reticulatae Viride).

➢ With profuse menstruation, add *yì mǔ cǎo* (Herba Leonuri) and remove *dāng guī* (Radix Angelicae Sinensis).

(Zhu Nan-sun, Zhu Rong-da, Dong Ping, et al. *Anthology of Zhu Xiaonan's Gynecological Experience* 朱小南妇科经验选. 1st edition. Beijing: People's Medical Publishing House, 1981: 118)

4. *Zhù Yùn Yī Hào Wán* (助孕Ⅰ号丸) AND *Zhù Yùn Èr Hào Wán* (助孕Ⅱ号丸) FOR INFERTILITY DUE TO KIDNEY DEFICIENCY AND BLOOD STASIS (LUO SONG-PING)

【Ingredients】

助孕Ⅰ号丸 *Zhù Yùn Yī Hào Wán*

菟丝子	*tù sī zǐ*	Semen Cuscutae
女贞子	*nǚ zhēn zǐ*	Fructus Ligustri Lucidi
金樱子	*jīn yīng zǐ*	Fructus Rosae Laevigatae
当归	*dāng guī*	Radix Angelicae Sinensis
地黄	*dì huáng*	Radix Rehmanniae
甘草	*gān cǎo*	Radix et Rhizoma Glycyrrhizae

助孕Ⅱ号丸 *Zhù Yùn Èr Hào Wán*

菟丝子	*tù sī zǐ*	Semen Cuscutae
淫羊藿	*yín yáng huò*	Herba Epimedii

金樱子	*jīn yīng zǐ*	Fructus Rosae Laevigatae
党参	*dǎng shēn*	Radix Codonopsis
丹参	*dān shēn*	Radix et Rhizoma Salviae Miltiorrhizae
甘草	*gān cǎo*	Radix et Rhizoma Glycyrrhizae

【Indications】

Zhù Yùn Yī Hào Wán (助孕Ⅰ号丸) for infertility with blood stasis and kidney yin deficiency.

Zhù Yùn Èr Hào Wán (助孕Ⅱ号丸) for infertility with blood stasis and kidney yang deficiency.

【Formula Analysis】

Zhù Yùn Yī Hào Wán (助孕Ⅰ号丸) and *Zhù Yùn Èr Hào Wán* (助孕Ⅱ号丸) can both regulate immune function and inhibit AsAb immune responses.

Medicinals that support the upright and secure the root can also benefit the immune system. For example, *dǎng shēn* (Radix Codonopsis) has been shown to promote phagocytosis and also to increase the functioning of the adrenal cortex.

However, yin-enriching blood-cooling medicinals such as *nǚ zhēn zǐ* (Fructus Ligustri Lucidi) and *dì huáng* (Radix Rehmanniae) can inhibit a hyperactive immune system. Blood-quickening stasis-transforming medicinals such as *dān shēn* (Radix et Rhizoma Salviae Miltiorrhizae) also inhibit the immune response through general inhibition and absorption of the antigen antibody complex. *Gān cǎo* (Radix et Rhizoma Glycyrrhizae) also displays hormone-like effects.

Zhù Yùn Yī Hào Wán (助孕Ⅰ号丸) and *Zhù Yùn Èr Hào Wán* (助孕Ⅱ号丸) both act to tonify the kidney, balance yin and yang, invigorate blood, and dispel stasis.

【Modifications】

➢ With blood stasis, add *táo rén* (Semen Persicae) and *hóng huā* (Flos Carthami).

> With phlegm, add *chén pí* (Pericarpium Citri Reticulatae) and *fǎ xià* (Rhizoma Pinelliae Praeparatum).

(Luo Song-ping, Zhang Yu-zhen. A Clinical and Empirical Study of Immune Miscarriage and Infertility 免疫性自然流产与免疫性不孕的临床与实验研究. *Journal of Traditional Chinese Medicine* (中医杂志), 1997, 38(6):353-354)

5. *Yú Shì Wēn Bǔ Fāng* (俞氏温补方) for Infertility due to Kidney Deficiency and Phlegm Turbidity
(Yu Jin)

【Ingredients】

俞氏温补方 *Yú Shì Wēn Bǔ Fāng*

熟地	*shú dì*	12g	Radix Rehmanniae Praeparata
黄精	*huáng jīng*	12g	Rhizoma Polygonati
仙灵脾	*xiān líng pí*	12g	Herba Epimedii
补骨脂	*bǔ gǔ zhī*	12g	Fructus Psoraleae
山甲	*shān jiǎ*	9g	Squama Manis
皂角刺	*zào jiǎo cì*	12g	Spina Gleditsiae
冰球子	*bīng qiú zǐ*	12g	Rhizoma Bletillae
贝母	*bèi mǔ*	12g	Bulbus Fritillaria

【Indications】

Infertility and PCOS associated with kidney yang insufficiency and exuberant phlegm turbidity.

【Formula Analysis】

The main actions of this formula are to warm and supplement. *Shú dì* (Radix Rehmanniae Praeparata), *xiān líng pí* (Herba Epimedii), and *bǔ gǔ zhī* (Fructus Psoraleae) can promote ovulation and also benefit conditions of dysfunctional uterine bleeding. Medicinals that enrich kidney yin such as *shú dì* (Radix Rehmanniae Praeparata) and *huáng jīng* (Rhizoma Polygonati) are selected to benefit yang since, "without yin, yang cannot arise". This formula can effectively regulate ovulation because kidney tonification methods also modulate gonad-stimulating hormone levels. Improved estrogen levels and biphasic BBT regulation may be expected in many cases.

Hardness-softening and phlegm-transforming medicinals such as *chuān shān jiǎ* (Squama Manis), *zào jiǎo cì* (Spina Gleditsiae), *bīng qiú zǐ* (Rhizoma Bletillae), and *bèi mǔ* (Bulbus Fritillariae) may also improve the testosterone-related symptoms of PCOS. This formula not only acts to directly regulate ovulation with hormone-like effects, but also promotes ovulation through regulation of the hypothalamus- hypophysis.

【Modifications】

➤ With fear of cold, add *fù zǐ* (Radix Aconiti Lateralis Praeparata) 9g and *ròu guì* (Cortex Cinnamomi) 3g.

➤ With liver constraint, add *dān pí* (Cortex Moutan) 9g, *chǎo shān zhī* (Fructus Gardeniae Frictus) 12g, *dāng guī* (Radix Angelicae Sinensis) 12g, *chái hú* (Radix Bupleuri) 6g and *qīng pí* (Pericarpium Citri Reticulatae Viride) 6g. Remove *zào jiǎo cì* (Spina Gleditsiae), *bīng qiú zǐ* (Rhizoma Bletillae) and *bèi mǔ* (Bulbus Fritillariae).

(Yang Si-shu, Yan Xiu-lan, Wang Xin-pei. *Collected Empirical Formulas of Renowned Physicians in Modern China* 中国现代名医验方荟海. 1st edition. Wuhan: Hubei Science and Technology Press, 1996: 1443)

Selected Case Studies

1. MEDICAL RECORDS OF LUO YUAN-KAI: INFERTILITY DUE TO SPLEEN AND KIDNEY DUAL DEFICIENCY WITH LIVER CONSTRAINT

Ms. Rao, age 36.

【Initial Visit】

April 15th, 1978.

The patient complained of being childless after more than 5 years of marriage. She had seen many doctors in the past with no result. Physical examination revealed no abnormality, and the semen analysis was also unremarkable. A recent endometrial biopsy taken 3 hours after menstruation revealed poor glandular secretion and a secretory endometrium.

Menarche arrived at age 15 with the appearance of regular cycles. However, following marriage in 1973, her menstruation became irregular and often delayed every 2 or 3 months. Her cycle had been artificially simulated for several months, but with no result.

Premenstrual breast distention was followed by the appearance of scant dark red menses. Other symptoms and signs included dizziness, fatigue, aching lumbus, cold limbs, long voidings of clear urine, and profuse vaginal discharge. Her complexion appeared sallow with dark macules, and the tongue dusky pale with a white coating. Pulses were deep and thready, weak at both *chi* positions.

【Pattern Differentiation】

Spleen and kidney dual deficiency with liver constraint.

【Treatment Principle】

Tonify kidney and fortify spleen, course the liver and resolve constraint.

【Medicinals】

菟丝子	*tù sī zǐ*	25g	Semen Cuscutae
覆盆子	*fù pén zǐ*	10g	Fructus Rubi
杞子	*qǐ zǐ*	15g	Fructus Lycii
金樱子	*jīn yīng zǐ*	25g	Fructus Rosae Laevigatae
当归	*dāng guī*	12g	Radix Angelicae Sinensis
川芎	*chuān xiōng*	6g	Rhizoma Chuanxiong
首乌	*shǒu wū*	25g	Radix Polygoni Multiflori
党参	*dǎng shēn*	20g	Radix Codonopsis
香附子	*xiāng fù zǐ*	10g	Rhizoma Cyperi

【Second Visit】

April 26th.

Her lumbar pain was relieved at dose 10. All other symptoms were unchanged.

【Ingredients】

菟丝子	tù sī zǐ	25g	Semen Cuscutae
淫羊藿	yín yáng huò	10g	Herba Epimedii
党参	dǎng shēn	20g	Radix Codonopsis
白术	bái zhú	15g	Rhizoma Atractylodis Macrocephalae
鸡血藤	jī xuè téng	30g	Caulis Spatholobi
白芷	bái zhǐ	6g	Radix Angelicae Dahuricae
香附子	xiāng fù zǐ	10g	Rhizoma Cyperi

One decocted daily dose.

【Third Visit】

May 3rd.

Premenstrual breast distention was relieved, and her spirit was improved. Treatment continued to tonify the kidney, fortify the spleen, and nourish blood.

【Ingredients】

菟丝子	tù sī zǐ	25g	Semen Cuscutae
淫羊藿	yín yáng huò	12g	Herba Epimedii
川断	chuān duàn	20g	Radix Dipsaci
金狗脊	jīn gǒu jǐ	20g	Rhizoma Cibotii
党参	dǎng shēn	20g	Radix Codonopsis
白术	bái zhú	15g	Rhizoma Atractylodis Macrocephalae
首乌	shǒu wū	30g	Radix Polygoni Multiflori
白芷	bái zhǐ	10g	Radix Angelicae Dahuricae

【Fourth Visit】

June 25th.

Menses appeared for one day on June 3rd, with increased menstrual flow. Dizziness and lumbar pain were relieved, and her appetite was normal. Her limbs were also somewhat warmer on this visit. Her tongue appeared pale red with a white coating. Pulses were deep and thready.

【Ingredients】

菟丝子	tù sī zǐ	25g	Semen Cuscutae
覆盆子	fù pén zǐ	10g	Fructus Rubi
党参	dǎng shēn	20g	Radix Codonopsis
杞子	qǐ zǐ	15g	Fructus Lycii
金樱子	jīn yīng zǐ	25g	Fructus Rosae Laevigatae
首乌	shǒu wū	25g	Radix Polygoni Multiflori
川芎	chuān xiōng	6g	Rhizoma Chuanxiong
当归	dāng guī	12g	Radix Angelicae Sinensis
香附子	xiāng fù zǐ	10g	Rhizoma Cyperi

4 doses per week; begin after menstruation.

The patient was advised to return after 2 or 3 months.

【Fifth Visit】

September 23rd.

Menstruation appeared on July 23rd for 4 days with a significantly increased menstrual flow, but then ceased for the next two months. She continued taking the formula until August 20th, at which time she experienced dizziness, nausea, poor appetite, and lassitude. A urine test at the local hospital revealed that she had become pregnant.

GYN examination revealed normal conditions consistent with a pregnancy of two months. The tongue appeared pale red with slightly greasy coating. Her pulses were thready, deep and slippery.

Further treatment was applied to tonify the kidney, fortify the spleen, and calm the fetus. The prescribed formula was *Shòu Tāi Wán* (寿胎丸) modified with *Sì Jūn Zǐ Tāng* (四君子汤).

Summary:

The basic cause of infertility in this case was deficiency of the kidney leading to failure to obtain essence. However, the patient presented with dual deficiency of the spleen and kidney, and also premenstrual tension resulting from liver constraint. The treatment principle here is to primarily tonify the kidney and fortify the spleen, and secondarily course the liver and resolve constraint. When the circulation of liver qi becomes normal, harmony returns to the qi and blood. With menstruation returning to normal, the chance of conception becomes much improved.

(Department of Gynecology and Obstetrics, Guangzhou University of TCM. *Anthology of Luo Yuan-kai's Medical Books* 罗元恺医著选 . 1ˢᵗ edition. Guangzhou: Guangdong Science & Technology Press, 1979: 218-222)

2. MEDICAL RECORDS OF CAI XIAO-SUN: INFERTILITY DUE TO KIDNEY DEFICIENCY

Ms. Wang, age 32.

【Initial Visit】

Oct 12ᵗʰ, 1987.

The patient complained of being childless after 4 years of marriage. Her period had arrived on time 3 days previously with scant, thin and pale menses. She now reported a profuse, clear and thin vaginal discharge. Other signs and symptoms included aching lumbus and limp knees, dizziness and tinnitus, and an occasional pulling pain in the lesser abdomen. The tongue coating appeared thin, and her pulses were thready. GYN exam and semen analysis revealed no abnormality in either partner.

【Pattern Differentiation】

Kidney yin insufficiency with insecurity of the girdling vessel.

【Treatment Principle】

Foster the kidney, free the collaterals, secure essence and check vaginal discharge.

【Medicinals】

| 菟丝子 | *tù sī zǐ* | 12g | Semen Cuscutae |
| 茯苓 | *fú líng* | 12g | Poria |

熟地	shú dì	12g	Radix Rehmanniae Praeparata
怀牛膝	huái niú xī	9g	Radix Achyranthis Bidentatae
路路通	lù lù tōng	9g	Fructus Liquidambaris
丁香	dīng xiāng	2.5g	Flos Caryophylli
仙灵脾	xiān líng pí	12g	Herba Epimedii
制黄精	huáng jīng	12g	Rhizoma Polygonati (prepared)
石楠叶	shí nán yè	9g	Folium Photiniae
山萸肉	shān yú ròu	9g	Fructus Corni
青皮	qīng pí	4.5g	Pericarpium Citri Reticulatae Viride
陈皮	chén pí	4.5g	Pericarpium Citri Reticulatae

7 doses.

【Second Visit】

Oct 19th.

The patient reported hypersensitive nipples and a reddish vaginal discharge appearing between periods. Her other symptoms were slightly improved. The tongue coating appeared thin, and her pulses were thready and wiry. The treatment principle here is to warm and foster the kidney.

【Medicinals】

茯苓	fú líng	12g	Poria
熟地	shú dì	9g	Radix Rehmanniae Praeparata
生地	shēng dì	9g	Radix Rehmanniae
石楠叶	shí nán yè	12g	Folium Photiniae
仙灵脾	xiān líng pí	12g	Herba Epimedii
肉苁蓉	ròu cōng róng	12g	Herba Cistanches
紫石英	zǐ shí yīng	12g	Fluoritum
旱莲草	hàn lián cǎo	12g	Herba Ecliptae
狗脊	gǒu jǐ	12g	Rhizoma Cibotii
葫芦巴	hú lú bā	9g	Semen Trigonellae
鹿角霜	lù jiǎo shuāng	9g	Cornu Cervi Degelatinatum

8 doses were prescribed.

Comments:

The kidney stores essence and governs reproduction. Therefore, kidney involvement is a primary consideration in all cases of infertility. Deficiency patterns are most common, with kidney tonification as the root principle in treatment.

This was a relatively simple case of kidney deficiency, so the approach to treatment in this case involved primarily fostering the kidney and freeing the collaterals.

Treatment began immediately following the menstrual period. *Fú líng* (Poria), *shú dì* (Radix Rehmanniae Praeparata), *shēng dì* (Radix Rehmanniae Recens), *huái niú xī* (Radix Achyranthis Bidentatae), *xiān líng pí* (Herba Epimedii) and *shí nán yè* (Folium Photiniae) were applied to harmonize yin and yang while tonifying the liver and kidney. *Dīng xiāng* (Flos Caryophylli) and *lù lù tōng* (Fructus Liquidambaris) were used to warm and free the uterine collaterals. *Tù sī zǐ* (Semen Cuscutae) and *shān yú ròu* (Fructus Corni) were used to secure essence and check vaginal discharge.

After 7 doses, the main focus of treatment was to warm and foster the kidney. *Dīng xiāng* (Flos Caryophylli) and *lù lù tōng* (Fructus Liquidambaris) were removed. *Zǐ shí yīng* (Fluoritum), *hú lú bā* (Semen Trigonellae), and *lù jiǎo shuāng* (Cornu Cervi Degelatinatum) were added to warm yang and foster the kidney to help the uterus obtain essence. *Shú dì* (Radix Rehmanniae Praeparata), *shēng dì* (Radix Rehmanniae Recens) and *hàn lián cǎo* (Herba Ecliptae) were prescribed to restrain yang from becoming hyperactive. *Hàn lián cǎo* (Herba Ecliptae) was also applied to address the reddish vaginal discharge and prevent intermenstrual bleeding.

After 8 doses, remaining symptoms and signs included scant, thin and pale menses due to qi and blood insufficiency. Modified *Bā Zhēn Tāng* (八珍汤) was prescribed to nourish blood and regulate menstruation.

After the menstrual period, the previous approach was applied for another four months. At this point, menstruation ceased and the patient tested positive for pregnancy.

(Cai Xiao-sun. *A Hundred Chinese Medicine Practitioners in a Hundred Years in China: Cai Xiao-sun*. 1st Edition. Beijing: China Press of Traditional Chinese Medicine, 2002, 145-146)

3. Case Studies of Han Bai-ling: Infertility due to Liver Constraint

Ms. Zhi Ji-zi. Initial visit: summer 1976.

The patient complained of infertility for several years. She also suffered lower abdominal discomfort and painful breast distention, which was typically relieved following menstruation. Menses appeared scant and dark purple with clots. Other symptoms and signs included a high clear voice, mental depression, impatience and irascibility, distention of the chest and rib-side, dry heat of the extremities, hiccup, no desire for food or drink, an aversion to greasy foods, constipation, and short voidings of reddish urine. Her complexion appeared dull, and the tongue coating was slightly yellow. Pulses were wiry, rough and forceful.

【Pattern Differentiation】

Liver qi constraint, inhibition of the collaterals, and obstruction of the uterine vessels.

【Treatment Principle】

Regulate the liver, regulate qi, and free the vessels and collaterals.

【Medicinals】

当归	dāng guī	9g	Radix Angelicae Sinensis
赤芍	chì sháo	9g	Radix Paeoniae Rubra
川牛膝	chuān niú xī	9g	Radix Cyathulae
川芎	chuān xiōng	6g	Rhizoma Chuanxiong
王不留行	wáng bù liú xíng	9g	Semen Vaccariae

通草	tōng cǎo	9g	Medulla Tetrapanacis
川楝	chuān liàn	9g	Fructus Toosendan
皂刺	zào cì	9g	Spina Gleditsiae
瓜蒌	guā lóu	9g	Fructus Trichosanthis
丹参	dān shēn	9g	Radix et Rhizoma Salviae Miltiorrhizae
香附	xiāng fù	9g	Rhizoma Cyperi

3 doses.

【Second Visit】

7 days after the initial visit.

Her appetite was improved, but all other symptoms and signs were unchanged. This presentation indicates a pattern of liver qi invading the spleen with spleen qi failing to move. To support the spleen, *bái zhú* (Rhizoma Atractylodis Macrocephalae) 9g and *shān yào* (Rhizoma Dioscoreae) 9g were added. 3 doses were prescribed.

【Third Visit】

The symptoms of breast distention and pain were relieved, and her appetite was improved. She also complained of an aching lumbus. To tonify the liver and kidney, *zào cì* (Spina Gleditsiae) and *guā lóu* (Fructus Trichosanthis) were removed from the basic formula, and *chuān duàn* (Radix Dipsaci) 9g and *sāng jì shēng* (Herba Taxilli) 9g were added. The patient was advised to continue taking the formula over a long period of time. She later reported giving birth to a female infant in the spring of 1978.

Comments:

Infertility conditions are often very tenacious, especially when associated with patterns of liver constraint. Long-term treatment is usually required. In this case, the condition was resolved with the application of an empirical formula composed by Dr. Han Bai-ling.

(Han Bai-ling. Bai-ling's *Gynecology* 百灵妇科 . 1st edition. Heilongjiang: Heilongjiang People's Publishing House, 1980: 161-162)

4. Case Studies of Ban Xiu-wen: Infertility due to Spleen Deficiency and Damp-turbidity

Ms. Cai, age 26.

【Initial Visit】

February 26th, 1974.

Infertility after 4 years of marriage. The patient reported long-term delayed menstruation, cramping and spasms in the lower abdomen during and after menstruation, and lumbar discomfort. Other symptoms and signs included a thick white vaginal discharge, and scant pale menses. Her appetite and elimination were normal. The tongue appeared with a moist white coating and teethmarks. Pulses were deep, thready and slow. GYN examination revealed a retroverted uterus, somewhat small in size.

【Pattern Differentiation】

Constrained damp-turbidity obstructing the qi dynamic.

【Treatment Principle】

Fortify the spleen, dry dampness, nourish blood, and regulate menstruation.

【Medicinals】

当归	dāng guī	9g	Radix Angelicae Sinensis
白芍	bái sháo	9g	Radix Paeoniae Alba
川芎	chuān xiōng	6g	Rhizoma Chuanxiong
茯苓	fú líng	15g	Poria
白术	bái zhú	9g	Rhizoma Atractylodis Macrocephalae
泽泻	zé xiè	9g	Rhizoma Alismatis
胆南星	dǎn nán xīng	9g	Arisaema cum Bile
法半夏	fǎ bàn xià	9g	Rhizoma Pinelliae Praeparatum
陈皮	chén pí	15g	Pericarpium Citri Reticulatae
益母草	yì mǔ cǎo	8g	Herba Leonuri
淫羊藿	yín yáng huò	9g	Herba Epimedii

甘草	gān cǎo	3g	Radix et Rhizoma Glycyrrhizae

6 daily decocted doses were prescribed.

【Second Visit】

April 6th.

The vaginal discharge resolved after 12 doses. Her previous menstrual period arrived March 17th. Menses appeared scant and dark red, but menstruation was otherwise normal. The tongue coating was thin white, and her pulses thready and moderate. The treatment principle was modified to emphasize tonification of the liver and kidney, while also regulating the penetrating and conception vessels.

【Medicinals】

菟丝子	tù sī zǐ	15g	Semen Cuscutae
川杞子	chuān qǐ zǐ	10g	Fructus Lycii
覆盆子	fù pén zǐ	10g	Fructus Rubi
车前子	chē qián zǐ	10g	Semen Plantaginis
五味子	wǔ wèi zǐ	5g	Fructus Schisandrae Chinensis
女贞子	nǚ zhēn zǐ	9g	Fructus Ligustri Lucidi
淫羊藿	yín yáng huò	9g	Herba Epimedii
当归身	dāng guī shēn	9g	Radix Angelicae Sinensis
黄精	huáng jīng	15g	Rhizoma Polygonati
淮山药	huái shān yào	15g	Rhizoma Dioscoreae
柴胡	chái hú	5g	Radix Bupleuri

【Third Visit】

Menstruation arrived April 17th with profuse red menses and no discomfort. The tongue coating appeared normal, and pulses were moderate. Since the patient was menstruating, a prescription was selected to primarily nourish blood.

【Medicinals】

当归身	dāng guī shēn	15g	Radix Angelicae Sinensis
川芎	chuān xiōng	5g	Rhizoma Chuanxiong

白芍	bái sháo	5g	Radix Paeoniae Alba
熟地	shú dì	15g	Radix Rehmanniae Praeparata
党参	dǎng shēn	15g	Radix Codonopsis
北芪	běi qí	15g	Radix Astragali Septentrionalis
坤草	kūn cǎo	12g	Herba Leonuri
艾叶	ài yè	2g	Folium Artemisiae Argyi
炙甘草	zhì gān cǎo	5g	Radix et Rhizoma Glycyrrhizae Praeparata cum Melle

3 decocted daily doses were prescribed.

【Fourth Visit】

May 30th.

Menstruation had been delayed for more than 10 days. She also complained of lassitude and a poor appetite. Her pulses were thready and slippery. The symptoms suggested pregnancy, so treatment was temporarily withdrawn and dietary guidelines were advised. She later gave birth to a healthy infant.

Comments:

Pathogenic damp is heavy, turbid and sticky. These qualities easily constrain the lower burner and uterus while also obstructing vital qi. This leads to failure of the penetrating vessel to govern the sea of blood, and the conception vessel failing to nourish the fetus. Delayed menstruation, scant pale menses, thick vaginal discharge, and infertility may result. All of these symptoms are caused by constraint and non-transformation of pathogenic damp. To benefit menstruation, first resolve the vaginal discharge. To resolve vaginal discharge, first dry the dampness.

According to the *Essential Prescriptions of the Golden Chamber* (金匮要略 , *Jīn Guì Yào Lüè*), "Phlegm-rheum should be harmonized with warming medicinals." In this case, *Dāng Guī Sháo Yào Sǎn* (当归芍药散) was combined with modified *Èr Chén Tāng* (二陈汤) to fortify the spleen, dry dampness, nourish blood, and regulate menstruation.

The signs and symptoms of internal dampness were resolved after 6 doses with the cessation of vaginal discharge. Menstruation also returned to normal. At the second visit, medicinals were applied to tonify the liver and kidney and also to regulate and nourish the penetrating and conception vessels. This approach aims to build up the root source of transformation so that essence becomes abundant, and qi and blood become sufficient. In this case, the application of this method resulted in a successful pregnancy.

(Ban Xiu-wen. *Anthology of Ban Xiu-wen's Gynecological Cases and Medical Treatises* 班秀文妇科医论医案选 . 1st edition. Beijing: People's Medical Publishing House, 1987: 205-206.)

5. MEDICAL RECORDS OF LI LI-YUN: INFERTILITY DUE TO QI DEFICIENCY AND BLOOD STASIS

Ms. Sang, age 32.

【Initial Visit】

July 25th, 1996.

Childless after 10 years of marriage. The patient reported that her menstruation was usually normal, but that her previous period on July 5 appeared with profuse menses and clots. She now complained of a sagging pain in the lesser abdomen, fatigued spirit, lack of strength, and a poor appetite. Urine and stool were reported normal. Her complexion was bright white, and her tongue appeared pale and dull with thin white coating. Pulses were thready and weak. GYN examination revealed a retroverted uterus of normal size, with thickening and tenderness of the uterosacral ligament.

【Pattern Differentiation】

Qi deficiency and blood stasis.

【Treatment Principle】

Supplement qi and dispel stasis.

【Formulas and Medicinals】

党参	dǎng shēn	15g	Radix Codonopsis
北芪	běi qí	15g	Radix Astragali Septentrionalis
白术	bái zhú	9g	Rhizoma Atractylodis Macrocephalae
炙甘草	zhì gān cǎo	6g	Radix et Rhizoma Glycyrrhizae Praeparata cum Melle
当归	dāng guī	9g	Radix Angelicae Sinensis
川芎	chuān xiōng	6g	Rhizoma Chuanxiong
鸡血藤	jī xuè téng	30g	Caulis Spatholobi
赤芍	chì sháo	12g	Radix Paeoniae Rubra

One decocted daily dose was prescribed.

【Second Visit】

August 5th.

After 10 doses, the lower abdominal discomfort had resolved, with her spirit and appetite both improved. The tongue and pulse signs were unchanged. Her previous menstrual period arrived on July 29th. Menses appeared bright red and moderate in volume. Hydrotubation revealed no obstruction of the oviduct, and ultrasound showed a normal uterus. No internal masses were found upon palpation.

Chuān duàn (Radix Dipsaci) 15g and *xiāng fù* (Rhizoma Cyperi) 9g were added to the formula. *Jī xuè téng* (Caulis Spatholobi) and *zhì gān cǎo* (Radix et Rhizoma Glycyrrhizae Praeparata cum Melle) were removed.

【Third Visit】

August 15th.

After 10 doses, all previous symptoms remained unchanged, but her basal body temperature indicated that she was about to ovulate. Medicinals were selected to mainly supplement qi and invigorate blood.

【Formulas and Medicinals】

白术	bái zhú	12g	Rhizoma Atractylodis Macrocephalae
党参	dǎng shēn	15g	Radix Codonopsis

北芪	běi qí	15g	Radix Astragali Septentrionalis
当归	dāng guī	9g	Radix Angelicae Sinensis
川芎	chuān xiōng	6g	Rhizoma Chuanxiong
丹参	dān shēn	9g	Radix et Rhizoma Salviae Miltiorrhizae
桂枝	guì zhī	6g	Ramulus Cinnamomi
艾叶	ài yè	6g	Folium Artemisiae Argyi

One decocted daily dose.

【Fourth Visit】

August 26th.

The patient reported that she had not menstruated for 50 days. She complained of dizziness, nausea, poor appetite, and lassitude. She had also tested positive for pregnancy, and ultrasound examination revealed the presence of a normal fetus. The treatment principle here is to tonify the kidney, fortify the spleen, and calm the fetus. The patient later gave birth to a healthy infant.

Comments:

The spleen is known as the root of the aquired constitution, and also the source of and qi and blood engendering and transformation. Spleen and stomach deficiency can also affect conception. When the source of qi and blood becomes insufficient, the sea of blood may become empty, and reproduction is affected. This can manifest with an empty or sagging sensation in the lower abdomen as a result of deficient qi failing to upraise. Furthermore, qi is the commander of the blood. Profuse menses with clots will manifest as a result of deficient qi failing to move blood. The formula prescribed in this case acts to fortify the spleen, supplement and regulate qi, engender and nourish blood, and dispel stasis. The chance of conception is greatly increased when the penetrating and conception vessels are well-nourished and regulated, and qi and blood become abundant.

(Li Li-yun, Wang Xiao-yun. *Gynecological Pattern Identification and*

Treatment of Chinese Medicine 中医妇科临证证治 . 1ˢᵗ edition. Guangzhou: Guangdong People's Publishing House, 1999: 288-289)

6. CASE STUDIES OF QIAN BO-XUAN: INFERTILITY DUE TO LIVER CONSTRAINT, KIDNEY DEFICIENCY AND DAMP-HEAT POURING DOWNWARD

Ms. Zhang, age 29.

【Initial Visit】

November 11ᵗʰ, 1972.

Infertility after 5 years of marriage. The patient reported a history of painful menstruation which had been effectively managed with Chinese medicinals. Her menstrual cycle arrived every 30 days, with a period of 7-8 days and moderate menstrual flow. Other signs and symptoms included distending pain of the lesser abdomen, aching lumbus, lack of strength, frequent vaginal discharge, profuse dreaming, vexation, and irascibility. The tongue coating appeared slimy and pale yellow with slight peeling in the center. Pulses were thin, thready and rapid. GYN examination revealed no abnormality.

【Pattern Differentiation】

Liver constraint, kidney deficiency, and damp-heat pouring downward.

【Treatment Principle】

Course the liver, benefit the kidney, clear heat, and eliminate dampness.

【Medicinals】

茯苓	fú líng	12g	Poria
山药	shān yào	12g	Rhizoma Dioscoreae
桑寄生	sāng jì shēng	15g	Ramus Loranthi seu Visci
川断	chuān duàn	20g	Radix Dipsaci
制香附	zhì xiāng fù	6g	Rhizoma Cyperi (prepared)
乌药	wū yào	6g	Radix Linderae
柴胡	chái hú	6g	Radix Bupleuri

薏苡仁	yì yǐ rén	12g	Semen Coicis
椿根皮	chūn gēn pí	12g	Cortex Ailanthi
贯众	guàn zhòng	12g	Rhizoma Cyrtomii
木香	mù xiāng	6g	Radix Aucklandiae
黄柏	huáng bǎi	3g	Cortex Phellodendri Chinensis

One daily decocted dose. 16 doses were prescribed.

【Second Visit】

The vaginal discharge was markedly reduced, and most of the other symptoms were also relieved. She still complained of lassitude with aching of the lower back. Her tongue appeared red with a slimy and pale yellow coating. Pulses were thin and soft on the left, and thin and wiry on the right.

The pattern of damp-heat seemed to be gradually resolving. The treatment principle here is to fortify the spleen, course the liver, and benefit the kidney.

【Medicinals】

党参	dǎng shēn	12g	Radix Codonopsis
白术	bái zhú	9g	Rhizoma Atractylodis Macrocephalae
茯苓	fú líng	12g	Poria
川断	chuān duàn	12g	Radix Dipsaci
山药	shān yào	12g	Rhizoma Dioscoreae
桑寄生	sāng jì shēng	12g	Ramus Loranthi seu Visci
柴胡	chái hú	6g	Radix Bupleuri
制香附	zhì xiāng fù	6g	Rhizoma Cyperi (prepared)
牛膝	niú xī	9g	Radix Achyranthis Bidentatae
艾叶	ài yè	6g	Folium Artemisiae Argyi
贯众	guàn zhòng	12g	Rhizoma Cyrtomii
川楝	chuān liàn	6g	Fructus Toosendan

One daily decocted dose. 16 doses were prescribed.

【Second Visit】

January 5th, 1973.

Menstruation arrived on December 19th for a period of 8 days. Menstrual symptoms included slight pain of lesser abdomen, fatigued spirit, and a lack of strength. Other symptoms and signs included nausea, torpid intake, cold and numbness of the feet, and disturbed sleep. The tongue coating was slightly yellow at the root. Pulses were thin, wiry and slippery.

These symptoms indicate a pattern of liver qi couterflowing upwards with liver and stomach disharmony. The treatment principle here is to course the liver, regulate qi, fortify the spleen, and harmonize the stomach.

【Medicinals】

白芍	bái sháo	9g	Radix Paeoniae Alba
柴胡	chái hú	6g	Radix Bupleuri
旋覆花	xuán fù huā	9g	Flos Inulae (wrapped)
茯苓	fú líng	12g	Poria
牛膝	niú xī	9g	Radix Achyranthis Bidentatae
橘皮	jú pí	9g	Pericarpium Citri Reticulatae
法半夏	fǎ bàn xià	9g	Rhizoma Pinelliae Praeparatum
佛手	fó shǒu	6g	Fructus Citri Sarcodactylis
木瓜	mù guā	6g	Fructus Chaenomelis
远志	yuǎn zhì	6g	Radix Polygalae

One daily decocted dose. 8 doses were prescribed.

The patient returned on March 28th to report that she had been pregnant for 3 months. However, she also suffered with lumbar pain due to an accidental fall on March 20th.

A formula was prescribed to secure the fetus and benefit the kidney.

【Medicinals】

干地黄	dì huáng	12g	Radix Rehmanniae (dried)
白芍	bái sháo	9g	Radix Paeoniae Alba
制香附	zhì xiāng fù	6g	Rhizoma Cyperi (prepared)
木香	mù xiāng	6g	Radix Aucklandiae

紫苏梗	zǐ sū gěng	6g	Caulis Perillae
木瓜	mù guā	9g	Fructus Chaenomelis
白术	bái zhú	9g	Rhizoma Atractylodis Macrocephalae
山药	shān yào	12g	Rhizoma Dioscoreae
川断	chuān duàn	12g	Radix Dipsaci
桑寄生	sāng jì shēng	12g	Ramus Loranthi seu Visci

One daily decocted dose. 8 doses were prescribed.

Comments:

This is a case of infertility associated with damp-heat brewing in the lower burner due to liver constraint, qi stagnation, and kidney yin depletion. Treatment methods were applied initially to course the liver, benefit the kidney, clear heat, and eliminate dampness. Later treatments emphasized harmonizing of qi and blood by coursing the liver, fortifying the spleen, and regulating the stomach. As a result, the patient was able to achieve a successful pregnancy.

(Edited by Xi Yuan Hospital of Chinese Medicine Institute of China. *Collected Works of Renowned Contemporary Physicians of Chinese Medicine: Volume 1: Gynecology Case Studies of Qian Bo-xuan* 现代著名老中医名著重刊丛书 . 第一辑 . 钱伯煊妇科医案 . Beijing: People's Medical Publishing House, 2005, 122-123)

7. CASE STUDIES OF HA LI-TIAN: INFERTILITY DUE TO KIDNEY YIN DEFICIENCY WITH BINDING OF PHLEGM AND HEAT

Ms. Sun, age 28.

【Initial Visit】

May 4th, 1972.

Infertility after 3 years of marriage. The patient reported regular menstruation until 1968, when she was also diagnosed with hyperthyroidism. Her presenting symptoms at that time included palpitation, insomnia, trembling hands, spontaneous sweating, and vexing heat. These symptoms were relieved following treatments with biomedicines and Chinese medicinal treatments, but her menstrual cycles remained irregular.

GYN examination revealed a small uterus. At the initial visit, the patient displayed an enlarged neck with a swollen thyroid. She also suffered from a constant feeling of suffocation, with facial heat sensations. Other signs and symptoms included aching lumbus, lack of strength, and a thick vaginal discharge. Menstruation was delayed, with scant dark menses. Her last period arrived on March 23rd. The tongue appeared red with a thin slimy coating. Pulses were wiry, thin and slightly rapid.

【Pattern Differentiation】

Binding of phlegm and heat affecting kidney yin.

【Treatment Principle】

Clear heat, resolve phlegm, soften hardness, dissipate binding, and benefit kidney yin.

【Medicinals】

山慈菇	*shān cí gū*	30g	Pseudobulbus Cremastrae seu Pleiones
黄药子	*huáng yào zǐ*	15g	Rhizoma Dioscoreae Bulbiferae
石楠叶	*shí nán yè*	12g	Folium Photiniae
女贞子	*nǚ zhēn zǐ*	12g	Fructus Ligustri Lucidi
旱莲草	*hàn lián cǎo*	9g	Herba Ecliptae
海藻	*hǎi zǎo*	9g	Sargassum
昆布	*kūn bù*	9g	Thallus Laminariae
穿山甲	*chuān shān jiǎ*	9g	Squama Manis

Grind into fine powder and take 3g, twice daily with brown sugar water. 15 days constitutes one course of treatment. The patient was advised to stop taking the formula for awhile following each one month period.

A twice daily medicinal bath containing *shé chuáng zǐ* (Fructus Cnidii) 12g, *huáng bǎi* (Cortex Phellodendri Chinensis) 6g, and *wú zhū yú* (Fructus

Evodiae) 3g was also prescribed.

After several months of treatment her neck and thyroid appeared normal, with her appetite and sleep also improved. The facial heat sensation and aching lumbus were completely relieved. Menstruation appeared normally except for some minor premenstrual discomfort.

The patient was instructed to take the same prescription once each morning, with one dose of *Bā Bǎo Kūn Shùn Dān* (八宝坤顺丹) before bed. After three months of treatment, the patient achieved a successful pregnancy.

Comments:

The *Yellow Emperor's Inner Classic* (黄帝内经 , *Huáng Dì Nèi Jīng*) states, "When reversal follows other symptoms, treat the root." Menstruation was initially normal in this case, with irregular menstruation and infertility occurring after a diagnosis of hyperthyroidism. As ancient physician Xiao Shen-zhai stated in *Principles for Women's Diseases* (女科 经纶 , *Nǚ Kē Jīng Lún*), "When treating irregular menstruation caused by other diseases, treat the other condition first. Menstruation will become regulated quite naturally."

An enlarged neck, a feeling of suffocation, swollen thyroid, thick vaginal discharge, facial heat sensation, and aching lumbus all indicate binding of phlegm and heat obstructing the qi passage, as well as damp-heat pouring downward affecting kidney yin.

Shān cí gū (Pseudobulbus Cremastrae seu Pleiones) and *huáng yào zǐ* (Rhizoma Dioscoreae Bulbiferae) were applied to resolve toxin, disperse swelling, and check vaginal discharge. *Hǎi zǎo* (Sargassum) and *kūn bù* (Thallus Laminariae) act to clear heat, disperse phlegm, soften hardness, and dissipate binding. *Chuān shān jiǎ* (Squama Manis) breaks blood, resolves stasis, and frees the channels and collaterals. *Shí nán yè* (Folium Photiniae), *nǚ zhēn zǐ* (Fructus Ligustri Lucidi) and *hàn lián cǎo* (Herba Ecliptae) were added to tonify kidney and essence, enrich water, and moisten wood.

Considering the long-term nature of the condition, a quick therapeutic effect could not be expected. Powdered medicinals were applied to produce a slow yet stable effect. Over time, menstruation became regular and pregnancy was acheived.

(Ha Li-tian. *Selected Gynecology Case Studies of Ha Li-tian.* 1st Edition. Tianjin: Tianjin Science and Technology Press, 1982, 192-194)

8. Case Studies of He Zi-huai: Infertility due to Phlegm-damp Obstruction

Ms. Hu, age 28.

【Initial Visit】

Infertility after 5 years of marriage. The patient reported delayed menstration for 10 to 15 days, and scant pale menses. Other symptoms and signs included obesity, nausea, and phlegm-drool.

【Pattern Differentiation】

Phlegm-damp obstruction with uterine congestion.

【Treatment Principle】

Warm and resolve phlegm-damp, soothe qi and blood.

【Medicinals】

苍术	cāng zhú	9g	Rhizoma Atractylodis
白术	bái zhú	9g	Rhizoma Atractylodis Macrocephalae
半夏（竹沥）	bàn xià (zhú lì)	9g	Rhizoma Pinelliae (prepared with Bambusae Succus)
泽兰	zé lán	9g	Herba Lycopi
泽泻	zé xiè	9g	Rhizoma Alismatis
陈胆星	chén dǎn xīng	9g	Arisaema cum Bile
茯苓	fú líng	12g	Poria
海浮石	hǎi fú shí	12g	Pumex
生山楂	shān zhā	30g	Fructus Crataegi
椒目	jiāo mù	1.5g	Pericarpium Zanthoxyli

肉桂	ròu guì	3g	Cortex Cinnamomi
六一散	Liù Yī Săn	9g	Six-to-One Powder

Menstruation was normal after one month of treatment. The patient also had lost weight; and her mental status was improved.

The treatment principle here is to nourish blood and warm the middle.

【Medicinals】

当归	dāng guī	9g	Radix Angelicae Sinensis
炒白术	chăo bái zhú	9g	Rhizoma Atractylodis Macrocephalae (dry-fried)
泽兰	zé lán	9g	Herba Lycopi
泽泻	zé xiè	9g	Rhizoma Alismatis
茯苓	fú líng	9g	Poria
制香附	xiāng fù	9g	Rhizoma Cyperi (prepared)
紫石英	zǐ shí yīng	30g	Fluoritum
丹参	dān shēn	12g	Radix et Rhizoma Salviae Miltiorrhizae
橘皮	jú pí	5g	Pericarpium Citri Reticulatae
橘络	jú luò	5g	Vascular Aurantii
炒小茴香	chăo xiăo huí xiāng	5g	Fructus Foeniculi (dry-fried)
炙甘草	zhì gān căo	5g	Radix et Rhizoma Glycyrrhizae Praeparata cum Melle

After 4 months of treatment, pregnancy testing showed that she had conceived. Treatment was withdrawn, and the patient later gave birth to a healthy infant.

Comments:

According to Zhu Dan-xi, infertility among obese women is generally associated with menstrual block due to fat congesting the uterus. The appearance of obesity often indicates spleen deficiency with failure to transport. As a result, phlegm-damp is engendered internally, which then leads to inhibition of the qi dynamic and also irregular menstruation.

The contemporary physician Zhu Xiao-nan has stated, "Blood moves through the spleen channel". When spleen deficiency with phlegm-damp involves the essence [of grain and water] failing to transform into blood, scant menstruation with shortened cycles may appear, or even menstrual block.

The *Compendium of Treating Females* (济阴纲目 , *Jì Yīn Gāng Mù*) states, "With obesity and fat filling the uterus, one cannot bear children even when menstruation appears normally. Uterus-opening medicinals must be applied to disperse the fat." Zhu Dan-xi's treatment method for excessive dampness and fat congestion is to dry dampness, eliminate phlegm, and move qi. Medicinals include *Dǎo Tán Tāng* (导痰汤), or *Èr Chén Tāng* (二陈汤) with added *cāng zhú* (Rhizoma Atractylodis), *bái zhú* (Rhizoma Atractylodis Macrocephalae), *mù xiāng* (Radix Aucklandiae), *xiāng fù* (Rhizoma Cyperi), *chuān xiōng* (Rhizoma Chuanxiong) and *dāng guī* (Radix Angelicae Sinensis).

In this case, the presenting signs and symptoms indicated a pattern of phlegm-damp obstruction. Following Zhu Dan-xi's treatment method, *cāng zhú* (Rhizoma Atractylodis), *bái zhú* (Rhizoma Atractylodis Macrocephalae), *fú líng* (Poria), *xiāng fù* (Rhizoma Cyperi), *bàn xià* (Rhizoma Pinelliae), *zé xiè* (Rhizoma Alismatis), *jú pí* (Pericarpium Citri Reticulatae), and *shān zhā* (Fructus Crataegi) were applied to dry dampness, eliminate phlegm, disperse fat, and regulate qi. *Jiāo mù* (Pericarpium Zanthoxyli) and *ròu guì* (Cortex Cinnamomi) act to warm the kidney and spleen, and also promote the transformation of dampness. *Chén dǎn xīng* (Arisaema cum Bile) and *hǎi fú shí* (Pumex) are applied to forcefully eliminate phlegm.

Medicinals should be applied to nourish blood and regulate menstruation only after the fat congestion has resolved. However, rich-flavored medicinals that replenish essence, tonify the kidney, and assist yang should be applied with caution. Their improper application may increase both internal dampness and pathogenic phlegm.

(Wen Le-xi. *Case Studies of Famous Gynecology Physicians.* 1st Edition.

Beijing: People's Military Surgeon Publishing House, 2007, 387-388)

9. CASE STUDIES OF PANG PAN-CHI: INFERTILITY DUE TO DAMP-HEAT AND STASIS OBSTRUCTION

Ms. Shen, age 29.

【Initial Visit】

November 30th, 1974.

Chief complaint: Infertility.

The patient had suffered from distending pain in the right lower abdomen for several months, especially during the premenstrual period. Other signs and symptoms included aching lumbus, vaginal discharge, emaciation, and poor appetite. The tongue coating appeared thin yellow and slimy. Pulses were wiry, thready and rapid.

GYN examination revealed minor cervicitis, and anteversion of the uterus. Palpation revealed a 2.5 cm × 3 cm mass present on the right side.

【Pattern Differentiation】

Damp-heat and stasis obstruction.

【Treatment Principle】

Regulate qi, dispel stasis, and clear damp-heat.

【Medicinals】

柴胡	chái hú	4.5g	Radix Bupleuri
当归	dāng guī	9g	Radix Angelicae Sinensis
赤芍	chì sháo	9g	Radix Paeoniae Rubra
白芍	bái sháo	9g	Radix Paeoniae Alba
川楝	chuān liàn	9g	Fructus Toosendan
延胡索	yán hú suǒ	9g	Rhizoma Corydalis
苍术	cāng zhú	9g	Rhizoma Atractylodis
红藤	hóng téng	30g	Caulis Sargentodoxae
小茴香	xiǎo huí xiāng	9g	Fructus Foeniculi
牡丹皮	mǔ dān pí	9g	Cortex Moutan
制香附	zhì xiāng fù	9g	Rhizoma Cyperi (prepared)

【**Second Visit**】

December 25th, 1974.

Menstruation arrived on the 14th. The patient reported less premenstrual pain, but the symptoms of lumbar pain and vaginal discharge were unchanged. The tongue appeared red at the margins, with a thin coating. Pulses were wiry, thready and rapid. This presentation indicates a pattern of qi stagnation and damp obstruction impairing the kidney qi. The previous formula was modified to more strongly tonify the kidney.

【**Medicinals**】

柴胡	*chái hú*	4.5g	Radix Bupleuri
当归	*dāng guī*	9g	Radix Angelicae Sinensis
赤芍	*chì sháo*	9g	Radix Paeoniae Rubra
白芍	*bái sháo*	9g	Radix Paeoniae Alba
川芎	*chuān xiōng*	9g	Rhizoma Chuanxiong
熟地黄	*shú dì huáng*	9g	Radix Rehmanniae Praeparata
生地黄	*shēng dì huáng*	9g	Radix Rehmanniae
肉苁蓉	*ròu cōng róng*	9g	Herba Cistanches
川断	*chuān duàn*	9g	Radix Dipsaci
菟丝子	*tù sī zǐ*	9g	Semen Cuscutae
牡丹皮	*mǔ dān pí*	9g	Cortex Moutan
红藤	*hóng téng*	30g	Caulis Sargentodoxae
薏苡仁	*yì yǐ rén*	12g	Semen Coicis

【**Third Visit**】

The patient complained of a dull pain in the right lower abdomen and lumbus. However, the amount of vaginal discharge had decreased. Her tongue was red with a thin slimy coating. Pulses were wiry, thready and rapid.

This presentation indicates a pattern of qi stagnation, stasis obstruction, and constrained fire brewing internally, so further tonification is contraindicated. The appropriate treatment method here is to regulate qi, dispel stasis, clear heat, and resolve constraint.

【Medicinals】

柴胡	chái hú	4.5g	Radix Bupleuri
当归	dāng guī	9g	Radix Angelicae Sinensis
赤芍	chì sháo	9g	Radix Paeoniae Rubra
牡丹皮	mǔ dān pí	9g	Cortex Moutan
制香附	zhì xiāng fù	9g	Rhizoma Cyperi (prepared)
炒栀子	chǎo zhī zǐ	9g	Fructus Gardeniae Praeparatus (stir-fried)
红藤	hóng téng	30g	Caulis Sargentodoxae
郁金	yù jīn	9g	Radix Curcumae
败酱草	bài jiàng cǎo	30g	Herba Patriniae
薏苡仁	yì yǐ rén	12g	Semen Coicis
桃仁	táo rén	12g	Semen Persicae
小茴香	xiǎo huí xiāng	9g	Fructus Foeniculi

【Fourth Visit】

January 14th, 1975

Menstruation arrived on January 8th, with scant bright red menses. Premenstrual pain of the lesser abdomen also persisted to some degree. Following menstruation, she experienced some intermittent stabbing lesser abdominal pain. No vaginal discharge or lumbar pain was reported. The pulse images and tongue appearance remained the same. The previous formula was slightly modified.

【Medicinals】

柴胡	chái hú	4.5g	Radix Bupleuri
郁金	yù jīn	9g	Radix Curcumae
牡丹皮	mǔ dān pí	9g	Cortex Moutan
炒栀子	chǎo zhī zǐ	9g	Fructus Gardeniae Praeparatus (stir-fried)
生薏苡仁	yì yǐ rén	9g	Semen Coicis (raw)
延胡索	yán hú suǒ	9g	Rhizoma Corydalis
川楝	chuān liàn	9g	Fructus Toosendan
红藤	hóng téng	30g	Caulis Sargentodoxae
败酱草	bài jiàng cǎo	30g	Herba Patriniae
川断	chuān duàn	9g	Radix Dipsaci

狗脊	*gǒu jǐ*	9g	Rhizoma Cibotii

【Fifth Visit】

January 17th, 1975.

The distending pain of the lower abdomen was greatly relieved. Lumbar pain had resolved, and the slimy tongue coating was also gone. Her pulses were wiry and thready. Since the previous prescription had taken effect, there was no need for modification.

【Medicinals】

柴胡	*chái hú*	4.5g	Radix Bupleuri
郁金	*yù jīn*	9g	Radix Curcumae
牡丹皮	*mǔ dān pí*	9g	Cortex Moutan
制香附	*zhì xiāng fù*	9g	Rhizoma Cyperi (prepared)
赤芍	*chì sháo*	9g	Radix Paeoniae Rubra
白芍	*bái sháo*	9g	Radix Paeoniae Alba
当归	*dāng guī*	9g	Radix Angelicae Sinensis
红藤	*hóng téng*	30g	Caulis Sargentodoxae
败酱草	*bài jiàng cǎo*	30g	Herba Patriniae
薏苡仁	*yì yǐ rén*	12g	Semen Coicis
桃仁	*táo rén*	12g	Semen Persicae

【Sixth Visit】

Along with the previous prescription, the patient received ten sessions of electrotherapy treatment. All symptoms were completely relieved, and treatment was discontinued. Her menstrual cycles had been regular for several months, with no abdominal pain. However, menstruation had been delayed for 11 days as of this visit. She also reported torpid intake, oppression of the chest, bland taste in the mouth, fatigue, lack of strength, and distending pain of the nipples. The tongue appeared red at the tip with a thin coating. Pulses were small, thready and rapid. Urine testing revealed that she had become pregnant. Medicinals were prescribed to harmonize the stomach and secure the fetus.

Comments:

Infertility can be caused by a variety of factors. The indiscriminate use of warming and tonifying medicinals is quite common, because many practitioners tend to incorrectly diagnose patterns of uterine cold. In this case, the pattern is clearly damp-heat and constrained fire congesting lower burner. Generally speaking, branch symptoms must be first eliminated in order to effectively address the root condition. Since infection was present in this case, cool and cold medicinals were applied to treat root and branch simultaneously. The red tongue and rapid pulses also confirmed the presence of internal heat. To promote conception, medicinals that regulate menstruation, dispel stasis, and promote the free flow of qi were also applied.

Cases of infertility presenting with patterns of constrained fire and obstruction due to damp and stasis will respond well to the formula *Dān Zhī Xiāo Yáo Sǎn* (丹栀逍遥散) with added *hóng téng* (Caulis Sargentodoxae) and *bài jiàng cǎo* (Herba Patriniae). Electrotherapy may also be applied to increase the therapeutic effect.

(Literature Graduate School of Shanghai Chinese Medicine University. *Collected Experience from Renowned Gynecologist Pang pan-chi*. 1st Edition. Shanghai: Shanghai TCM University Publishing House, 2004, 28-30)

10. CASE STUDIES OF LIU FENG-WU: INFERTILITY DUE TO QI AND BLOOD DUAL DEFICIENCY

Ms. Ren, age 35.

【Initial Visit】

April 5th, 1973.

Chief complaint: Infertility for 5 years.

Menarche arrived at age 17, with the appearance of regular cycles. The patient reported a history of premenstrual dizziness, nausea and vomiting, and menstrual pain of the lumbus and abdomen. These symptoms were generally managed with Chinese medicine and other prescription medications. However, after giving birth in 1968, her menstrual cycles became irregular with scant pale menses. She also reported menstrual pain of the lumbus and abdomen which was somewhat relieved by warmth and pressure. Other symptoms and signs included flusteredness, shortness of breath, lack of strength, and profuse dreaming. After the first childbirth, she had been not able to conceive for 5 years. Her tongue appeared dark with a thin white coating. Pulses were thready and moderate. GYN examination revealed a retroverted uterus of reduced size.

【Pattern Differentiation】

Qi and blood dual deficiency with heart and spleen insufficiency.

【Treatment Principle】

Supplement qi and blood, tonify heart and spleen.

【Medicinals】

当归	dāng guī	15g	Radix Angelicae Sinensis
白芍	bái sháo	9g	Radix Paeoniae Alba
川芎	chuān xiōng	4.5g	Rhizoma Chuanxiong
益母草	yì mǔ cǎo	9g	Herba Leonuri
党参	dǎng shēn	12g	Radix Codonopsis
炒白术	chǎo bái zhú	15g	Rhizoma Atractylodis Macrocephalae (dry-fried)
黄芪	huáng qí	15g	Radix Astragali
茯苓	fú líng	12g	Poria
甘草	gān cǎo	6g	Radix et Rhizoma Glycyrrhizae
山药	shān yào	12g	Rhizoma Dioscoreae
龙眼肉	lóng yǎn ròu	9g	Arillus Longan
酸枣仁	suān zǎo rén	12g	Semen Ziziphi Spinosae

8 doses were prescribed along with 20 pills of *Kūn Shùn Dān* (坤顺丹).

The patient later reported normal menstruation and also relief from her lumbar and abdominal pain.

On July 12th she reported that her cycle had been delayed for over one month. She then tested positive for pregnancy, and later gave birth to a healthy infant.

Comments:

This infertility case was associated with patterns of qi and blood dual deficiency with heart and spleen insufficiency. The deficiency pattern initially appeared after the patient gave birth to her first child, manifesting with irregular menstruation and scant pale menses. She also experienced menstrual pain due to emptiness of the sea of blood and malnourishment of the uterine collaterals.

The pattern of heart and spleen insufficiency manifested with flusteredness, shortness of breath, lack of strength, and profuse dreaming. When the sea of blood becomes empty and the uterine vessels are in lack of nourishment, pregnancy cannot be expected.

Modified *Guī Pí Tāng* (归脾汤) was selected.

Dāng guī (Radix Angelicae Sinensis), *bái sháo* (Radix Paeoniae Alba) and *chuān xiōng* (Rhizoma Chuanxiong) together nourish blood. *Huáng qí* (Radix Astragali) also tonifies blood. *Dǎng shēn* (Radix Codonopsis), *chǎo bái zhú* (dry-fried Rhizoma Atractylodis Macrocephalae), *fú líng* (Poria), *gān cǎo* (Radix et Rhizoma Glycyrrhizae) and *shān yào* (Rhizoma Dioscoreae) fortify the spleen and tonify qi. *Lóng yǎn ròu* (Arillus Longan) and *suān zǎo rén* (Semen Ziziphi Spinosae) nourish the heart and calm the spirit. *Yì mǔ cǎo* (Herba Leonuri) was selected to invigorate blood and regulate menstruation. The basic formula was combined with with *Kūn Shùn Dān* (坤顺丹).

After more than 2 months of tonification, pain of the lumbus and abdomen was relieved, and menstruation appeared normally. The penetrating and conception vessels became well-nourished, and the patient became pregnant.

(Beijing Chinese Medicine School and Beijing Chinese Medicine

Hospital. *Liu Feng-wu's Experience in Gynecology*. 1st Edition. Beijing: People's Medical Publishing House, 1977, 186-187)

Discussions

1. Luo Yuan-kai

Disorders involving infertility often present with complex patterns, so the clinical methods of treatment are various. In order to determine the proper approach to treatment, accurate pattern identification and a clear understanding of the pathomechanism is essential. That being said, Dr. Luo tends to emphasize methods that focus on regulation of the menstrual cycle. When the menses become regular, the chance of conception is greatly increased. Dr. Luo asserts that cases involving female infertility may be divided into five general patterns. These include kidney deficiency, qi and blood deficiency, liver constraint, blood stasis, and phlegm-damp.

(1) Infertility due to Kidney Deficiency

Kidney deficiency presentations include patterns of kidney yang deficiency, kidney yin deficiency, and kidney yin and yang dual deficiency.

A. Kidney yang deficiency

The symptoms and signs here include menstrual irregularities, delayed menstruation, oligomenorrhea, clear thin menses, aching lumbus and knees, cold in the abdomen, lack of warmth in the limbs, devitalized spirit, fear of cold, fatigue and lack of strength, somber facial complexion, dark perilabial macules, dark color around the eyes, frigidity, long voidings of clear urine, nocturia, and loose stools. The tongue appears soft and pale with a white moist coating. Pulses are deep and slow or forceless and thready, especially in the *chi* positions.

The treatment principle here is to warm the kidney and uterus, and invigorate yang.

Yòu Guī Wán (右归丸) is indicated.

右归丸 *Yòu Guī Wán*

附子	*fù zǐ*	Radix Aconiti Lateralis Praeparata
熟地	*shú dì*	Radix Rehmanniae Praeparata
菟丝子	*tù sī zǐ*	Semen Cuscutae
枸杞子	*gǒu qǐ zǐ*	Fructus Lycii
杜仲	*dù zhòng*	Cortex Eucommiae
鹿角胶	*lù jiǎo jiāo*	Colla Cornus Cervi
当归	*dāng guī*	Radix Angelicae Sinensis
肉桂	*ròu guì*	Cortex Cinnamomi
山萸肉	*shān yú ròu*	Fructus Corni
淮山药	*huái shān yào*	Rhizoma Dioscoreae

B. Kidney yin deficiency

The symptoms and signs here include scant or delayed menstruation with red menses, vexing heat in the five hearts, restless sleep, insomnia, dry mouth, night sweats, emaciation, aching lumbus and limp knees, and a dry bound stool. The tongue appears red with little or no coating, or peeled. Pulses are thready, weak and slightly rapid.

The treatment principle here is to enrich the kidney, nourish yin, and supplement blood. Select the formula *Zuǒ Guī Yǐn* (左归饮).

左归饮 *Zuǒ Guī Yǐn*

地黄	*dì huáng*	Radix Rehmanniae
山萸肉	*shān yú ròu*	Fructus Corni
枸杞	*gǒu qǐ*	Fructus Lycii
山药	*shān yào*	Rhizoma Dioscoreae
茯苓	*fú líng*	Poria
炙甘草	*zhì gān cǎo*	Radix et Rhizoma Glycyrrhizae Praeparata cum Melle

C. Kidney yin and yang dual deficiency

The treatment principle here is to tonify both yin and yang with careful modifications of the aforementioned formulas. This may be accomplished by following the principle, "When tonifying yin, do not neglect yang. When tonifying yang, do not neglect yin. In this way, yin and yang will grow together".

(2) Infertility due to Qi and Blood Deficiency

Classical Chinese medical texts state that the vital activities of the female are governed by blood. This means that menstruation, pregnancy, delivery and lactation can occur only when the condition of the blood remains normal. Qi and blood deficiency can lead to the penetrating and conception vessels becoming deprived of nourishment, resulting in menstrual irregularities and infertility. Qi and blood deficiency patterns may be associated with constitutional deficiency, and also chronic disease.

Patients with this pattern usually display irregular menstruation with thin pale menses. Those with blood deficiency will present with scant menses. When qi deficiency results in failure to contain blood, the menses may be profuse, but also thin and pale. Other signs and symptoms include dull lower abdominal pain following menstruation, dizziness, blurred vision, palpitation, fearful throbbing, fatigue, numbness, and a somber yellow or sallow yellow facial complexion. The tongue appears pale with a white thin coating. Pulses are thready and weak.

The treatment principle here is to strongly tonify qi and blood while also warming the kidney.

Select *Yù Lín Zhū* (毓麟珠) from *Jingyue's Complete Compendium* (景岳全书 , *Jing-yue Quán Shū*).

毓麟珠 *Yù Lín Zhū*

党参	*dǎng shēn*	Radix Codonopsis
白术	*bái zhú*	Rhizoma Atractylodis Macrocephalae
云苓	*yún líng*	Poria
炙甘草	*zhì gān cǎo*	Radix et Rhizoma Glycyrrhizae Praeparata cum Melle
当归	*dāng guī*	Radix Angelicae Sinensis

白芍	*bái sháo*	Radix Paeoniae Alba
川芎	*chuān xiōng*	Rhizoma Chuanxiong
熟地	*shú dì*	Radix Rehmanniae Praeparata
菟丝子	*tù sī zǐ*	Semen Cuscutae
杜仲	*dù zhòng*	Cortex Eucommiae
鹿角霜	*lù jiǎo shuāng*	Cornu Cervi Degelatinatum

(3) Infertility due to Qi Stagnation and Blood Stasis

Qi stagnation can result in blood stagnation, and blood stagnation can lead to blood stasis. Irregular and ungratifying or painful menstruation occurs when the penetrating and conception vessels become inhibited. Qi stagnation and blood stasis patterns are often associated with infertility secondary to pelvic inflammatory disease (PID), endometriosis, and salpingemphraxis.

Symptoms and signs include menstrual irregularities, painful menstruation, pelvic pain, and dark purple menses with clots. The tongue appears dusky red with stasis maculae at the tip and margin, and the lips may appear dusky purple with maculae. Pulses are deep and wiry.

The treatment principle here is to move qi and invigorate blood, transform stasis, and regulate menses.

With predominant heat, combine *Dān Zhī Xiāo Yáo Sǎn* (丹栀逍遥散) with *Jīn Líng Zǐ Sǎn* (金铃子散) and remove *bái zhú* (Rhizoma Atractylodis Macrocephalae). Add *qīng pí* (Pericarpium Citri Reticulatae Viride) and *wǔ líng zhī* (Faeces Togopteri).

With predominant cold, select *Shào Fù Zhú Yū Tāng* (少腹逐瘀汤) from *Correction of Errors in the Medical Classics* (医林改错 , *Yī Lín Gǎi Cuò*).

干姜	*gān jiāng*	Rhizoma Zingiberis
桂枝	*guì zhī*	Ramulus Cinnamomi
没药	*mò yào*	Myrrha
小茴香	*xiǎo huí xiāng*	Fructus Foeniculi
川芎	*chuān xiōng*	Rhizoma Chuanxiong

当归	*dāng guī*	Radix Angelicae Sinensis
芍药	*sháo yào*	Radix Paeoniae Alba
延胡索	*yán hú suǒ*	Rhizoma Corydalis
五灵脂	*wǔ líng zhī*	Faeces Togopteri
蒲黄	*pú huáng*	Pollen Typhae

(4) Infertility due to Liver Qi Constraint

Mental and emotional factors can also seriously influence reproductive function. Menstrual irregularities often result from stress, excessive thinking, rumination, melancholy, and other mental states. This is because emotional disturbances lead to patterns of liver qi constraint, which also result in the inhibited movement of qi and blood. Psychological counseling is very useful in the treatment of infertility.

Symptoms and signs of this pattern include distending pain of the lesser abdomen, vexation, agitation, irascibility, depression, disquieted spirit, and sadness with a desire to weep. Menstruation is irregular or inhibited, with menses appearing dusky red with clots. The tongue appears dusky red with thin white coating. Pulses are thin and wiry.

The treatment principle here is to course the liver, resolve depression, move qi, and nourish blood.

Select *Kāi Yù Zhòng Yù Tāng* (开郁种玉汤) from *Fu Qing-zhu's Gynecology* (傅青主女科 , *Fu Qing-zhu Nǔ Kē*).

开郁种玉汤 *Kāi Yù Zhòng Yù Tāng*

当归	*dāng guī*	Radix Angelicae Sinensis
香附	*xiāng fù*	Rhizoma Cyperi
茯苓	*fú líng*	Poria
丹皮	*dān pí*	Cortex Moutan
花粉	*huā fěn*	Radix Trichosanthis

(5) Infertility due to Internal Phlegm-damp Obstruction

Patients presenting with this pattern often appear overweight with a somber white complexion. The main mechanisms here involve qi deficiency failing to move dampness, water-damp collecting internally, and phlegm congealing in the lower burner which obstructs the channels; uterus, and uterine collaterals. The accumulation of phlegm-damp can also lead to disharmony of the penetrating and conception vessels.

Patients with this pattern often report inhibited menstrual flow, oligomenorrhea, or amenorrhea. Other symptoms and signs include profuse vaginal discharge, fatigue, profuse sweating, aversion to cold, thoracic oppression, nausea, torpid intake, and loose sloppy stools. The tongue appears swollen and pale with a white slimy coating. Pulses are deep, moderate and slippery.

The treatment principle here is to dry dampness and transform phlegm while tonifying blood.

Select Ye Tian-shi's *Cāng Fù Dǎo Tán Wán* (苍附导痰丸).

苍附导痰丸 *Cāng Fù Dǎo Tán Wán*

苍术	*cāng zhú*	Rhizoma Atractylodis
香附	*xiāng fù*	Rhizoma Cyperi
茯苓	*fú líng*	Poria
胆南星	*dǎn nán xīng*	Arisaema cum Bile
橘红	*jú hóng*	Exocarpium Citri Rubrum
甘草	*gān cǎo*	Radix et Rhizoma Glycyrrhizae
枳壳	*zhǐ qiào*	Fructus Aurantii
神曲	*shén qū*	Massa Medicata Fermentata
姜汁	*jiāng zhī*	Rhizoma Zingiberis Recens Succus

(Department of Gynecology and Obstetrics, Guangzhou University of TCM. *Anthology of Luo Yuan-kai's Medical Books* 罗元恺医著选 . 1st edition. Guangzhou: Guangdong Science & Technology Press, 1979: 118-125)

2. HAN BAI-LING

Disorders involving the liver, spleen, and kidney can lead to infertility, as well as simple disharmonies of qi and blood, or yin and yang. The clinical presentation is often more complex than this, however. According to the experience of Dr. Han, cases involving female infertility may be divided into into twelve general patterns.

(1) Kidney Yin Deficiency

Symptoms and signs include advanced menstruation, scant thick red menses, emaciation, palpitation, insomnia, aching lumbus, and limp knees. The tongue appears red with a thin white coating. Pulses are rapid and thready.

The treatment principle here is to enrich yin, tonify the kidney, and secure the penetrating and conception vessels.

Select the following medicinals:

熟地	*shú dì*	Radix Rehmanniae Praeparata
杜仲	*dù zhòng*	Cortex Eucommiae
山茱萸	*shān zhū yú*	Fructus Corni
怀牛膝	*huái niú xī*	Radix Achyranthis Bidentatae
川断	*chuān duàn*	Radix Dipsaci
山药	*shān yào*	Rhizoma Dioscoreae
寄生	*jì shēng*	Herba Taxilli
牡蛎	*mǔ lì*	Concha Ostreae
龟板	*guī bǎn*	Carapax et Plastrum Testudinis
白芍	*bái sháo*	Radix Paeoniae Alba
海螵蛸	*hǎi piāo xiāo*	Endoconcha Sepiae

(2) Kidney Yang Deficiency

Symptoms and signs include delayed menstruation, scant pale red menses with clots, cold pain in the lower abdomen, aching lumbus and weak legs, clear profuse vaginal discharge, and frigidity. The tongue appears with a thin white coating. Pulses are thready.

The treatment principle here is to warm the kidney, support yang, and secure the penetrating and conception vessels.

Select the following medicinals:

山药	shān yào	Rhizoma Dioscoreae
云苓	yún líng	Poria
白术	bái zhú	Rhizoma Atractylodis Macrocephalae
熟地	shú dì	Radix Rehmanniae Praeparata
菟丝子	tù sī zǐ	Semen Cuscutae
泽泻	zé xiè	Rhizoma Alismatis
巴戟天	bā jǐ tiān	Radix Morindae Officinalis
仙茅	xiān máo	Rhizoma Curculiginis
芡实	qiàn shí	Semen Euryales
破故纸	pò gù zhǐ	Fructus Psoraleae
鹿角	lù jiǎo	Cornu Cervi
肉桂	ròu guì	Cortex Cinnamomi

(3) Spleen Yang Deficiency

Symptoms and signs include advanced and profuse menstruation, light red menses, shortness of breath, reticence, lassitude, weak limbs, poor appetite, sloppy stools, and profuse watery vaginal discharge. The tongue appears pale with a thin white coating. Pulses are weak and thready.

The treatment principle here is to fortify the spleen, supplement qi, and eliminate dampness.

Select the following medicinals:

党参	dǎng shēn	Radix Codonopsis
白术	bái zhú	Rhizoma Atractylodis Macrocephalae
云苓	yún líng	Poria
陈皮	chén pí	Pericarpium Citri Reticulatae
砂仁	shā rén	Fructus Amomi
扁豆	biǎn dòu	Semen Lablab Album
苡仁	yǐ rén	Semen Coicis
芡实	qiàn shí	Semen Euryales
苍术	cāng zhú	Rhizoma Atractylodis

车前子	*chē qián zǐ*	Semen Plantaginis
半夏	*bàn xià*	Rhizoma Pinelliae
山药	*shān yào*	Rhizoma Dioscoreae

(4) Spleen Blood Deficiency

Symptoms and signs include scant pale menses, palpitation, fearful throbbing, dizziness, insomnia, and profuse dreaming. The tongue appears pale with a thin white coating. Pulses are thready.

The treatment principle here is to fortify the spleen, enrich yin, and engender blood.

Select the following medicinals:

云苓	*yún líng*	Poria
白术	*bái zhú*	Rhizoma Atractylodis Macrocephalae
山药	*shān yào*	Rhizoma Dioscoreae
熟地	*shú dì*	Radix Rehmanniae Praeparata
当归	*dāng guī*	Radix Angelicae Sinensis
枸杞	*gǒu qǐ*	Fructus Lycii
女贞子	*nǚ zhēn zǐ*	Fructus Ligustri Lucidi
龟板	*guī bǎn*	Carapax et Plastrum Testudinis
木瓜	*mù guā*	Fructus Chaenomelis
阿胶	*ē jiāo*	Colla Corii Asini
白芍	*bái sháo*	Radix Paeoniae Alba
黄芪	*huáng qí*	Radix Astragali

(5) Liver Constraint and Qi Stagnation

Symptoms and signs include irregular menstruation, profuse or scant dark purple menses, distention of the chest and rib-side, distending lower abdominal pain, and frequent sighing. The tongue appears red with a thin white coating. Pulses are rough and wiry.

The treatment principle here is to course the liver, regulate qi, and free the collaterals.

Select the following medicinals:

当归	*dāng guī*	Radix Angelicae Sinensis
枳壳	*zhǐ qiào*	Fructus Aurantii
川楝	*chuān liàn*	Fructus Toosendan
川牛膝	*chuān niú xī*	Radix Cyathulae
炮山甲	*pào shān jiǎ*	Squama Manis
瓜蒌	*guā lóu*	Fructus Trichosanthis
王不留行	*wáng bù liú xíng*	Semen Vaccariae
通草	*tōng cǎo*	Medulla Tetrapanacis
皂刺	*zào cì*	Spina Gleditsiae
白芍	*bái sháo*	Radix Paeoniae Alba

(6) Liver Constraint Transforming into Heat

Symptoms and signs include advanced or irregular menstruation, profuse red menses, distending breast pain, vexation, agitation, irascibility, and lower abdominal pain and distention. The tongue appears red with a thin yellow coating. Pulses are wiry, thready and rapid.

The treatment principle here is to regulate the liver, clear heat, and cool blood.

Select the following medicinals:

白芍	*bái sháo*	Radix Paeoniae Alba
生地	*shēng dì*	Radix Rehmanniae
枳壳	*zhǐ qiào*	Fructus Aurantii
地骨皮	*dì gǔ pí*	Cortex Lycii
栀子	*zhī zǐ*	Fructus Gardeniae
丹皮	*dān pí*	Cortex Moutan
夏枯草	*xià kū cǎo*	Spica Prunellae
川楝	*chuān liàn*	Fructus Toosendan
川牛膝	*chuān niú xī*	Radix Cyathulae
银柴胡	*yín chái hú*	Radix Stellariae
甘草	*gān cǎo*	Radix et Rhizoma Glycyrrhizae

(7) Liver and Kidney Yin Deficiency

Symptoms and signs include delayed menstruation, scant or dusky red menses, emaciation, vexing heat in the five hearts, poor sleep, dizziness, tinnitus, dryness of the mouth and eyes, night sweating, and an aching lumbus with weak knees. The tongue appears red with little coating. Pulses are thready and rapid.

The treatment principle here is to enrich the liver and kidney.

Select the following medicinals:

熟地	*shú dì*	Radix Rehmanniae Praeparata
山茱萸	*shān zhū yú*	Fructus Corni
淮山药	*huái shān yào*	Rhizoma Dioscoreae
丹皮	*dān pí*	Cortex Moutan
云苓	*yún líng*	Poria
泽泻	*zé xiè*	Rhizoma Alismatis

(8) Liver Constraint and Kidney Deficiency

Symptoms and signs include delayed or irregular menstruation, scant or profuse dark menses with clots, breast distention, oppression of the chest, and lumbar pain. The tongue appears dusky with thin white coating. Pulses are thready and wiry.

The treatment principle here is to regulate the liver, tonify the kidney, and regulate qi.

Select the following medicinals:

当归	*dāng guī*	Radix Angelicae Sinensis
枳壳	*zhǐ qiào*	Fructus Aurantii
川楝	*chuān liàn*	Fructus Toosendan
川牛膝	*chuān niú xī*	Radix Cyathulae
佛手	*fó shǒu*	Fructus Citri Sarcodactylis
山药	*shān yào*	Rhizoma Dioscoreae
王不留行	*wáng bù liú xíng*	Semen Vaccariae
通草	*tōng cǎo*	Medulla Tetrapanacis
皂刺	*zào cì*	Spina Gleditsiae
白芍	*bái sháo*	Radix Paeoniae Alba

| 川断 | chuān duàn | Radix Dipsaci |
| 寄生 | jì shēng | Herba Taxilli |

(9) Liver Constraint and Spleen Deficiency

Symptoms and signs include delayed menstruation, scant or profuse menses, breast distention, palpitation, sloppy stools, and facial puffiness. The tongue appears pale with a white coating. Pulses are wiry and thready.

The treatment principle here is to regulate the liver, regulate qi and fortify the spleen.

Select the following medicinals:

当归	dāng guī	Radix Angelicae Sinensis
枳壳	zhǐ qiào	Fructus Aurantii
川楝	chuān liàn	Fructus Toosendan
川牛膝	chuān niú xī	Radix Cyathulae
山药	shān yào	Rhizoma Dioscoreae
王不留行	wáng bù liú xíng	Semen Vaccariae
通草	tōng cǎo	Medulla Tetrapanacis
柴胡	chái hú	Radix Bupleuri
白芍	bái sháo	Radix Paeoniae Alba
川断	chuān duàn	Radix Dipsaci
寄生	jì shēng	Herba Taxilli

(10) Spleen and Kidney Yang Deficiency

Symptoms and signs include delayed menstruation or amenorrhea, scant pale menses, somber complexion, lumbar pain, weak legs, aversion to cold, cold limbs, frigidity, clear vaginal discharge, long voidings of clear urine, and sloppy stools. The tongue appears enlarged with tooth marks on the margins and a thin white coating. Pulses are deep and weak.

The treatment principle here is to warm the kidney, support yang, and fortify the spleen.

Select the following medicinals:

山药	*shān yào*	Rhizoma Dioscoreae
云苓	*yún líng*	Poria
熟地	*shú dì*	Radix Rehmanniae Praeparata
白术	*bái zhú*	Rhizoma Atractylodis Macrocephalae
泽泻	*zé xiè*	Rhizoma Alismatis
巴戟天	*bā jǐ tiān*	Radix Morindae Officinalis
菟丝子	*tù sī zǐ*	Semen Cuscutae
芡实	*qiàn shí*	Semen Euryales
仙灵脾	*xiān líng pí*	Herba Epimedii
破故纸	*pò gù zhǐ*	Fructus Psoraleae
肉桂	*ròu guì*	Cortex Cinnamomi

(11) Qi Stagnation and Blood Stasis

Symptoms and signs include irregular menstruation or amenorrhea, dysmenorrhea, thick menses with clots, and fixed pain of the lesser abdomen. The tongue appears dusky with stasis maculae. Pulses are rough.

The treatment principle here is to course the liver, regulate qi, dispel stasis, and free the collaterals.

Select the following medicinals:

白芍	*bái sháo*	Radix Paeoniae Alba
当归	*dāng guī*	Radix Angelicae Sinensis
云苓	*yún líng*	Poria
白术	*bái zhú*	Rhizoma Atractylodis Macrocephalae
郁金	*yù jīn*	Radix Curcumae
丹皮	*dān pí*	Cortex Moutan
枳壳	*zhǐ qiào*	Fructus Aurantii
川楝	*chuān liàn*	Fructus Toosendan
玄胡	*xuán hú*	Rhizoma Corydalis
川牛膝	*chuān niú xī*	Radix Cyathulae
丹参	*dān shēn*	Radix et Rhizoma Salviae Miltiorrhizae

(12) Phlegm-damp Obstructing the Collaterals

Symptoms and signs include infrequent menstruation or amenorrhea, inhibited menses, obesity, slimy sensation in the mouth, heaviness of the head, listlessness, frigidity, and poor appetite. The tongue appears enlarged and pale. Pulses are moderate, deep and slippery.

The treatment principle here is to fortify the spleen, dry dampness, dispel stasis and free the collaterals.

Select the following medicinals:

山药	shān yào	Rhizoma Dioscoreae
苍术	cāng zhú	Rhizoma Atractylodis
白术	bái zhú	Rhizoma Atractylodis Macrocephalae
半夏	bàn xià	Rhizoma Pinelliae
枳壳	zhǐ qiào	Fructus Aurantii
厚朴	hòu pò	Cortex Magnoliae Officinalis
神曲	shén qū	Massa Medicata Fermentata
陈皮	chén pí	Pericarpium Citri Reticulatae
炮甲珠	pào jiǎ zhū	Squama Manis
茯苓	fú líng	Poria
滑石	huá shí	Talcum
皂刺	zào cì	Spina Gleditsiae

(Wang Hui-dong. Han Bai-ling's Treatment of Infertility 韩百灵辨治不孕症 . *China Journal of Traditional Chinese Medicine and Pharmacy* (中国医药学报), 1995, (4): 31)

3. XIA GUI-CHENG

Disorders of the immune system contribute to female infertility in a number of ways.

The formulas *Zī Yīn Yì Kàng Tāng* (滋阴抑抗汤) and *Zhù Yáng Yì Kàng Tāng* (助阳抑抗汤) are both effective in the treatment of female infertility associated with immune responses.

(1) *Zī Yīn Yì Kàng Tāng* (滋阴抑抗汤), **also known as** *Kàng Jīng Yī Hào Fāng* (抗精Ⅰ号方)

The indications of this formula include advanced menstruation, profuse or scant thick red menses, dizziness, tinnitus, palpitation, insomnia, aching lumbus and weak legs, vexation, agitation, and dry mouth. The tongue appears red with a greasy yellow coating. Pulses are thready, wiry and rapid. The above symptoms and signs are generally associated with patterns of effulgent yin deficiency fire.

The formula contains the following medicinals:

炒当归	*chǎo dāng guī*	Radix Angelicae Sinensis (dry-fried)
赤芍	*chì sháo*	Radix Paeoniae Rubra
白芍	*bái sháo*	Radix Paeoniae Alba
山药	*shān yào*	Rhizoma Dioscoreae
丹皮	*dān pí*	Cortex Moutan
地黄	*dì huáng*	Radix Rehmanniae
山茱萸	*shān zhū yú*	Fructus Corni
甘草	*gān cǎo*	Radix et Rhizoma Glycyrrhizae
钩藤	*gōu téng*	Ramulus Uncariae Cum Uncis

Application: One daily decocted dose, beginning after menstruation.

Modification: For 7 days of the ovulation period, add *chuān duàn* (Radix Dipsaci) 10g, *tù sī zǐ* (Semen Cuscutae) 10g, and *lù jiǎo piàn* (Cornu Cervi) 10g.

The use of condoms is recommended when taking this formula.

(2) *Zhù Yáng Yì Kàng Tāng* (助阳抑抗汤), **also known as** *Kàng Jīng Zǐ Èr Hào Fāng* (抗精子Ⅱ号方)

The indications of this formula include delayed menstruation, aching lumbus and weak legs, lower abdominal cold, sloppy stools, fatigue, and lack of strength. The tongue appears pale with a white coating. Pulses are thready. The above symptoms and signs are generally associated with patterns of yang deficiency and stasis turbidity.

The formula contains the following medicinals:

黄芪	huáng qí	Radix Astragali
党参	dǎng shēn	Radix Codonopsis
鹿角片	lù jiǎo piàn	Cornu Cervi
丹参	dān shēn	Radix et Rhizoma Salviae Miltiorrhizae
赤芍	chì sháo	Radix Paeoniae Rubra
白芍	bái sháo	Radix Paeoniae Alba
云苓	yún líng	Poria
川断	chuān duàn	Radix Dipsaci
山楂	shān zhā	Fructus Crataegi

Application: One daily decocted dose. This formula should be taken from the beginning of ovulation to day one of menstruation.

Note: *Huáng qí* (Radix Astragali) and *lù jiǎo piàn* (Cornu Cervi) are medicinals that "tonify yang within qi", and are also effective in the treatment of AsAb immune infertility.

The use of condoms is recommended when taking this formula.

(3) For infertility with predominant yin deficiency, select *Sì Wù Tāng* (四物汤) and add *shān zhū yú* (Fructus Corni) and remove *chuān xiōng* (Rhizoma Chuanxiong). This formula is also called *Yǎng Jīng Zhòng Yù Tāng* (养精种玉汤), as referred to in *Fu Qing-zhu's Gynecology* (傅青主女 科 , *Fu Qing-zhu Nǚ Kē*).

This modification follows the principle of "using sweet and sour to transform yin". *Yǎng Jīng Zhòng Yù Tāng* has also been shown to increase pregnancy rates in patients testing positive for AsAb.

(Xia Gui-cheng. Identification and Treatment in 50 Cases of Immune Infertility 辨治免疫性不孕 50 例 . *China Journal of Traditional Chinese Medicine and Pharmacy* (中国医药学报), 1990, (6): 43)

4. BAN XIU-WEN

Dr. Ban Xiu-wen's experience in the treatment of infertility can be summarized with the following three main points.

First, select formulas to resolve vaginal discharge and regulate menstruation.

Representative formulas include *Zuǒ Guī Yǐn* (左归饮), *Yòu Guī Yǐn* (右归饮), *Wǔ Zǐ Yǎn Zōng Wán* (五子衍宗丸), *Guī Pí Wán* (归脾丸), *Rén Shēn Yǎng Róng Tāng* (人参养荣汤) and *Dāng Guī Sháo Yào Sǎn* (当归芍药散).

Second, focus on regulation and tonification of the liver and kidney. Failure to ovulate is most often associated with disorders of the liver and kidney.

Apply warming formulas that free the vessels such as *Wǔ Zǐ Yǎn Zōng Wán* (五子衍宗丸) and *Guī Sháo Dì Huáng Tāng* (归芍地黄汤).

Third, combine pattern identification with disease identification. Adjust the treatment approach according to changes in the presenting pattern.

For infertility secondary to salpingemphraxis:

鸡血藤	*jī xuè téng*	Caulis Spatholobi
当归	*dāng guī*	Radix Angelicae Sinensis
川芎	*chuān xiōng*	Rhizoma Chuanxiong
桂枝	*guì zhī*	Ramulus Cinnamomi
香附	*xiāng fù*	Rhizoma Cyperi
刘寄奴	*liú jì nú*	Herba Artemisiae Anomalae
路路通	*lù lù tōng*	Fructus Liquidambaris
皂角刺	*zào jiǎo cì*	Spina Gleditsiae
急性子	*jí xìng zǐ*	Semen Impatientis
王不留行	*wáng bù liú xíng*	Semen Vaccariae
穿破石	*chuān pò shí*	Radix seu Vanieriae Caulis
猫爪草	*māo zhuǎ cǎo*	Radix Ranunculi Ternati

With qi stagnation and blood stasis, select *Chái Hú Shū Gān Sǎn* (柴胡疏肝散).

With uterine fibroids and endometriosis, add blood-invigorating and stasis-transforming medicinals such as *é zhú* (Rhizoma Curcumae), *yì mǔ cǎo* (Herba Leonuri), *sū mù* (Lignum Sappan), *zé lán* (Herba Lycopi), *jī xuè téng* (Caulis Spatholobi), *mǔ dān pí* (Cortex Moutan), *chì sháo* (Radix Paeoniae Rubra) and *liú jì nú* (Herba Artemisiae Anomalae).

(Lu Hui-ling. Abstracts of Ban Xiu-wen's Experience in the Treatment of Infertility 班秀文教授治疗不孕证的经验撮要. *Guangxi Journal of Traditional Chinese Medicine* (广西中医药), 1995, (1):18)

5. Xu Run-san

From Dr. Xu Run-san's perspective, ovulation failure is the fundamental issue in most cases of infertility. "The kidney governing reproduction" includes functional relationships involving the brain, uterus, *tian gui*, and the penetrating and conception vessels. This Chinese medical perspective corresponds to the biomedical view of reproduction as related to the functions of the hypothalamus, pituitary gland, and ovaries. Infertility due to anovulation may therefore be viewed as a manifestation of kidney deficiency.

Dr. Xu recognizes four main patterns:

(1) Kidney Deficiency

Symptoms and signs include delayed menstruation with scant menses, aching lumbus and weak knees, reduced libido, scant vaginal discharge, and cold limbs. The tongue appears pale, and pulses are deep and thready. BBT is typically monophase or diphase.

The treatment principle here is to tonify the kidney and nourish blood.

Select the following medicinals:

仙茅	*xiān máo*	Rhizoma Curculiginis
仙灵脾	*xiān líng pí*	Herba Epimedii
巴戟天	*bā jǐ tiān*	Radix Morindae Officinalis
肉苁蓉	*ròu cōng róng*	Herba Cistanches

当归	*dāng guī*	Radix Angelicae Sinensis
甘草	*gān cǎo*	Radix et Rhizoma Glycyrrhizae
沙苑子	*shā yuàn zǐ*	Semen Astragali Complanati
党参	*dǎng shēn*	Radix Codonopsis
枸杞	*gǒu qǐ*	Fructus Lycii
菟丝子	*tù sī zǐ*	Semen Cuscutae

(2) Kidney Deficiency and Liver Constraint

Symptoms and signs include irregular menstruation, profuse or scant menses, and premenstrual breast distention. Pulses are thready and wiry.

The treatment principle here is to tonify the kidney and regulate the liver.

Select the following medicinals:

山茱萸	*shān zhū yú*	Fructus Corni
紫河车	*zǐ hé chē*	Placenta Hominis
柴胡	*chái hú*	Radix Bupleuri
当归	*dāng guī*	Radix Angelicae Sinensis
白芍	*bái sháo*	Radix Paeoniae Alba
制香附	*zhì xiāng fù*	Rhizoma Cyperi (prepared)
益母草	*yì mǔ cǎo*	Herba Leonuri

(3) Kidney Deficiency and Phlegm Excess

Symptoms and signs include include obesity, excessive bodyhair, scant menstruation or amenorrhea, and slight edema. Pulses are soggy and thready.

The treatment principle here is to tonify the kidney, support the spleen, dispel stasis and invigorate blood.

Select the following medicinals:

鹿角霜	*lù jiǎo shuāng*	Cornu Cervi Degelatinatum
巴戟天	*bā jǐ tiān*	Radix Morindae Officinalis
半夏	*bàn xià*	Rhizoma Pinelliae

昆布	kūn bù	Thallus Laminariae
川芎	chuān xiōng	Rhizoma Chuanxiong
白术	bái zhú	Rhizoma Atractylodis Macrocephalae
生黄芪	shēng huáng qí	Radix Astragali Cruda
当归	dāng guī	Radix Angelicae Sinensis
益母草	yì mǔ cǎo	Herba Leonuri
枳壳	zhǐ qiào	Fructus Aurantii

(4) Kidney Deficiency and Blood Stasis

Symptoms and signs include irregular menstruation, prolonged menstruation, and a pale tongue. Pulses are rough and thready. BBT is typically monophase.

The treatment principle here is to tonify the kidney, regulate the liver, and invigorate blood.

Select the following medicinals:

柴胡	chái hú	Radix Bupleuri
当归	dāng guī	Radix Angelicae Sinensis
白芍	bái sháo	Radix Paeoniae Alba
熟地	shú dì	Radix Rehmanniae Praeparata
山茱萸	shān zhū yú	Fructus Corni
鹿角胶	lù jiǎo jiāo	Colla Cornus Cervi
香附	xiāng fù	Rhizoma Cyperi
丹参	dān shēn	Radix et Rhizoma Salviae Miltiorrhizae
党参	dǎng shēn	Radix Codonopsis
益母草	yì mǔ cǎo	Herba Leonuri

One decocted daily dose, beginning after menstruation.

Excessive menstrual bleeding may be treated with the addition of blood-cooling medicinals. Apply the following medicinals until the end of the bleeding stage:

玳瑁	dài mào	10g	Carapax Eretmochelydis
生地	shēng dì	30g	Radix Rehmanniae

白芍	*bái sháo*	20g	Radix Paeoniae Alba
丹皮	*dān pí*	15g	Cortex Moutan
三七粉	*sān qī fěn*	3g	Pulverata Radix et Rhizoma Notoginseng
太子参	*tài zǐ shēn*	30g	Radix Pseudostellariae

(Xu Run-san. The Kidney in the Treatment of Anovulatory Infertility 从肾论治无排卵性不孕症 . *The Practical Journal of Integrating Chinese Medicine with Modern Medicine* (实用中西医结合杂志), 1990, (10): 298)

6. Wang Zi-yu

(1) Kidney Qi Deficiency

Symptoms and signs include delayed menstruation, scant pale menses, dark facial complexion, aching lumbus and knees, frigidity, frequent night urination, and sloppy stools. The tongue appears pale with a white coating. Pulses are deep and slow.

The treatment principle here is to warm the kidney, benefit essence, and regulate the penetrating and conception vessels.

Commonly selected medicinals include:

仙灵脾	*xiān líng pí*	Herba Epimedii
巴戟天	*bā jǐ tiān*	Radix Morindae Officinalis
石楠叶	*shí nán yè*	Folium Photiniae
当归	*dāng guī*	Radix Angelicae Sinensis
熟地	*shú dì*	Radix Rehmanniae Praeparata
川芎	*chuān xiōng*	Rhizoma Chuanxiong
白芍	*bái sháo*	Radix Paeoniae Alba
五味子	*wǔ wèi zǐ*	Fructus Schisandrae Chinensis
菟丝子	*tù sī zǐ*	Semen Cuscutae
覆盆子	*fù pén zǐ*	Fructus Rubi
紫河车	*zǐ hé chē*	Placenta Hominis

(2) Liver Constraint and Qi Stagnation

Symptoms and signs include irregular menstruation, menstrual pain, inhibited menstruation with clots, distending pain of the breasts and rib-side, depression, vexation, agitation, and irascibility. The tongue appears dusky red with a thin white coating.

The treatment principle here is to course the liver, resolve constraint, nourish blood, and regulate the penetrating vessel.

The representative formula contains the following:

柴胡	*chái hú*	Radix Bupleuri
香附	*xiāng fù*	Rhizoma Cyperi
娑罗子	*suō luó zǐ*	Semen Aesculi
郁金	*yù jīn*	Radix Curcumae
合欢皮	*hé huān pí*	Cortex Albiziae
川芎	*chuān xiōng*	Rhizoma Chuanxiong
当归	*dāng guī*	Radix Angelicae Sinensis
熟地	*shú dì*	Radix Rehmanniae Praeparata
白芍	*bái sháo*	Radix Paeoniae Alba
橘核	*jú hé*	Semen Citri Reticulatae
橘络	*jú luò*	Vascular Aurantii
路路通	*lù lù tōng*	Fructus Liquidambaris

(3) Phlegm-damp Obstruction

Symptoms and signs include obesity, delayed menstruation or amenorrhea, profuse, thick and sticky vaginal discharge, bright white facial complexion, dizziness, palpitation, oppression of the chest, and abdominal distention. The tongue coating appears white and slimy. Pulses are slippery.

The treatment principle here is to warm the kidney, invigorate yang, resolve phlegm, and eliminate dampness.

The representative formula contains the following:

仙灵脾	*xiān líng pí*	Herba Epimedii
仙茅	*xiān máo*	Rhizoma Curculiginis
鹿角霜	*lù jiǎo shuāng*	Cornu Cervi Degelatinatum

菟丝子	*tù sī zǐ*	Semen Cuscutae
覆盆子	*fù pén zǐ*	Fructus Rubi
胆南星	*dǎn nán xīng*	Arisaema cum Bile
苍术	*cāng zhú*	Rhizoma Atractylodis
茯苓	*fú líng*	Poria
半夏	*bàn xià*	Rhizoma Pinelliae
白术	*bái zhú*	Rhizoma Atractylodis Macrocephalae
枳壳	*zhǐ qiào*	Fructus Aurantii
川芎	*chuān xiōng*	Rhizoma Chuanxiong
泽兰	*zé lán*	Herba Lycopi
山楂	*shān zhā*	Fructus Crataegi

(4) Blood Deficiency with Malnourishment of the Uterine Collaterals

Symptoms and signs include delayed menstruation, scant pale menses, dizziness, blurred vision, withered-yellow facial complexion, fatigue, palpitation, and insomnia. The tongue appears pale with a thin coating. Pulses are deep and thready.

The treatment principle here is to nourish the liver and kidney, tonify blood, and regulate menstruation.

Commonly selected medicinals include:

熟地	*shú dì*	Radix Rehmanniae Praeparata
川芎	*chuān xiōng*	Rhizoma Chuanxiong
当归	*dāng guī*	Radix Angelicae Sinensis
紫河车	*zǐ hé chē*	Placenta Hominis
山茱萸	*shān zhū yú*	Fructus Corni
茺蔚子	*chōng wèi zǐ*	Fructus Leonuri
鹿角胶	*lù jiǎo jiāo*	Colla Cornus Cervi

(5) Blood Stasis

Symptoms and signs include menstrual pain with lower abdominal distention, dark-colored menses with clots, headache, painful breast distention, and premenstrual abdominal pain. Dark spots on the face may also be observed. The tongue appears dark purple or with static maculae. Pulses are wiry and rough.

The treatment principle here is to invigorate blood, resolve stasis, soften hardness, and dissipate binding.

Commonly selected medicinals include:

桂枝	guì zhī	Ramulus Cinnamomi
茯苓	fú líng	Poria
桃仁	táo rén	Semen Persicae
三棱	sān léng	Rhizoma Sparganii
莪术	é zhú	Rhizoma Curcumae
海藻	hǎi zǎo	Sargassum
赤芍	chì sháo	Radix Paeoniae Rubra
丹参	dān shēn	Radix et Rhizoma Salviae Miltiorrhizae
刘寄奴	liú jì nú	Herba Artemisiae Anomalae
石见穿	shí jiàn chuān	Herba Salviae Chinensis

With profuse menses, remove *sān léng* (Rhizoma Sparganii) and *é zhú* (Rhizoma Curcumae), and add *sān qī fěn* (Pulverata Radix et Rhizoma Notoginseng), *mǎ chǐ xiàn* (Herba Portulacae) and *chǎo mián zǐ* (dry-fried Semen Gossypium Grboreum).

With ovarian swelling, add *zhū líng* (Polyporus) and *cù chǎo yuán huā* (vinegar-fried Flos Genkwa).

With static blood obstructing the oviduct, select the following medicinals:

当归尾	dāng guī wěi	Radix Angelicae Sinensis
川芎	chuān xiōng	Rhizoma Chuanxiong
赤芍	chì sháo	Radix Paeoniae Rubra
丹参	dān shēn	Radix et Rhizoma Salviae Miltiorrhizae
柞木枝	zuò mù zhī	Xylosma Congestum
穿山甲	chuān shān jiǎ	Squama Manis
海藻	hǎi zǎo	Sargassum
路路通	lù lù tōng	Fructus Liquidambaris

皂角刺	zào jiǎo cì	Spina Gleditsiae
血竭	xuè jié	Sanguis Draconis
柴胡	chái hú	Radix Bupleuri
广木香	guǎng mù xiāng	Radix Aucklandiae

(Wang Yao-yun. Professor Wang Zi-yu's Five Methods of Treating Infertility 王子瑜教授辨治不孕症五法 . *Journal of Beijing University of Traditional Chinese Medicine* (北京中医药大学学报), 1994, (17) 1: 40)

7. QIU XIAO-MEI

(1) Kidney Deficiency and Uterine Cold

Symptoms and signs include delayed menarche, amenorrhea, scant thin pale menses, aching lumbus and weak knees, cold limbs, lower abdominal cold, and frigidity. The tongue appears moist. Pulses are deep and slow.

The treatment principle here is to warm yang, replenish kidney essence, and warm the uterus.

Guì Xiān Tāng (桂仙汤) is indicated.

仙灵脾	xiān líng pí	Herba Epimedii
仙茅	xiān máo	Rhizoma Curculiginis
肉桂末	ròu guì mò	Cortex Cinnamomi (ground)
巴戟天	bā jǐ tiān	Radix Morindae Officinalis
肉苁蓉	ròu cōng róng	Herba Cistanches
紫石英	zǐ shí yīng	Fluoritum

(2) Liver Constraint and Blood Stasis

Symptoms and signs include advanced or delayed menstruation with profuse or scant menses, inhibited dark red menses with clots, distending breast pain, lower abdominal pain and distention, depression, and irascibility. The tongue appears red or purple. Pulses are wiry and thready.

The treatment principle here is to course the liver, regulate qi, dispel stasis and free the collaterals.

Select *Jí Lí Săn* (蒺藜散) combined with *Xiāo Yáo Săn* (逍遥散).

蒺藜散 *Jí Lí Săn*

白蒺藜	*bái jí lí*	Fructus Tribuli
青皮	*qīng pí*	Pericarpium Citri Reticulatae Viride
橘核	*jú hé*	Semen Citri Reticulatae
橘络	*jú luò*	Vascular Aurantii
八月扎	*bā yuè zhā*	Fructus Akebiae
蒲公英	*pú gōng yīng*	Herba Taraxaci

(3) Blood Deficiency and Malnourishment of the Uterine Collaterals

Symptoms and signs include scant pale menses, amenorrhea, a withered-yellow complexion, dizziness, blurred vision, lassistude, palpitation, and insomnia. The tongue appears light red. Pulses are deep and thready.

The treatment principle here is to nourish blood, regulate menstruation, and tonify the liver and kidney.

Commonly selected medicinals include:

当归	*dāng guī*	Radix Angelicae Sinensis
山茱萸	*shān zhū yú*	Fructus Corni
黄芪	*huáng qí*	Radix Astragali
菟丝子	*tù sī zǐ*	Semen Cuscutae
炒白术	*chǎo bái zhú*	Rhizoma Atractylodis Macrocephalae (dry-fried)
熟地	*shú dì*	Radix Rehmanniae Praeparata
白芍	*bái sháo*	Radix Paeoniae Alba
党参	*dǎng shēn*	Radix Codonopsis
枸杞	*gǒu qǐ*	Fructus Lycii
紫河车	*zǐ hé chē*	Placenta Hominis
巴戟天	*bā jǐ tiān*	Radix Morindae Officinalis
玫瑰花	*méi guī huā*	Flos Rosae Rugosae

(4) Phlegm-damp Obstructing the Uterus

Symptoms and signs include irregular menstruation, amenorrhea, obesity, profuse vaginal discharge, palpitation, shortness of breath, and a bright white facial complexion. The tongue appears soft with teethmarks. Pulses are wiry, thready and slippery.

The treatment principle here is to move qi, eliminate phlegm, warm the kidney, and fortify the spleen.

Select *Cāng Fù Dǎo Tán Wán* (苍附导痰丸) modified with *Guì Xiān Tāng* (桂仙汤).

(Zheng Jian-wei. A Brief Introduction to Dr. Qiu Xiao-mei's Experience in the Treatment of Infertility 裘笑梅主任医师治疗不孕症经验简介 . *New Journal of Traditional Chinese Medicine* (新中医), 1998, 30 (12): 5-6)

8. PANG PAN-CHI

(1) Freeing the Oviduct

Secret Records from the Stone Chamber (石室秘录 , *Shí Shì Mì Lù*) states, "When mounting-conglomeration affects the conception and governing vessels, essence will not pass through, due to outside obstruction." Dr. Pang considers "mounting-conglomeration" here as referring to those accumulations, gatherings, concretions, and conglomerations which obstruct the vessels and collaterals. The passage of essence is obstructed, blood cannot be contained, and infertility results.

The presenting patterns are usually associated with the liver and kidney. Symptoms and signs include aching lumbus and weak knees, and painful distention or dull pain of the lesser abdomen. Premenstrual symptoms of breast distention, vexation, agitation, and irascibility may also appear. Menstrual symptoms include clotted menses, dizziness, tinnitus, poor memory, and stabbing or distending pains of the lesser abdomen which become aggravated at night. The tongue appears dark with static spots. Pulses are thin and wiry, or thin and rough.

The treatment principle here is to regulate qi and invigorate blood.

Select *Táo Hóng Sì Wù Tāng* (桃红四物汤) as the basic formula.

熟地黄	*shú dì huáng*	Radix Rehmanniae Praeparata
当归	*dāng guī*	Radix Angelicae Sinensis
川芎	*chuān xiōng*	Rhizoma Chuanxiong
白芍	*bái sháo*	Radix Paeoniae Alba
香附	*xiāng fù*	Rhizoma Cyperi
桃仁	*táo rén*	Semen Persicae
红花	*hóng huā*	Flos Carthami
路路通	*lù lù tōng*	Fructus Liquidambaris
石菖蒲	*shí chāng pú*	Rhizoma Acori Tatarinowii
皂角刺	*zào jiǎo cì*	Spina Gleditsiae
薏苡仁	*yì yǐ rén*	Semen Coicis
海螵蛸	*hǎi piāo xiāo*	Endoconcha Sepiae

(2) Promoting Ovulation

The pathomechanism of ovulatory dysfunction primarily involves disorders of the kidney, according to Dr. Pang. The presenting patterns are usually associated with liver and kidney insufficiency with uterine deficiency cold.

Symptoms and signs include infertility with delayed or scant menses, amenorrhea, dizziness, tinnitus, clear thin vaginal discharge, aching lumbus and weak legs, fullness and oppression of the chest and rib-side, fatigue, taxation, frigidity, obesity, and menstrual dripping. The tongue appears soft and pale with a thin or white slimy coating. Pulses are deep and thready, or soggy and thready.

The treatment principle here is to tonify the kidney and regulate the penetrating vessel.

Select modified *Sì Wù Tāng* (四物汤).

熟地黄	shú dì huáng	Radix Rehmanniae Praeparata
当归	dāng guī	Radix Angelicae Sinensis
川芎	chuān xiōng	Rhizoma Chuanxiong
白芍	bái sháo	Radix Paeoniae Alba
杜仲	dù zhòng	Cortex Eucommiae
仙灵脾	xiān líng pí	Herba Epimedii
王不留行	wáng bù liú xíng	Semen Vaccariae
黄精	huáng jīng	Rhizoma Polygonati
肉苁蓉	ròu cōng róng	Herba Cistanches
菟丝子	tù sī zǐ	Semen Cuscutae
茺蔚子	chōng wèi zǐ	Fructus Leonuri
泽兰	zé lán	Herba Lycopi
紫石英	zǐ shí yīng	Fluoritum
石楠叶	shí nán yè	Folium Photiniae
牛膝	niú xī	Radix Achyranthis Bidentatae

(3) Invigorating the Corpus Luteum

Infertility due to dysfunction of the corpus luteum can be viewed as an imbalance of yin and yang transformation, liver and kidney insufficiency, and depletion of essence and blood. When resulting from spleen and kidney yang debilitation, symptoms and signs include profuse pale menses, aversion to cold, cold limbs, fatigue, torpid intake, and loose stools. The tongue appears pale with a thin coating. Pulses are deep and thready.

The treatment principle here is to tonify the spleen and kidney and regulate qi and blood.

Select *Shèng Yù Tāng* (圣愈汤) as the basic formula.

熟地黄	shú dì huáng	Radix Rehmanniae Praeparata
白芍	bái sháo	Radix Paeoniae Alba
当归	dāng guī	Radix Angelicae Sinensis
川芎	chuān xiōng	Rhizoma Chuanxiong
黄精	huáng jīng	Rhizoma Polygonati
肉苁蓉	ròu cōng róng	Herba Cistanches

菟丝子	*tù sī zǐ*	Semen Cuscutae
茺蔚子	*chōng wèi zǐ*	Fructus Leonuri
泽兰	*zé lán*	Herba Lycopi
人参	*rén shēn*	Radix et Rhizoma Ginseng
黄芪	*huáng qí*	Radix Astragali

(Liu Ai-wu. Pang Pan-chi's Experience in Treating Infertility 通管、促排卵、健黄体、庞泮池治疗不孕症的经验. *Shanghai Journal of Traditional Chinese Medicine* (上海中医药杂志), 1995, 12: 1-2)

9. ZHU NAN-SUN

(1) Deficiency Patterns

A. *Kidney yang deficiency*

Signs and symptoms include irregular menstruation with scant pale menses, amenorrhea, fatigue, torpid intake, aversion to cold, aching lumbus, frigidity, abdominal cold, and loose stools. The tongue appears enlarged and pale with a thick coating. Pulses are slow and thready, deep at the *chi* positions.

Treatment may be divided into 3 phases.

Phase One: Fortify the spleen, harmonize the stomach, nourish blood, and regulate menstruation.

Medicinals:

当归	*dāng guī*	Radix Angelicae Sinensis
焦党参	*jiāo dǎng shēn*	Radix Codonopsis (scorch-fried)
茯苓	*fú líng*	Poria
白芍	*bái sháo*	Radix Paeoniae Alba
赤芍	*chì sháo*	Radix Paeoniae Rubra
焦白术	*jiāo bái zhú*	Rhizoma Atractylodis Macrocephalae (scorch-fried)
陈皮	*chén pí*	Pericarpium Citri Reticulatae
姜半夏	*jiāng bàn xià*	Rhizome Pinelliae Praeparata
炙甘草	*zhì gān cǎo*	Radix et Rhizoma Glycyrrhizae Praeparata cum Melle
煨木香	*wēi mù xiāng*	Radix Aucklandiae (roasted)

| 砂仁（后下） | shā rén | Fructus Amomi (decocted later) |
| 补骨脂 | bǔ gǔ zhī | Fructus Psoraleae |

Phase Two: Nourish and warm the penetrating and conception vessels, replenish essence and marrow.

党参	dǎng shēn	Radix Codonopsis
黄芪	huáng qí	Radix Astragali
当归	dāng guī	Radix Angelicae Sinensis
熟地黄	shú dì huáng	Radix Rehmanniae Praeparata
白芍	bái sháo	Radix Paeoniae Alba
川芎	chuān xiōng	Rhizoma Chuanxiong
肉苁蓉	ròu cōng róng	Herba Cistanches
紫河车（研末吞）	zǐ hé chē	Placenta Hominis (ground for swallowing)
菟丝子	tù sī zǐ	Semen Cuscutae
覆盆子	fù pén zǐ	Fructus Rubi
巴戟天	bā jǐ tiān	Radix Morindae Officinalis
鹿角霜（包煎）	lù jiǎo shuāng	Cornu Cervi Degelatinatum (wrapped)

Phase Three: Warm the kidney to benefit conception.

党参	dǎng shēn	Radix Codonopsis
黄芪	huáng qí	Radix Astragali
当归	dāng guī	Radix Angelicae Sinensis
熟地黄	shú dì huáng	Radix Rehmanniae Praeparata
鹿角霜（包煎）	lù jiǎo shuāng	Cornu Cervi Degelatinatum (wrapped)
巴戟天	bā jǐ tiān	Radix Morindae Officinalis
仙灵脾	xiān líng pí	Herba Epimedii
仙茅	xiān máo	Rhizoma Curculiginis
石楠叶	shí nán yè	Folium Photiniae
蛇床子	shé chuáng zǐ	Fructus Cnidii
四制香附丸（包煎）	sì zhì xiāng fù wán	sì zhì xiāng fù wán (wrapped)

B. Kidney yin deficiency

Symptoms and signs include irregular menstruation, scant purple menses, amenorrhea, dizziness, insomnia, palpitation, painful dry throat, bitter taste in the mouth, oral putrescence, dry bound stools, and aching lumbus with weak limbs. The complexion appears withered-yellow or with dark spots. The tongue appears red with a thin or peeled coating. Pulses are weak at the *chi* positions.

Treatment may be divided into 2 phases.

Phase One: Tonify the liver and kidney, nourish blood, and regulate menstruation.

白芍	*bái sháo*	Radix Paeoniae Alba
赤芍	*chì sháo*	Radix Paeoniae Rubra
巴戟天	*bā jǐ tiān*	Radix Morindae Officinalis
熟地黄	*shú dì huáng*	Radix Rehmanniae Praeparata
山茱萸	*shān zhū yú*	Fructus Corni
黄精	*huáng jīng*	Rhizoma Polygonati
肉苁蓉	*ròu cōng róng*	Herba Cistanches
沙参	*shā shēn*	Radix Adenophorae
麦冬	*mài dōng*	Radix Ophiopogonis
生地	*shēng dì*	Radix Rehmanniae
丹参	*dān shēn*	Radix et Rhizoma Salviae Miltiorrhizae
脐带	*qí dài*	umbilical cord (1 piece)

Phase Two: Tonify the kidney to benefit conception.

巴戟天	*bā jǐ tiān*	Radix Morindae Officinalis
熟地黄	*shú dì huáng*	Radix Rehmanniae Praeparata
山茱萸	*shān zhū yú*	Fructus Corni
菟丝子	*tù sī zǐ*	Semen Cuscutae
覆盆子	*fù pén zǐ*	Fructus Rubi
紫石英	*zǐ shí yīng*	Fluoritum
石楠叶	*shí nán yè*	Folium Photiniae
枸杞	*gǒu qǐ*	Fructus Lycii

(2) Excess Patterns

A. Penetrating and conception vessel damage with damp-heat brewing internally

Signs and symptoms include irregular menstruation, premenstrual stabbing pain of the lesser abdomen, low-grade fever, and premenstrual breast distention. The tongue appears red with a slimy coating. Pulses are wiry and rapid.

The treatment principle here is to clear heat, disinhibit dampness, course the liver, and regulate menstruation.

生地	*shēng dì*	Radix Rehmanniae
赤芍	*chì sháo*	Radix Paeoniae Rubra
蒲公英	*pú gōng yīng*	Herba Taraxaci
柴胡	*chái hú*	Radix Bupleuri
红藤	*hóng téng*	Caulis Sargentodoxae
牡丹皮	*mǔ dān pí*	Cortex Moutan
郁金	*yù jīn*	Radix Curcumae
延胡索	*yán hú suǒ*	Rhizoma Corydalis
知母	*zhī mǔ*	Rhizoma Anemarrhenae
黄柏	*huáng bǎi*	Cortex Phellodendri Chinensis
川楝子	*chuān liàn zǐ*	Fructus Toosendan

B. Obstruction of the penetrating and conception vessels with uterine collateral blockage

Signs and symptoms include premenstrual breast distention, emotional constraint, abdominal distention, aching lumbus, and frigidity. The tongue coating appears slimy. Pulses are wiry and thready, or soggy and thready.

The treatment principle here is to disinhibit qi and free stagnation.

制香附	*zhì xiāng fù*	Rhizoma Cyperi (prepared)
石菖蒲	*shí chāng pú*	Rhizoma Acori Tatarinowii
王不留行	*wáng bù liú xíng*	Semen Vaccariae
枳壳	*zhǐ qiào*	Fructus Aurantii
紫苏子	*zǐ sū zǐ*	Fructus Perillae
路路通	*lù lù tōng*	Fructus Liquidambaris
沉香（研末吞）	*chén xiāng*	Lignum Aquilariae Resinatum (ground for swallowing)

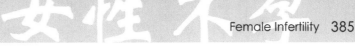
| 小茴香 | xiǎo huí xiāng | Fructus Foeniculi |
| 月季花 | yuè jì huā | Flos Rosae Chinensis |

(Tang Wan-wu. Doctor Zhu Nan-sun's Experience in Treating Infertility 朱南孙老中医治疗不孕症的经验. *Journal of Anhui Traditional Chinese Medical College* (安徽中医学院学报), 1993, (12) 4: 10)

PERSPECTIVES OF INTEGRATIVE MEDICINE

Challenges and Solutions

The clinical treatment of female infertility is particularly challenging. The associated pathomechanisms are typically complex, with specific causes often remaining unclear. There a number of difficult issues to consider in the diagnosis and treatment of these conditions.

CHALLENGE #1: PREVENTION

Although infertility conditions are generally associated with a number of factors, the cause may be congenital, and thus unpreventable. Ming dynasty physician Wan Quan recognized five forms of female infertility, or "five unwomanlinesses". They include deformity of the vagina, constricted vagina, imperforate hymen, excessively developed clitoris, and menstrual irregularities such as absent menses, flooding, or vaginal discharge.

Some diseases that appear duing adolescence may also result in infertility later in life. Other conditions that may contribute to infertility include tuberculosis, mumps, pubertal dysfunctional uterine bleeding, PCOS, amenorrhea, amenorrhea galactorrhea syndrome, pituitary microadenoma, premature ovarian failure, Sheehan's disease, abortion, salpingemphraxis, pelvic inflammation, cervicitis, vaginitis, uterine submucous myoma, endometrial polyps, endometrial tuberculosis, endometriosis, hyperthyroidism, hypothyroidism, diabetes, hyperinsulinemia, psychic trauma, severe malnutrition, and chromosomal disease. Although each of these conditions can be treated effectively or even prevented in many cases, effective methods of prevention and treatment for infertility are significantly less clear. Furthermore, many symptoms associated with infertility are similar to those of other diseases. Causes may be viewed as congenital, systemic, or gynecological in nature. To prevent infertility and maintain reproductive health, all abnormal systemic or gynecological conditions must be addressed as early as possible.

CHALLENGE #2: IDENTIFYING THE ETIOLOGY

It is relatively simple to make a diagnosis of infertility according to its basic definition. However, it is much more difficult to discover specific causes based on clinical evidence. Symptomatic treatments are often ineffective because the underlying cause remains unclear. Some couples are infertile even though examination results are normal. It also seems that many cases are clearly associated with mental and emotional factors. Ironically, some couples will conceive only after they give up trying. In any event, uncovering the causes and making an accurate diagnosis may prove difficult. Pattern identification based on information obtained from the four examinations is most useful when combined with a clear understanding of the physiological and pathological factors involved.

(1) Evaluating Ovulation

There are a number of methods to evaluate ovulatory function, but due to their individual limitations, a combination of testing methods is recommended. For example, measurement of BBT and progesterone during the mid-luteal phase is of limited value since both levels rise following ovulation. Urine LH testing and ultrasonic examination are more useful because ovulation can be predicted in advance. Ovulation generally occurs within 24 hours after urine LH levels reach their peak. Ultrasound examination may be used to monitor both ovulation and follicular development, but endocrine function and estrogen levels cannot be determined with this method. Although cervical scores may reflect estrogen levels, this information alone is insufficient for a complete evaluation.

Laparoscopy is the most reliable method to accurately confirm ovulation, next to a positive pregnancy test. A number of well-coordinated events occur locally within the ovarian follicle during the periovulatory interval, and laparoscopy is currently the routine method to evaluate this process.

Hormone levels may also be evaluated through testing of peritoneal fluid taken after ovulation. These levels may be contrasted with the results of serum testing. A higher concentration of estrogen in the abdominal cavity indicates improved egg quality. However, invasive procedures like laparoscopy should not be performed repeatedly.

(2) Evaluating Tubal Obstruction

Hysterosalpingography and laparoscopy are the principal examinations for evaluating infertility conditions. However, hysterosalpingography can result in misdiagnosis of patients presenting with spasmodic uterine contractions. An unobstructed oviduct can be accurately confirmed through laparoscopy, which can also reveal the presence of endometriosis and uterine adhesions. Treatment of these conditions may require surgical intervention.

(3) Hysteroscopy and Intrauterine Causes

Hysteroscopy allows for the observation of intrauterine diseases such as uterine fibroids, endometrial polyps, endometrial tuberculosis, and intrauterine adhesions.

(4) Reproductive Immunology

Unexplained infertility may indicate the need for immunological screening. Between 20 and 25 percent of all repeated miscarriages are due to immunological problems. Testing includes screening for a number of factors including anti-phospholipid, anti-cardiolipid, and anti-sperm antibodies.

CHALLENGE #3: THE TREATMENT OF DIFFICULT CASES

Jingyue's Complete Compendium (景岳全书 , *Jǐng Yuè Quán Shū*) states, "There is no routine treatment for infertility. Vary the medicinals to suit the individual." When pattern identification is the basis of diagnosis, a number of treatment possibilities exist. There are also a number of basic treatment principles to follow. These include, "first seek the root", "deficiency patterns require tonification", "excess patterns require drainage", "for cold conditions, apply heat" and "for heat conditions, apply cold".

Other guidelines for the treatment of difficult cases are listed below.

Use both disease identification and pattern differentiation

Disease identification and pattern differentiation are two distinct methods for understanding the nature of the condition and its clinical manifestations. The combining of these perspectives is the most effective approach to determining treatment.

A. Infertility due to ovulation failure

Regular menstruation results from the harmonious transformations of kidney yin and kidney yang. Irregular menstruation, anovulia, and luteal phase defects require the regulation of kidney yin and yang to allow for the "planting of seeds", or conception. According to our experience, the transformation of kidney yin into yang occurs predominately during the post-menstrual and ovulation periods. At these times, the harmony of the qi and blood of the penetrating and conception vessels and uterus are restored. In cases of ovulation failure, the basic treatment principle is to enrich the kidney and nourish yin.

Select *Zī Shèn Zhòng Zǐ Tāng* (滋肾种子汤) or *Zuǒ Guī Wán* (左归丸) to nourish *tian gui* and secure the penetrating and conception vessels. For congenital kidney yang deficiency, apply modifications of *Yòu Guī Wán* (右归丸).

During the ovulatory phase, add *dān shēn* (Radix et Rhizoma Salviae Miltiorrhizae), *dāng guī* (Radix Angelicae Sinensis) and *wū yào* (Radix Linderae) to move qi and invigorate blood. This modification acts to stimulate the dominant follicle.

From ovulation through the premenstrual period, apply *Guī Shèn Wán* (归肾丸) to neutrally tonify yin and yang.

With BBT in diphase lasting for 14 to 16 days, select *Shòu Tāi Wán* (寿胎丸) with added *bái sháo* (Radix Paeoniae Alba), *shú dì huáng* (Radix Rehmanniae Praeparata) and *shā rén* (Fructus Amomi) to nourish yin-blood and foster the fetus.

When fertilization is unsuccessful, the BBT will drop, and the the sea of blood will fill and discharge. With scant menses, apply medicinals to invigorate blood and free the menses. For profuse menstruation with stasis, stanch bleeding and eliminate stasis. For profuse menstruation due to qi deficiency, secure the penetrating vessel and supplement qi to contain blood.

B. Infertility caused by salpingemphraxis

Obstruction of the fallopian tube is often associated with PID, salpingitis, genital tuberculosis, endometriosis, and post-surgical adhesions. The pathogenesis generally involves stasis obstructing the vessels and collaterals with qi stagnation, cold-damp, or damp-heat.

Apply *Tōng Guǎn Tāng* (通管汤) to invigorate blood, dispel stasis, dissipate bind, and free the collaterals.

通管汤 *Tōng Guǎn Tāng*

炮山甲	*pào shān jiǎ*	9g	Squama Manis
皂角刺	*zào jiǎo cì*	15g	Spina Gleditsiae
三棱	*sān léng*	9g	Rhizoma Sparganii
莪术	*é zhú*	9g	Rhizoma Curcumae
制乳香	*zhì rǔ xiāng*	9g	Olibanum (prepared)
制没药	*zhì mò yào*	9g	Myrrha (prepared)
赤芍	*chì sháo*	9g	Radix Paeoniae Rubra
丹参	*dān shēn*	30g	Radix et Rhizoma Salviae Miltiorrhizae
桃仁	*táo rén*	9g	Semen Persicae
路路通	*lù lù tōng*	15g	Fructus Liquidambaris
昆布	*kūn bù*	9g	Thallus Laminariae
海藻	*hǎi zǎo*	9g	Sargassum
益母草	*yì mǔ cǎo*	30g	Herba Leonuri
夏枯草	*xià kū cǎo*	9g	Spica Prunellae

Wēn Guǎn Tāng (温管汤) may also be applied to invigorate blood, dispel stasis, warm the channels, and free the collaterals.

温管汤 *Wēn Guǎn Tāng*

炮山甲	*pào shān jiǎ*	9g	Squama Manis
皂角刺	*zào jiǎo cì*	15g	Spina Gleditsiae
三棱	*sān léng*	9g	Rhizoma Sparganii
莪术	*é zhú*	9g	Rhizoma Curcumae
制乳香	*zhì rǔ xiāng*	9g	Olibanum (prepared)
制没药	*zhì mò yào*	9g	Myrrha (prepared)
赤芍	*chì sháo*	9g	Radix Paeoniae Rubra
丹参	*dān shēn*	30g	Radix et Rhizoma Salviae Miltiorrhizae
桃仁	*táo rén*	9g	Semen Persicae
路路通	*lù lù tōng*	15g	Fructus Liquidambaris
当归	*dāng guī*	9g	Radix Angelicae Sinensis
附子	*fù zǐ*	6g	Radix Aconiti Lateralis Praeparata
肉桂	*ròu guì*	1.5g	Cortex Cinnamomi
小茴香	*xiǎo huí xiāng*	6g	Fructus Foeniculi
茯苓	*fú líng*	9g	Poria

仙灵脾	xiān líng pí	15g	Herba Epimedii
紫石英	zǐ shí yīng	30g	Fluoritum
蜈蚣	wú gōng	2pieces	Scolopendra

Qīng Guǎn Tāng (清管汤) may be applied to invigorate blood, transform stasis, clear heat, and free the collaterals.

清管汤 *Qīng Guǎn Tāng*

炮山甲	pào shān jiǎ	9g	Squama Manis
皂角刺	zào jiǎo cì	15g	Spina Gleditsiae
三棱	sān léng	9g	Rhizoma Sparganii
莪术	é zhú	9g	Rhizoma Curcumae
制乳香	zhì rǔ xiāng	9g	Olibanum (prepared)
制没药	zhì mò yào	9g	Myrrha (prepared)
赤芍	chì sháo	9g	Radix Paeoniae Rubra
丹参	dān shēn	30g	Radix et Rhizoma Salviae Miltiorrhizae
桃仁	táo rén	9g	Semen Persicae
路路通	lù lù tōng	15g	Fructus Liquidambaris
益母草	yì mǔ cǎo	30g	Herba Leonuri
夏枯草	xià kū cǎo	9g	Spica Prunellae
丹皮	dān pí	9g	Cortex Moutan
黄柏	huáng bǎi	9g	Cortex Phellodendri Chinensis
银花	yín huā	30g	Flos Lonicerae Japonicae
连翘	lián qiào	15g	Fructus Forsythiae
公英	gōng yīng	18g	Herba Taraxaci
败酱草	bài jiàng cǎo	24g	Herba Patriniae

C. Infertility caused by polycystic ovarian syndrome (PCOS)

PCOS is an endocrine disorder associated with abnormally high levels of male hormones that very often result in anovulation. Common symptoms include oligomenorrhea, amenorrhea, irregular vaginal bleeding, excessive bodyhair, obesity, and ovarian cysts. PCOS usually presents with patterns of kidney qi depletion, spleen deficiency, stasis obstructing the penetrating and conception vessels, and phlegm-damp gathering and congealing.

The proper treatment method is to tonify and attack simultaneously to address both branch and root. For excess branch patterns, emphasize attacking methods while also applying tonification, dispelling stasis, and eliminating dampness.

With obvious deficiency, primarily tonify and warm the spleen and kidney yang while also resolving phlegm and moving stagnation. Apply the empirical formula *Dǎo Tán Zhòng Zǐ Tāng* (导痰种子汤).

With obviously enlarged ovaries, add *sān léng* (Rhizoma Sparganii) 9g, *é zhú* (Rhizoma Curcumae) 9g, and *biē jiǎ* (Carapax Trionycis) 12g. Rich and greasy, or raw and cold-natured foods are also prohibited.

导痰种子汤 *Dǎo Tán Zhòng Zǐ Tāng*

胆南星	*dǎn nán xīng*	9g	Arisaema cum Bile
茯苓	*fú líng*	12g	Poria
白术	*bái zhú*	9g	Rhizoma Atractylodis Macrocephalae
陈皮	*chén pí*	12g	Pericarpium Citri Reticulatae
法半夏	*fǎ bàn xià*	12g	Rhizoma Pinelliae Praeparatum
当归	*dāng guī*	6g	Radix Angelicae Sinensis
川芎	*chuān xiōng*	6g	Rhizoma Chuanxiong
黄芪	*huáng qí*	15g	Radix Astragali
淫羊藿	*yín yáng huò*	9g	Herba Epimedii
巴戟天	*bā jǐ tiān*	12g	Radix Morindae Officinalis
鸡血藤	*jī xuè téng*	12g	Caulis Spatholobi
香附	*xiāng fù*	6g	Rhizoma Cyperi

D. Infertility caused by amenorrhea galactorrhea syndrome

Amenorrhea galactorrhea syndrome refers to persistent lactation with amenorrhea in a woman who is not breastfeeding or has stopped nursing for over a year. It is most often associated with elevated levels of prolactin in the blood. Associated factors and causes include pituitary dysfunction or tumor, hypothyroidism, antidepressant medications, and oral contraceptives. Manifestations include amenorrhea, galactorrhea, infertility, and climacteric symptoms. When due to pituitary tumor, the optic nerve may become compressed causing headache, and impaired or double-vision. Bromocriptine is generally prescribed to reduce PRL and galactorrhea. In these cases, the combining of Chinese medicinals with bromocriptine may significantly reduce side effects.

In Chinese medicine, this syndrome is referred to as "menstrual block" with "galactorrhea". This syndrome usually presents with patterns of liver constraint, qi stagnation, and liver-stomach disharmony. The proper treatment method is to soothe the liver, resolve depression, suppress lactation, conduct menses, and benefit conception.

Select *Kāi Yù Zhòng Zǐ Tāng* (开郁种子汤) or *Chái Hú Shū Gān Sǎn* (柴胡疏肝散) with added *chǎo mài yá* (dry-fried Fructus Hordei Germinatus), *dàn dòu chǐ* (Semen Sojae Praeparatum), *fú líng* (Poria), *chuān niú xī* (Radix Cyathulae), *māo zhuǎ cǎo* (Radix Ranunculi Ternati) and *zhǐ qiào* (Fructus Aurantii).

E. Infertility caused by endometriosis

Endometriosis is often associated with dysmenorrhea, chronic pelvic pain, and infertility, being diagnosed in up to 50% of infertile women. Reproductive performance is typically poorer among women with endometriosis, especially in those with severe pelvic adhesions which block the oviduct. Other associated conditions include ovulation failure, salpingemphraxis, hyperprolactinemia, luteinized unruptured follicle syndrome, and immune reactions. The symptoms associated with endometriosis get worse when exposed to estrogen and improve with hypoestrogenism.

In Chinese medicine, blood that accumulates outside the vessels is referred to as static blood. Static blood can give rise to palpable masses that indicate concretion in the lower abdomen, and obstruction of the penetrating and conception vessels and uterine vessels. During the non-bleeding stages, the proper treatment method is to invigorate blood, transform stasis, disperse concretions and dissipate bind.

Individual medicinals include *sān léng* (Rhizoma Sparganii), *é zhú* (Rhizoma Curcumae), *zhǐ shí* (Fructus Aurantii Immaturus), *biē jiǎ* (Carapax Trionycis), *guī jiǎ* (Carapax et Plastrum Testudinis), *zhēn zhū mǔ* (Concha Margaritifera), *jī nèi jīn* (Endothelium Corneum Gigeriae Galli), *dāng guī* (Radix Angelicae Sinensis), *dān shēn* (Radix et Rhizoma Salviae Miltiorrhizae), *sān qī* (Radix et Rhizoma Notoginseng), and *dà huáng* (Radix et Rhizoma Rhei).

Selected formulas include *Tōng Yū Yī Hào* (通瘀一号) and *Xiāo Zhēng Chōng Jì*.

通瘀一号 *Tōng Yū Yī Hào*

丹参	*dān shēn*	Radix et Rhizoma Salviae Miltiorrhizae
威灵仙	*wēi líng xiān*	Radix et Rhizoma Clematidis
三棱	*sān léng*	Rhizoma Sparganii
莪术	*é zhú*	Rhizoma Curcumae
当归	*dāng guī*	Radix Angelicae Sinensis
川芎	*chuān xiōng*	Rhizoma Chuanxiong

10g, three times daily, dissolved in boiling water.

During the bleeding period, apply medicinals to regulate qi, invigorate blood, dispel stasis, and clear the penetrating vessel.

These medicinals include *dān shēn* (Radix et Rhizoma Salviae Miltiorrhizae), *mǔ dān pí* (Cortex Moutan), *dāng guī* (Radix Angelicae Sinensis), *sān qī* (Radix et Rhizoma Notoginseng), *wǔ líng zhī* (Faeces Togopteri), *pú huáng* (Pollen Typhae), *hóng huā* (Flos Carthami) and *yì mǔ cǎo* (Herba Leonuri).

Tōng Yū Èr Hào (通瘀二号) may be applied to absorb static blood.

通瘀二号 *Tōng Yū Èr Hào*

红花	*hóng huā*	Flos Carthami
赤芍	*chì sháo*	Radix Paeoniae Rubra
丹参	*dān shēn*	Radix et Rhizoma Salviae Miltiorrhizae

牡丹皮	mǔ dān pí	Cortex Moutan
郁金	yù jīn	Radix Curcumae
枳实	zhǐ shí	Fructus Aurantii Immatu rus
夏枯草	xià kū cǎo	Spica Prunellae

10g three times daily, dissolved in boiling water.

With severe menstrual pain, add *guǎng mù xiāng* (Radix Aucklandiae) and *xiāng fù* (Rhizoma Cyperi).

With profuse menstruation, remove *dān shēn* (Radix et Rhizoma Salviae Miltiorrhizae) and *hóng huā* (Flos Carthami) and add *dì yú* (Radix Sanguisorbae), *mò hàn lián* (Herba Ecliptae), *hǎi piāo xiāo* (Endoconcha Sepiae) and *zhǐ qiào* (Fructus Aurantii).

Clinical and empirical studies have shown that blood-invigorating stasis-transforming medicinals can benefit hemorheological conditions, reduce pathological lesions, and also improve immunity. This treatment approach can improve the chance of conception in cases associated with pelvic endometriosis.

F. Infertility caused by lutenized unruptured follicle syndrome

In a small percentage of women, the dominant follicle will undergo the luteinization process without rupturing. Lutenized unruptured follicle syndrome often presents with regular menstruation and midcycle anovulia with unruptured follicles.

In Chinese medicine, this condition is generally associated with patterns of deficiency affecting the kidney, essence and blood, and the penetrating and conception vessels. Patterns of stasis obstructing the uterine vessels and collaterals can also prevent fertilization.

The general treatment principle here is to tonify the kidney and dispel stasis.

Select the following medicinals:

| 熟地 | shú dì | 12g | Radix Rehmanniae Praeparata |
| 山茱萸 | shān zhū yú | 9g | Fructus Corni |

巴戟天	bā jǐ tiān	9g	Radix Morindae Officinalis
菟丝子	tù sī zǐ	9g	Semen Cuscutae
淫羊藿	yín yáng huò	15g	Herba Epimedii
紫石英	zǐ shí yīng	30g	Fluoritum
三棱	sān léng	9g	Rhizoma Sparganii
莪术	é zhú	9g	Rhizoma Curcumae
穿山甲	chuān shān jiǎ	12g	Squama Manis
昆布	kūn bù	9g	Thallus Laminariae
海藻	hǎi zǎo	9g	Sargassum
桃仁	táo rén	9g	Semen Persicae
红花	hóng huā	9g	Flos Carthami

With hyperthyroidism, remove *hǎi zǎo* (Sargassum) and *kūn bù* (Thallus Laminariae). This formula acts to tonify the kidney and invigorate blood and may also promote regulation of the hypothalamus-pituitary-ovarian axis. Medicinals that break stasis, free the collaterals, and dissipate binding can also promote follicular wall rupture and release.

G. Immune infertility

Immune infertility results from an antigenic autoimmune response of the reproductive system. Sperm, seminal plasma, and ovarian cells which produce steroid hormones all contain specific antigens. Immune reactions associated with these antibodies directly effect reproduction, often leading to infertility.

In Chinese medicine, this condition generally presents with failure of the spleen and kidney, and yin deficiency of the liver and kidney with stasis.

Qiáng Tǐ Zhòng Zǐ Fāng (强体种子方) is selected to tonify the kidney, fortify the spleen, and supplement qi.

Zī Shèn Tián Jīng Fāng (滋肾填精方) is selected to enrich yin and tonify blood.

Patients should abstain from sexual intercourse for 2 to 3 months, or use condoms.

Treatment for both partners is indicated when the male tests positive for AsAb.

强体种子方 *Qiáng Tǐ Zhòng Zǐ Fāng*

女贞子	*nǚ zhēn zǐ*	20g	Fructus Ligustri Lucidi
黄精	*huáng jīng*	15g	Rhizoma Polygonati
茯苓	*fú líng*	15g	Poria
山药	*shān yào*	15g	Rhizoma Dioscoreae
黄芪	*huáng qí*	15g	Radix Astragali
防风	*fáng fēng*	9g	Radix Saposhnikoviae
丹参	*dān shēn*	9g	Radix et Rhizoma Salviae Miltiorrhizae
丹皮	*dān pí*	9g	Cortex Moutan

滋肾填精方 *Zī Shèn Tián Jīng Fāng*

生地	*shēng dì*	12g	Radix Rehmanniae
山茱萸	*shān zhū yú*	9g	Fructus Corni
麦冬	*mài dōng*	9g	Radix Ophiopogonis
白芍	*bái sháo*	9g	Radix Paeoniae Alba
墨旱莲	*mò hàn lián*	12g	Herba Ecliptae
龟板	*guī bǎn*	30	Testudinis Plastrum
鳖甲	*biē jiǎ*	30	Carapax Trionycis
丹皮	*dān pí*	9g	Cortex Moutan
丹参	*dān shēn*	30	Radix et Rhizoma Salviae Miltiorrhizae
黄芪	*huáng qí*	30	Radix Astragali
制黄精	*zhì huáng jīng*	15g	Rhizoma Polygonati (prepared)
黄芩	*huáng qín*	9g	Radix Scutellariae
徐长卿	*xú cháng qīng*	9g	Radix et Rhizoma Cynanchi Paniculati
生甘草	*shēng gān cǎo*	9g	Radix et Rhizoma Glycyrrhizae (raw)

Note: The empirical formulas *Zhù Yùn Yī Hào* (助孕 Ⅰ 号) and *Zhù Yùn Èr Hào* (助孕 Ⅱ 号) are also commonly prescribed for this condition, as mentioned earlier in this text.

H. Infertility caused by Sheehan's syndrome

Sheehan's syndrome is associated with hypofunction and necrosis of the anterior pituitary caused by insufficient blood supply to the gland due to severe blood loss or intravascular clotting and hemorrhage during childbirth. Other associated conditions include amenorrhea, reduced libido, atrophy of the breasts and genital organs, hypothyroidism, and hypoadrenalism.

In Chinese medicine, this condition generally presents with blood desiccation menstrual block.

The general treatment principle here is to warm kidney yang and tonify qi and blood.

Select modified *Èr Xiān Tāng* (二仙汤).

二仙汤 *Èr Xiān Tāng*

淫羊藿	*yín yáng huò*	Herba Epimedii
仙茅	*xiān máo*	Rhizoma Curculiginis
附子	*fù zǐ*	Radix Aconiti Lateralis Praeparata
炙甘草	*zhì gān cǎo*	Radix et Rhizoma Glycyrrhizae Praeparata cum Melle
人参	*rén shēn*	Radix et Rhizoma Ginseng
熟地	*shú dì*	Radix Rehmanniae Praeparata
当归	*dāng guī*	Radix Angelicae Sinensis
川芎	*chuān xiōng*	Rhizoma Chuanxiong

With distending pain in the lower abdomen and inhibited menses, select *Táo Hóng Sì Wù Tāng* (桃红四物汤) with added *yín yáng huò* (Herba Epimedii), *bā jǐ tiān* (Radix Morindae Officinalis), *yì mǔ cǎo* (Herba Leonuri), *xiāng fù* (Rhizoma Cyperi) and *wáng bù liú xíng* (Semen Vaccariae) to conduct blood and free menstruation.

When applying formulas to tonify the spleen and kidney and supplement qi and blood, low dosages of synthetic hormones such as thyroxine may also be prescribed.

I. Infertility caused by anorexia nervosa

Anorexia nervosa is a psychiatric disorder characterized by a persistent unwillingness to eat, most often occurring in adolescent women. The main symptoms include severe emaciation and amenorrhea. Amenorrhea may occur before or after the patient becomes emaciated. Laboratory examinations may show no apparent abnormality.

The general treatment principle here is to fortify the spleen, harmonize the stomach, enrich the kidney, and replenish essence. For non-compliant patients, acupuncture may be a more appropriate therapy. Over time, tonifying medicinals may be included in the treatment plan. Psychotherapy is also generally indicated.

Insight from Empirical Wisdom

Infertility often appears as a symptom that can be associated with a variety of medical conditions. The classical literature often refers to this condition under the headings of *reproduction, offspring,* or *planting seeds*. In order to properly diagnosis and treat this condition, we should take an approach which combines pattern identification with a clear understanding of the disease characteristics. The diagnostic methods of modern medicine are most useful for identifying the underlying causes. Pattern differentiation should then be employed to distinguish the chief pattern from secondary and concurrent patterns. Proper treatment should take all of this into consideration.

1. REGULATING MENSTRUATION

The classics state, "To promote conception, first regulate menstruation".

Dan-xi's Heart-Approach (丹溪心法 , *Dān xī Xīn Fǎ*) also points out, "A fetus cannot be formed without regular menstruation." [7]

Secrets of Gynecology, (妇人秘科, *Fù Rén Mì Kē*) points out: "Childlessness among women usually results from menstrual irregularities." [8]

When regulating the menstruation to promote conception, we should

---

[7] 见《丹溪心法》："经水不调，不能成胎。"
[8] 见《妇人秘科》："女人无子，多以经候不调。"

also emphasize regulation of the kidney, liver and spleen. The kidney is considered as the root of earlier heaven, original qi, and the penetrating and conception vessels. It stores the essence of both earlier and later heaven, governs reproduction, and is also the source of *tian gui*.

The classic literature states that, "Menses emanate from the kidney" and "The uterine vessel is connected to the kidney." Furthermore, the *Treatise on the Six Periods and Visceral Manifestation from the Plain Questions* (素问·六节藏象论, *Sù Wèn. Liù Jié Zàng Xiàng Lùn*) states, "The kidney governs hibernation. It is the root of storage and the location of essence." A woman can become pregnant only when the kidney essence and qi are abundant, the conception vessel is free, the penetrating vessel is exuberant, and the menstrual vessels are regular.

The liver stores blood, and also governs free coursing. Furthermore, essence and blood are of the same source. Normal menstruation and fertility are maintained by the free coursing function of the liver and the storage function of the kidney.

The spleen is the source of qi and blood formation. When the spleen qi is abundant, later heaven qi can then nourish the qi of earlier heaven. When regulating the kidney, spleen and liver, also pay close attention to the state of qi and blood. It is said that the vital activities of women are governed by blood, with blood being the material foundation of menstruation.

Also consider the close relationship between qi and blood. It is said that blood is the mother of qi, and that qi is the commander of blood. Therefore, when qi moves, the blood also moves. When qi stagnates, the blood becomes static.

To regulate menstruation and promote conception, the treatment principles may include tonifying kidney qi, supplementing kidney essence, regulating and nourishing the penetrating and conception vessels, coursing liver qi, nourishing liver yin, fortifying the spleen and stomach, transforming phlegm and dampness, and regulating qi and blood.

Commonly used formulas to tonify kidney qi, supplement essence and blood, and regulate the penetrating and conception vessels include *Zuǒ Guī Wán* (左归丸), *Yòu Guī Wán* (右归丸), *Shèn Qì Wán* (肾气丸), *Èr Xiān Tāng* (二仙汤), *Liù Wèi Dì Huáng Wán* (六味地黄丸), *Wǔ Zǐ Yǎn Zōng Tāng* (五子衍宗汤) and *Guī Shèn Wán* (归肾丸).

Individual medicinals include *shú dì* (Radix Rehmanniae Praeparata), *tù sī zǐ* (Semen Cuscutae), *nǔ zhēn zǐ* (Fructus Ligustri Lucidi), *gǒu qǐ zǐ* (Fructus Lycii), *yín yáng huò* (Herba Epimedii), *ròu cōng róng* (Herba Cistanches), *bā jǐ tiān* (Radix Morindae Officinalis), *lù jiǎo shuāng* (Cornu Cervi Degelatinatum) and *zǐ hé chē* (Placenta Hominis).

Commonly used formulas to course liver qi and nourish liver yin include *Xiāo Yáo Wán* (逍遥丸), *Chái Hú Shū Gān Tāng* (柴胡疏肝汤), *Kāi Yù Zhòng Yù Tāng* (开郁种玉汤), *Sì Nì Sǎn* (四逆散), *Dìng Jīng Tāng* (定经汤), *Tiáo Gān Tāng* (调肝汤) and *Èr Zhì Wán* (二至丸).

Individual medicinals include *bái sháo* (Radix Paeoniae Alba), *chái hú* (Radix Bupleuri), *yù jīn* (Radix Curcumae), *qīng pí* (Pericarpium Citri Reticulatae Viride), *zhǐ qiào* (Fructus Aurantii), *fó shǒu* (Fructus Citri Sarcodactylis), *shān zhū yú* (Fructus Corni), *nǔ zhēn zǐ* (Fructus Ligustri Lucidi), *mò hàn lián* (Herba Ecliptae), *sāng shèn* (Fructus Mori), *gǒu qǐ zǐ* (Fructus Lycii), and *sāng jì shēng* (Herba Taxilli).

Commonly used formulas to fortify the spleen and stomach and resolve phlegm and dampness include *Guī Pí Tāng* (归脾汤), *Wán Dài Tāng* (完带汤), *Cāng Fù Dǎo Tán Wán* (苍附导痰丸) and *Chén Xià Lìu Jūn Zǐ Tāng* (陈夏六君子汤).

Individual medicinals include *shān yào* (Rhizoma Dioscoreae), *fú líng* (Poria), *dǎng shēn* (Radix Codonopsis), *bái zhú* (Rhizoma Atractylodis Macrocephalae), *huáng qí* (Radix Astragali), *qiàn shí* (Semen Euryales), *chén pí* (Pericarpium Citri Reticulatae), *cāng zhú* (Rhizoma Atractylodis), *pèi lán* (Herba Eupatorii) and *hòu pò* (Cortex Magnoliae Officinalis).

Commonly used formulas to tonify qi and blood include *Bā Zhēn Tāng* (八珍汤), *Yù Lín Zhū* (毓麟珠), *Sì Wù Tāng* (四物汤), *Shèng Yù Tāng* (圣愈汤), *Dāng Guī Bǔ Xuè Tāng* (当归补血汤), *Rén Shēn Yǎng Róng Tāng* (人参养荣汤) and *Wēn Jīng Tāng* (温经汤).

Individual medicinals include *shú dì* (Radix Rehmanniae Praeparata), *dāng guī* (Radix Angelicae Sinensis), *shǒu wū* (Radix Polygoni Multiflori), *bái sháo* (Radix Paeoniae Alba), *chuān xiōng* (Rhizoma Chuanxiong), *dǎng shēn* (Radix Codonopsis), *huáng qí* (Radix Astragali), *huáng jīng* (Rhizoma Polygonati), *dà zǎo* (Fructus Jujubae) and *jī xuè téng* (Caulis Spatholobi).

Commonly used formulas to invigorate blood and transform stasis include *Shào Fù Zhú Yū Tāng* (少腹逐瘀汤), *Xuè Fǔ Zhú Yū Tāng* (血府逐瘀汤), *Gé Xià Zhú Yū Tāng* (膈下逐瘀汤), *Dà Huáng Mǔ Dān Tāng* (大黄牡丹汤), *Jiě Dú Huó Xuè Tāng* (解毒活血汤) and *Táo Hóng Sì Wù Tāng* (桃红四物汤).

Individual medicinals include *dān shēn* (Radix et Rhizoma Salviae Miltiorrhizae), *dān pí* (Cortex Moutan), *táo rén* (Semen Persicae), *hóng huā* (Flos Carthami), *yù jīn* (Radix Curcumae), *xuè jié* (Sanguis Draconis), *dāng guī* (Radix Angelicae Sinensis), and *jī xuè téng* (Caulis Spatholobi).

2. Treating Leukorrhea

Normal vaginal discharges are considered to be a kind of yin-humor. Its appearance is white, slightly thick, and odorless. During the intermenstrual period, it appears clear and bright and of greater volume. Normal discharge acts to nourish and lubricate the vagina, and it can also counteract pathogens. The ancient physician Wang Meng-ying stated, "Vaginal discharge is a congenital condition for women. It is a humor that constantly moistens. Originally, it is not a disease."

Women are unique in that they display menstruation, vaginal discharge, pregnancy, childbirth and the production of breastmilk.

They may also suffer with conditions of birth injury, flooding, spotting, and turbid vaginal discharges. Also, the lower genital tract opens to the external environment and may thus be affected by a variety of pathogens. The warm temperature and humidity of the vagina provides pathogens with an ideal climate for growth. Vaginal discharges may become abnormal in color, volume, thickness, or odor. Vaginitis, cervicitis and endometritis may generate a turbid yellow vaginal discharge that can impair the movement of sperm. Purulent white blood cells and trichomonas vaginalis can also affect sperm quality and motility.

To promote conception, first identify the specific location of the disease, and then determine the nature of the pathogen. Abnormal vaginal discharge may be associated with patterns of cold, heat, deficiency or excess. However, infertility conditions associated with vaginal discharge are most often related to patterns of dampness.

The Qing dynasty physician Fu Qing-zhu stated, "Vaginal discharge generally indicates a pattern of dampness." External dampness can easily invade the uterus and uterine vessels via the genitourinary tract. Internal dampness may result from the bowels and viscera being deprived of nourishment, especially when associated with dysfunction of the kidney, liver, and spleen. In severe cases, dampness may transfom into pathogenic phlegm and lead to infertility.

The general treatment principle here is to transform dampness, eliminate turbidity, support the upright and dispel evil. Apply methods that clear and disinhibit, warm and transform, or drain and tonify. Other methods may be indicated, depending on the nature of the vaginal discharge. These include dispelling dampness, eliminating turbidity, regulating and tonifying the bowels and viscera, regulating the penetrating and conception vessels, and fortifying and securing the governing and girdling vessels. Conception may be further promoted with medicinals that warm, transform, disinhibit, percolate, upbear yang, and free the vessels.

Commonly used formulas to clear, disinhibit, and transform dampness include modified *Bì Xiè Shèn Shī Tāng* (萆薢渗湿汤), *Zhǐ Dài Tāng* (止带汤) and *Chén Xià Liù Jūn Zǐ Tāng* (陈夏六君子汤).

Individual medicinals include *bù zhā yè* (Microcos Paniculata), *yīn chén* (Herba Artemisiae Scopariae), *pèi lán* (Herba Eupatorii), *yì yǐ rén* (Semen Coicis), *zé xiè* (Rhizoma Alismatis), *tōng cǎo* (Medulla Tetrapanacis), *bì xiè* (Rhizoma Dioscoreae Septemlobae), *chē qián cǎo* (Herba Plantaginis) and *jīn yín huā* (Flos Lonicerae Japonicae).

For exuberant damp-heat and toxin, apply *Lóng Dǎn Xiè Gān Tāng* (龙胆泻肝汤), *Wǔ Wèi Xiāo Dú Yǐn* (五味清毒饮) and *Huáng Lián Jiě Dú Tāng* (黄连解毒汤).

Individual medicinals include *pú gōng yīng* (Herba Taraxaci), *yú xīng cǎo* (Herba Houttuyniae), *bái huā shé shé cǎo* (Herba Hedyotis), *jīn yín huā* (Flos Lonicerae Japonicae), *dà huáng* (Radix et Rhizoma Rhei), *bài jiàng cǎo* (Herba Patriniae), *huáng qín* (Radix Scutellariae), *huáng lián* (Rhizoma Coptidis) and *zhī zǐ* (Fructus Gardeniae).

For cold dampness, apply *Jiàn Gù Tāng* (健固汤), *Líng Guì Zhú Gān Tāng* and *Zhēn Wǔ Tāng* (真武汤).

Individual medicinals include *guì zhī* (Ramulus Cinnamomi), *fú líng* (Poria), *bái zhú* (Rhizoma Atractylodis Macrocephalae), *wēi líng xiān* (Radix et Rhizoma Clematidis), *shú fù zǐ* (Radix Aconiti Lateralis Praeparata), and *bā jǐ tiān* (Radix Morindae Officinalis).

Commonly used formulas to upbear yang and eliminate dampness include *Wán Dài Tāng* (完带汤) and *Shēn Líng Bái Zhú Sǎn* (参苓白术散). These act to regulate the qi dynamic and eliminate dampness while also tonifying qi.

Individual medicinals include *dǎng shēn* (Radix Codonopsis), *huáng qí* (Radix Astragali), *shān yào* (Rhizoma Dioscoreae), *bái zhú* (Rhizoma Atractylodis Macrocephalae), and *chén pí* (Pericarpium Citri Reticulatae).

Commonly used formulas to transform dampness and sweep phlegm include *Cāng Fù Dǎo Tán Wán* (苍附导痰丸), *Chén Xià Liù Jūn Zǐ Tāng* (陈夏六君子汤) and *Èr Chén Tāng* (二陈汤).

Individual medicinals include *chén pí* (Pericarpium Citri Reticulatae), *fǎ bàn xià* (Rhizoma Pinelliae Praeparatum), *dǎn nán xīng* (Arisaema cum Bile), *fú líng* (Poria), *bái zhú* (Rhizoma Atractylodis Macrocephalae), *hòu pò* (Cortex Magnoliae Officinalis), *xiāng fù* (Rhizoma Cyperi) and *kūn bù* (Thallus Laminariae).

Combined therapies are often applied to improve therapeutic effects and shorten the course of treatment. Adjunctive treatments may include acupuncture, moxibustion, ear needling, plum-blossom needling, retention enema, external compress, intrauterine douche, intervenous drip infusion, intramuscular injection, herbal baths, point injection, picking therapy, and catgut embedding methods.

3. MALE REPRODUCTIVE HEALTH

The reproductive health of the male partner is a factor in many cases of infertility. This refers to normal seminal fluid constituents, endocrine and prostatic secretions, genital structure, and sexual function.

Male infertility can result from structural abnormalities, physiological causes, and a number of organic diseases. In ancient times, the "five unmanlinesses" referred to congenital eunuchism, seminal discharge, castration, impotence, and hermaphroditism. Six kinds of disorders were recorded: essence deficiency, qi deficiency, excessive phlegm, effulgent ministerial fire, lack of essence, and qi constraint. Associated biomedical conditions include prostatitis, varicocele, and immune disorders. These often result in azoospermia, necrospermia, oligospermatism, asthenospermia, nonliquefaction of semen, and poor sperm penetration. Unhealthy lifestyle choices also impact male reproductive function. Smoking, alcohol, and drug abuse are known risk factors, and psychological stress also seems to be a factor.

The combining of accurate disease identification with pattern differentiation is the most effective approach for the treatment of male infertility. Treatments include medicinals that tonify the kidney, invigorate yang, enrich the kidney, replenish essence, fortify the spleen, supplement qi, clear the liver, discharge heat, transform stasis, or eliminate turbidity. Lifestyle and infertility counseling has also been shown effective for improving clinical results.

4. Timed Intercourse

The *Canon of gynecology* (女科经纶 , *Nǚ Kē Jīng Lún*) quotes physician Yuan Liao-fan: "The female menses appear once a month. There is one day in between menstruation periods that contains a "vaporization period". For two hours, the steaming of qi with heat, clouding, and oppression appear. The woman shows a strong desire for intercourse that seems impossible to resist. This is "the time". Follow this good timing, and it will be easier to conceive." [9]

Standards of Gynecology (妇 科 玉 尺 , *Fù Kē Yù Chǐ*) also states: "This only occurs one day each month, and for only two hours of that day." [10]

This time was also known as the "true dynamic" period. Normally, ovulation begins 14 days before menstruation, plus or minus 2 days. During this period, women display thicker vaginal fluids and some distention of the lower abdomen. The chance of conception may be improved by determining the ovulation period and planning for sexual intercourse at the proper time. The date of ovulation can also be predicted through measurement of the basal body temperature.

---

[9] 《女科经纶》引袁了凡言："凡妇人一月经行一度，必有一日氤氲之候……次此的候也……顺而施之，则成胎矣。"

[10] 《妇科玉尺》："一月止有一日，一日止有一时。"

5. Emotions and Conception

Optimistic attitudes and positive mental states can certainly improve reproductive health. However, many infertile couples suffer with poor appetite, restless sleep, devitalized essence-spirit, anxiety, tension, depression, and fear. These difficulties can impact ovarian function through the neuroendocrine system, often resulting in a failure to ovulate. Psychological issues can contribute to general poor health, affecting the immune system in particular. Unbalanced emotions can cause disharmonies of qi and blood affecting the penetrating and conception vessels, as well as the bowels and viscera. Mental-emotional factors are important considerations in many cases of infertility.

Secrets of Gynecology (妇人秘科 , *Fù Rén Mì Kē*) states, "For the planting of seeds, it is essential for women to be calm at heart and settled in qi. Anxiety causes qi to bind, over-thinking causes qi depression, anger causes qi to rise, and resentment causes qi obstruction. Blood follows qi, therefore qi counterflow leads to blood counterflow. It is most important for women to be calm at heart and settled in qi."

The liver is yin in substance and yang in function. When liver qi is stagnated, liver yin becomes insufficient, and the liver function of orderly reaching is affected. The treatment principle is to course the liver and resolve constraint. In these cases, it is most important to help the patient maintain a positive attitude.

6. The Importance of a Proper Diet

Medicinals and foods are of the same source, so a proper diet can certainly promote fertility. In fact, patients in the clinic often seek out dietary advice and nutritional counseling. The following medicinal recipes and dietary guidelines are based on differentiation of the presenting pattern.

For infertility caused by kidney yang deficiency, *Fù Zǐ Bāo Gǒu Ròu* (附子煲狗肉), *Dāng Guī Yáng Ròu Tāng* (当归羊肉汤), *Lù Róng Dùn Gōng Jī* (鹿茸炖公鸡), *Hé Táo Bāo Zhū Yāo* (核桃煲猪腰), *Jī Zǐ Nuò Mǐ Jiǔ* (鸡子糯米酒) and *Běi Qí Niú Ròu Tāng* (北芪牛肉汤) are recommended to warm the kidney and uterus and invigorate yang. Avoid raw or cold-natured foods and drinks, especially bananas and pears.

For infertility caused by deficiency of kidney essence affecting the penetrating and conception vessels, *Huā Jiāo Shòu Ròu Tāng* (花胶瘦肉汤), *Chóng Cǎo Dùn Shuǐ Yā* (虫草炖水鸭) and *Yàn Wō Jī Sī Gēng* (燕窝鸡丝羹) are recommended. Avoid warming, supplementing, or dry and hot medicinals.

For infertility caused by qi and blood deficiency, *Dāng Guī Dà Zǎo Jī Dàn Chá* (当归大枣鸡蛋茶), *Zhú Sī Jī Nuò Mǐ Zhōu* (竹丝鸡糯米粥), *Shú Dì Qǐ Zǐ Shòu Ròu Zhōu* (熟地杞子瘦肉汤), *Pái Gǔ Yuán Ròu Tāng* (排骨元肉汤) and *Lián ǒu Hóng Dòu Jì Yú Tāng* (莲藕红豆鲫鱼汤) are recommended.

For infertility caused by spleen deficiency with dampness, *Lián Zǐ Jī Dàn Chá* (莲子鸡蛋茶), *Huái Shān Jì Yú Tāng* (淮山鲫鱼汤), *Qiàn Shí Yì Mǐ Gēng* (芡实薏米羹), *Lián Zǐ Nuò Mǐ Dà Zǎo Zhōu* (莲子糯米大枣粥) and *Fú Líng Běi Qí Shòu Ròu Zhōu* (茯苓北芪瘦肉粥) are recommended. Avoid greasy, sweet, raw and cold foods.

For infertility caused by liver constraint, *Bǎi Hé Jī Dàn Chá* (百合鸡蛋茶), *Mài Ròu Dà Zǎo Nuò Mǐ Zhōu* (麦肉大枣糯米粥), *Xiān Nǎi Dùn Jī Dàn* (鲜奶炖鸡蛋) and *Huáng Huā Jì Yú Tāng* (黄花鲫鱼汤) are recommended. Avoid spicy and fried foods.

For infertility caused by concretions and conglomerations, *Wū Guī Dùn Tǔ Fú Líng Tāng* (乌龟煲土茯苓汤), *Biē Jiǎ Dùn Shān Yào Tāng* (鳖甲炖山药汤), *Tián Qī Huā Qí Shēn Chá* (田七花旗参茶), *Kūn Bù Hǎi Zǎo Shòu Ròu Tāng* (昆布海藻瘦肉汤) and *Hǎi Dài Lǜ Dòu Tāng* (海带绿豆汤) are recommended.

For infertility associated with malnutrition, anemia, and vitamin deficiencies, diet becomes even more important. Many women diet in order to lose weight and remain attractive, but they do so improperly. Anorexia is also rapidly increasing in today's society, causing anemia and even severe malnutrition in many cases. Reproductive health is naturally affected as well. It is most essential for these patients to receive both nutritional counseling and psychological support.

Summary

1. INTEGRATIVE DIAGNOSTIC METHODS

(1) Disease Identification and Pattern Differentiation

In diagnosis, Chinese medicine employs pattern differentiation, whereas the biomedical approach emphasizes accurate disease identification. Pattern differentiation and disease identification each have their own respective advantages and disadvantages. With gynecological conditions in particular, the most effective method includes a combination of these two perspectives. Furthermore, we must take into account the age of the individual, as well as environmental and social factors. The diagnostic method used in contemporary China generally includes a biomedical assessment combined with Chinese medical pattern identification. By adopting the strong points of each system, we may avoid their respective shortcomings while also improving therapeutic effects.

Female infertility is not itself an independent disease, but rather often a result of many factors including ovarian dysfunction, salpingitis, salpingemphraxis, endometritis, endometriosis, cervicitis, or vaginitis. Salpingitis and salpingemphraxis can be associated with patterns of qi deficiency blood stasis, spleen and kidney yang deficiency, damp-heat pouring downwards, and damp-toxin congestion. Ovarian dysfunction may be associated with kidney qi deficiency, kidney yin deficiency, liver qi stagnation, liver constraint transforming into fire, phegm-damp brewing internally and qi deficiency blood stasis. A more complete diagnosis and treatment plan can be developed through the proper combining of disease identification and pattern differentiation methods.

(2) Emphasizing Disease Identification

In clinic, a number of diseases can be diagnosed at a relatively early stage of development. However, when the traditional four examinations are unremarkable, no associated pattern of disharmony can be identified. In cases where the patient presents with regular menstruation and normal vaginal discharges, diagnosis and treatment should be based on contemporary gynecological examination and treatment methods.

(3) Emphasizing Pattern Identification

GYN examinations are generally unremarkable in cases of idiopathic infertility, so an immediate and definitive biomedical diagnosis is sometimes not possible. With cases of infertility due to unknown origin, we must then rely on accurate pattern differentiation. Treatments may be applied to address the presenting patterns, which in these cases generally include kidney deficiency, liver constraint, blood stasis, and phlegm dampness.

2. INTEGRATIVE TREATMENT METHODS

(1) Disease Identification and Pattern Differentiation

Pattern differentiation and disease identification are based on a different set of principles, each with their own unique characteristics. Treatment based on pattern differentiation is applied according to the nature, location, and specific patterns of manifestation. The most effective approach is to develop a treatment plan based on pattern differentiation, while also applying contemporary diagnostic theory and pharmaceutical treatment methods.

In Chinese medicine, menstrual irregularities are considered as a primary etiology in most cases of infertility. The classics state, "To promote conception, first regulate menstruation". Furthermore, "reproduction is governed by the kidney". Regulating menstruation to promote conception involves regulation of the kidney, uterus, *tian gui*, and the penetrating and conception vessels. This perspective parallels the functional regulation of hypothalamus-pituitary-ovarian axis in contemporary biomedicine.

Cycle therapy in Chinese medicine obtains a superior therapeutic effect when used to regulate menstruation. However, since this method cannot effectively stimulate ovulation, fertility drugs such as clomiphene may be applied. On the other hand, clomiphene may also negatively impact the endometrium and cervical mucus.

Chinese medicinals that supplement the kidney and nourish yin may also increase estrogen levels and improve the quality of the cervical mucus and endometrium. Therefore, an integrative approach to treatment may be more effective at recovering ovarian function and normalizing menstruation, resulting in higher rates of conception.

In addition, it is also useful to apply methods that supplement the kidney, assist yang, nourish blood, and warm the uterus in order to raise the levels of LH during the intermenstrual and premenstrual periods. For cases of immune infertility, Chinese medicinals that enrich yin may also act to repress antibodies. In addition to eliminating immune factors, Chinese medicinals can also improve ART and IVF success rates. An integrative approach to treatment can reduce pharmaceutical side effects, and also shorten the course of treatment.

(2) Chinese Medicine and Biomedical Treatment

Many patients respond to treatment based on the applications of laparoscopy and hysteroscopy, and also because of recent developments in ART and IVF-ET methods. However, the overall conception rates using these techniques are still relatively low. They also display certain side effects, and are often prohibitively expensive. On the other hand, by combining these methods with Chinese medicinal therapy, infertility can be effectively treated in most cases. For example, the application of Chinese medicinals following laparoscopic salpingotomy and hydrotubation can help avoid postoperative adhesions. Also, the use of Chinese medicinals when stimulating ovulation can also relieve ovarian hyperstimulation syndrome to some degree.

3. REFERRING TO BIOMEDICAL TREATMENT

(1) With uterine malformations such as septated uterus, surgery is recommended.

(2) With uterine polyps and uterine myoma, hysteroscopy and therapeutic laparoscopy are recommended.

(3) With fibroids larger than 4cm, surgery is recommended.

(4) With ovarian cysts larger than 4cm, surgery is also recommended.

(5) With polycystic ovarian syndrome, if after 3 months of treatment, there is still no ovulation, therapeutic laparoscopy and ART methods are recommended.

(6) When pituitary microadenoma impacts ovulation, surgery is recommended.

(7) With twisted fallopian tubes or with severe adhesions, if there is no response after 3 to 6 months of treatment, therapeutic laparoscopy and ART methods are recommended.

(8) With oligospermia, asthenospermia, retrograde ejaculation, and immune infertility, artificial insemination is recommended.

SELECTED QUOTES FROM CLASSICAL TEXTS

Danxi's Heart-Approach:Gynecology:Part Nine:Offspring (丹溪治法心要·妇人科·子嗣第九, *Dān Xī Zhì Fǎ Xīn Yào. Fù Rén Kē. Zǐ Sì Dì Jiǔ*)

"肥者不孕，因躯脂闭塞子宫，而致经事不行，用导痰之类；瘦者不孕，因子宫无血，精气不聚故也，用四物养血、养阴等药。予侄女形气俱实，得子之迟，服神仙聚宝丹，背发痈疽，证候甚危。诊其脉数大而涩，急以四物汤加减，百余帖补其阴血，幸其质厚，易于收救，质之薄者，悔将何及！"

"Infertility among the obese due to menstrual block is caused by bodyfat blocking and congesting the uterus. Medicinals that conduct phlegm are indicated. Infertility among the thin is due to an absence of blood in the uterus and essential qi failing to gather. Medicinals that nourish blood and yin such as *Sì Wù Tāng* (四物汤) are indicated. My niece is abundant in both physical constitution and qi, but she had never been able to become pregnant. After taking *Shén Xiān Jù Bǎo Dān* (神仙聚宝丹), welling-abscesses and flat-abscesses appeared on her back. The condition became very critical. Her pulses were rapid, large and rough. Urgently, I administered more than one hundred doses of modified *Sì Wù Tāng* (四物汤). Luckily, the abscesses were easy to treat because of her good physical condition. If the patient were someone in poor physical condition, the situation would have become full of sorrow."

The Orthodox Tradition of Medicine:Gynecology:Antepartum (医学正传·妇人科中·胎前, *Yī Xué Zhèng Zhuàn. Fù Rén Kē Zhōng. Tāi Qián*)

"夫人欲求嗣，必先视其妇之经脉调否，其或未调，必以药而调之，经脉既调，宜以人事副之，按其法而行之，庶不失其候也。"

"To seek fertility, first determine if the women's menstrual periods are regular. If not, first regulate them with medicinals, then assist [conception] with the correct approach and appropriate timing."

Compendium to Save Yin:Conception:Treatise on Miscellaneous Methods of Pregnancy (济阴纲目 · 求子门 · 论孕子杂法 , *Jì Yīn Gāng Mù. Qiú Zǐ Mén. Lùn Yùn Zǐ Zá Fǎ*)

"薛氏曰：妇人之不孕，亦有因六淫七情之邪，有伤冲任；或宿疾淹留，传遗脏腑；或子宫虚冷，或气旺血衰，或血中伏热；又有脾胃虚损，不能营养冲任（求责极当，诚哉言也）。审此更当察其男子之形质虚实何如，有肾虚精弱，不能融育成胎者；有禀赋元弱，气血虚损者；有嗜欲无度，阴精衰惫者，各当求其原而治之。至于大要，则当审男女之尺脉。若左尺微细，或虚大无力者，用八味丸；左尺洪大，按之无力者，用六味丸；两尺俱微细，或浮大者，用十补丸（岂此三方所能尽，宜扩充之）。若误用辛热燥血，不惟无益，反受其害。"

"Dr. Xue once said, 'female infertility can result from the six pathogenic excesses and seven affects which damage the penetrating and conception vessels; long-standing diseases affecting the organs; deficiency cold of the uterus; qi effulgence with blood debilitation; latent heat in the blood; damage and deficiency of the spleen and stomach which fails to nourish the penetrating and conception vessels.' These words are the truth. He also said, 'in addition to those factors, we should also distinguish the status of the male's condition. Male infertility can be caused by kidney essence deficiency; congenital qi and blood deficiency; and yin-essence debilitation due to over-indulgent sexual activity. Treatment should be based on the root. The basic formulas should be applied according to the pulse images at the *chi* position. When the pulse is faint and thready, or deficient, large and forceless, *Bā Wèi Wán* (八味丸) is indicated. When the pulse is surging and large yet forceless under pressure, *Liù Wèi Wán* (六味丸) is indicated. When the pulse is faint and thready, or floating and large at both *chi* positions, *Shí Bǔ Wán* (十补丸) is indicated. The improper application of acrid and hot medicinals which dry the blood would aggravate, rather than benefit the condition."

The Level-Line of Gynecological Pattern Identification and Treatment: *Antepartum:Conception* (女科证治准绳·胎前门·求子, *Nǚ Kē Zhèng Zhì Zhǔn Shéng. Tāi Qián Mén. Qiú Zǐ*)

"胎前之道，始于求子。求子之法，莫先调经。每见妇人之无子者，其经必或前或后，或多或少，或将行作痛，或行后作痛，或紫或黑或淡，或凝而不调，不调则血气乖争，不能成孕矣，详夫不调之由，其或前或后，及行后作痛者虚也。其少而淡者血虚也，多者气虚也。其将行作痛及凝块不散者，滞也。紫黑色者，滞而挟热也。治法：血虚者四物，气虚者四物加参、芪。滞者香附、缩砂、木香、槟榔、桃仁、玄胡。滞久而沉痼者，吐之下之。脉证热者，四物加芩、连。脉证寒者，四物加桂、附及紫石英之类是也。直至积去、滞行、虚回，然后血气和平，能孕子也。予每治经不调者，只一味香附末，醋为丸服之，亦百发百中也。"

"Conception leads to pregnancy, and regulated menstruation leads to conception. Women with infertility are commonly seen with advanced, delayed, profuse or scant menstruation that is purplish, dark or pale in color, congealed in nature, and with pain appearing before or after menstruation. Irregular menstruation indicates a disorder of qi and blood which can also lead to conception failure. The main causes are as follows."

"Menstruation at irregular arrivals with pain afterwards indicates deficiency. Scant pale menses indicate blood deficiency. Profuse menses indicate qi deficiency. Pain before menstruation with congealed clottting indicates stagnation. Purplish and dark menses indicate stagnation with heat. The treatment methods are as follows."

"For blood deficiency, select *Sì Wù Tāng* (四物汤). For qi deficiency, select *Sì Wù Tāng* (四物汤) with added *rén shēn* (Radix et Rhizoma Ginseng) and *huáng qí* (Radix Astragali). With stagnation, select *xiāng fù* (Rhizoma Cyperi), *suō shā* (Fructus Amomi), *mù xiāng* (Radix Aucklandiae), *bīng láng* (Semen Arecae), *táo rén* (Semen Persicae) and *xuán hú* (Rhizoma Corydalis). With long-standing stagnation that becomes stubborn, apply ejection and precipitation methods. With pulses and patterns indicating heat, select *Sì Wù Tāng* (四物汤) with added *huáng qín* (Radix Scutellariae) and *huáng lián* (Rhizoma Coptidis). With pulses and patterns indicating cold, select *Sì Wù Tāng* (四物汤) with added *guì zhī* (Ramulus Cinnamomi), *fù zǐ* (Radix Aconiti Lateralis) and *zǐ shí yīng* (Fluoritum). Once the accumulation has been eliminated, the stagnation has been moved, and the deficiency has been supplemented, then the blood and qi will be in harmony, and conception will occur. When I treat irregular menstruation, *xiāng fù* (Rhizoma Cyperi) powder made into pills with vinegar has always shown great effect."

Gathered Blooms of Acupuncture and Moxibustion:Subtle Treastise on The Jade Swivel, Identification and Treatment with Acupuncture and Moxibustion: Women (针灸聚英 · 玉机微义针灸证治 · 妇人, *Zhēn Jiū Jù Yīng. Yù Jī Wēi Yì Zhēn Jiū Zhèng Zhì. Fù Rén*)

"女子不月。灸会阴三壮。妇人月水不利。难产。子上冲心。痛不得息。灸气冲七壮。妇人月事不利。利即多。心下满。目不能远视。腹中痛。灸水泉五壮。妇人月事不调。带下崩中。因产恶露不止。绕脐痛。灸气海。妇人不孕。月不调匀。赤白带下。气转连背引痛不可忍。灸带脉二穴。产后恶露不止。及诸淋注。灸气海。产后两胁急痛不可忍。灸石关五十壮。女子月事不调。产后恶露不止。绕脐冷痛。灸阴交百壮。带下癥瘕。因产恶露不止。断产绝孕。经冷。灸关元百壮。妇人卒口噤。语音不出。风痫。灸承浆五壮。妇人产后。血气俱虚。灸血海百壮。妇人疝气。脐腹冷疼。相引胁下痛不可忍。先灸中庭三七壮。"

"For menstrual block, burn three cones of moxa at *hui yin*. For inhibited menses, difficult delivery, and the fetus surging up into the heart with unceasing pain, burn seven cones of moxa at *qi chong*. For inhibited menstruation which becomes profuse after disinhibiting, fullness below the heart, inability to see at a distance, and abdominal pain, burn five cones of moxa at *shui quan*. For irregular menstruation, vaginal discharge, flooding, persistent postpartum flow of lochia, and pain around the umbilicus, moxa *qi hai*. For female infertility, irregular menstruation, red and white vaginal discharge, and intolerable pulling pain of the back, moxa two points on the girdling vessel."

The Classified Canon, Disease of Bowels:Viscera, Channels and Network Vessels (类经 · 脏腑经络病 , *Lèi Jīng. Zàng Fǔ Jīng Luò Bìng*)

"任脉为病，男子内结七疝，女子带下瘕聚。冲脉为病，逆气里急。督脉为病，脊强反折。此生病，从少腹上冲心而痛，不得前后，为冲疝。其女子不孕，癃痔遗溺嗌干。"

"Diseases of the conception vessel cause internal binding of the seven mountings in males; and vaginal discharge, conglomerations, and gatherings in the female. Diseases of the penetrating vessel cause qi counterflow and abdominal urgency. Diseases of the governing vessel cause the spine to become rigid and bend backward."

"This disease manifests with pain surging upward from the lesser abdomen into the heart, and an inability to bend forward or backwards. This is called surging mounting. Women with this disease will display infertility, dribbling block, hemorrhoids, enuresis, and dry throat."

Heart-Approach and Essential Rhymes for Gynecology:Menstruation Regulation:The Causes of Female Infertility (妇科心法要诀 · 调经门 · 妇人不孕之故 , *Fù Kē Xīn Fǎ Yào Jué. Tiáo Jīng Mén. Fù Rén Bù Yùn Zhī Gù*)

"不孕之故伤任冲，不调带下经漏崩，或因积血胞寒热，痰饮脂膜病子宫。"

"Infertility that is caused by damage to the penetrating and conception vessels manifests with irregular menstruation, vaginal discharge, and flooding and spotting. Other causes include blood accumulation, cold or hot uterus, and phlegm-rheum or fat in the uterus."

Canon of Gynecology:Offspring:Intercourse at the appropriate age when yin and yang are both complete and fulfilled (女科经纶 · 嗣育门 · 合男女必当其年欲阴阳之完实 , *Nǚ Kē Jīng Lùn. Sì Yù Mén. Hé Nán Nǚ Bì Dāng Qí Nián Yù Yīn Yáng Zhī Wán Shí*)

"褚澄曰：合男女必当其年，男虽十六而精通，必三十而娶。女虽十四而天癸至，必二十而嫁。皆欲阴阳完实，然后交而孕，孕而育，育而为子坚壮强寿。今未笄之女，天癸始至，已近男色，阴气早泄，未完而伤，未实而动，是以交而不孕，孕而不育，育而子脆不寿。"

"Physician Chu Cheng said, 'Intercourse between men and women should occur at the appropriate age. Although the essence of a man becomes free at age sixteen, he should not get married before age thirty. Although the *tian gui* of a woman arrives at age fourteen, she should not get married before age twenty.' Wait until yin and yang have both become complete and fulfilled; then have intercourse to conceive and deliver. The child will become strong and have a long life. Nowadays, before a girl turns fifteen, when *tian gui* has just arrived, she has already been with men. Yin qi has been discharged too early, meaning that it becomes damaged even before it has become fulfilled, and disturbed before it has become replete. Therefore, intercourse will not lead to conception, conception will not lead to delivery, and delivery will lead to weak and short-lived children."

Essentials of Gynecology:Offspring:Introduction (女科精要 · 嗣育门 · 绪论 *Nǚ Kē Jīng Yào. Sì Yù Mén. Xù Lùn*)

"妇人无子者，或经不匀，或血不足，或有疾病，或交不时，四者而已。调其经而补其血，去其病而节其欲，无疾病而交有时，岂有不妊娠者乎。然更有二，凡肥盛妇人，禀受甚厚，恣于酒食，不能有胎，谓之躯脂满溢，闭塞子宫，宜燥湿痰，如星、半、苍术、台芎、香附、陈皮，或导痰汤之类；若是瘦怯性急之人，经水不调，不能成胎，谓之子宫干涩无血，不能摄受精气，宜凉血降火。如四物加黄芩、香附，养阴补血及六味地黄丸之类。"

"Female infertility may be caused by irregular menstruation, blood deficiency, [chronic] diseases or improper timing. Regulate the menstruation, tonify the blood, eliminate disease, and control desire. With a healthy constitution and proper timing, conception will certainly occur. However, there are two other factors. When obese women with a strong physical constitution indulge themselves in excessive drinking and eating, conception becomes impossible. This condition is called excessive bodyfat blocking and congesting the uterus. The drying of dampness and phlegm is indicated. Select *dǎn nán xīng* (Arisaema cum Bile), *bàn xià* (Rhizoma Pinelliae), *cāng zhú* (Rhizoma Atractylodis), *chuān xiōng* (Rhizoma Chuanxiong), *xiāng fù* (Rhizoma Cyperi), *chén pí* (Pericarpium Citri Reticulatae) or *Dǎo Tán Tāng* (导痰汤)."

"In those with emaciation, shyness and irascibility who have irregular menstruation resulting in infertility, the condition is referred to as dry and bloodless uterus failing to obtain the essence. The cooling of blood and downbearing of fire is indicated. Select *Sì Wù Tāng* (四物汤) with added *huáng qín* (Radix Scutellariae) and *xiāng fù* (Rhizoma Cyperi), or *Yǎng Yīn Bǔ Xuè Tāng* (养阴补血汤) and *Liù Wèi Dì Huáng Wán* (六味地黄丸)."

Bamboo Grove Gynecological Pattern Identification and Treatment:Desiring Offspring (part one):Female Infertility due to Deficiency (竹林女科证治 · 求嗣上 · 妇人虚弱不孕 , *Zhú Lín Nǚ Kē Zhèng Zhì. Qiú Sì Shàng. Fù Rén Xū Ruò Bù Yùn*)

"妇人气血俱虚，经脉不调，或断续，或带浊，或腹痛，或腰酸，或饮食不甘，瘦弱不孕，宜服毓麟珠一、二斤，即可受胎。凡种子诸方无以加此。毓麟珠：人参　白术（蜜炙）　茯苓　白芍（酒炒，各二两）　川芎　炙甘草（各一两）　当归　熟地黄（各四两）　菟丝子（制,四两）　杜仲（酒炒）　鹿角霜　川椒（各二两,去目）。上为末,蜜丸弹子大。空心嚼服一、二丸,白汤下，或作小丸吞服。如经迟腹痛，加破故纸（酒炒）、肉桂各一两，甚则再加吴茱萸（汤泡炒）五钱。如带多腹痛，加破故纸（酒炒）一两、北五味五钱，或加龙骨（醋煅）一两。如子宫寒甚，或泄或痛，加附子（制熟）、干姜（炮）各数钱。如血热多火、经早内热者，加川续断、地骨皮各二两，或另以汤剂暂清其火，而后服此，或以汤引，酌宜送下。"

"Women with qi and blood dual deficiency will suffer from irregular menstruation with turbid vaginal discharge, abdominal pain, aching lumbus, and poor appetite or emaciation, all of which lead to infertility. This can be treated by administering 1 or 2 *jin* of *Yù Lín Zhū* (毓麟珠). There is no better formula for the treatment of infertility than this. The [formula] includes the following ingredients."

"2 *liang* each of *rén shēn* (Radix et Rhizoma Ginseng), *bái zhú* (Rhizoma Atractylodis Macrocephalae, honey-fried), *fú líng* (Poria), and *bái sháo* (Radix Paeoniae Alba, stir-fried with wine), *lù jiǎo shuāng* (Cornu Cervi Degelatinatum) and *chuān jiāo* (Pericarpium Zanthoxyli, without seeds), 1 *liang* each of *chuān xiōng* (Rhizoma Chuanxiong) and *zhì gān cǎo* (Radix et Rhizoma Glycyrrhizae Praeparata cum Melle), and 4 *liang* each of *dāng guī* (Radix Angelicae Sinensis), *shú dì huáng* (Radix Rehmanniae Praeparata) and prepared *tù sī zǐ* (Semen Cuscutae). Grind all of the ingredients into powder, and make honey pills of the size of a marble. Chew and swallow 1 or 2 pills at a time with hot water, or make smaller pills to swallow."

"With delayed menstruation and abdominal pain, add 1 *liang* each of *pò gù zhǐ* (Fructus Psoraleae, stir-fried with wine) and *ròu guì* (Cortex Cinnamomi); in severe cases, add 5 *qian* of *wú zhū yú* (Fructus Evodiae, soaked and fried)."

"With excessive vaginal discharge and abdominal pain, add 1 *liang* of *pò gù zhǐ* (Fructus Psoraleae, stir-fried with wine), 5 *qian* of *běi wǔ wèi* (Fructus Schisandrae Chinensis), or 1 *liang* of *lóng gǔ* (Os Draconis, calcined with vinegar)."

"With extreme cold in the uterus presenting with diarrhea or pain, add several *qian* of *shú fù zǐ* (Radix Aconiti Lateralis Praeparata) and *pào jiāng* (Rhizoma Zingiberis Praeparatum)."

"With blood heat and excessive fire, or advanced menstruation with internal heat, add 2 *liang* each of *xù duàn* (Radix Dipsaci) and *dì gǔ pí* (Cortex Lycii), or apply another decoction to clear the fire before taking *Yù Lín Zhū* (毓麟珠). Taking the pills along with the [fire-clearing] decoction is also permissible."

The Warp and Woof of Warm Heat:Chapter of Damp-heat Disease by Xue Sheng-bai (温热经纬·薛生白湿热病篇 , *Wēn Rè Jīng Wěi. Xue Sheng-bai Shī Rè Bìng Piān*)

"何报之云：子和治病，不论何证，皆以汗吐下三法取效，此有至理存焉。盖万病非热则寒，寒者气不运而滞，热者气亦壅而不运，气不运则热郁痰生，血停食积，种种阻塞于中矣。人身气血，贵通而不贵塞，非三法何由通乎？又去邪即所以补正，邪去则正自复，但以平淡之饮食调之，不数日而精神勃发矣。故妇人不孕者，此法行后即孕，阴阳和畅也，男子阳道骤兴，非其明验乎。后人不明其理而不敢用，但以温补为稳，杀人如麻，可叹也！ "

"Physician He Bao-zhi said, 'Physician Zhang Zi-he treated all diseases with sweating, ejection, and precipitation methods, regardless of the pattern. There is ultimate truth to this. All diseases are conditions of either heat or cold. Cold leads to qi failing to transport, causing stagnation. Heat leads to qi congestion which also fails to transport. With qi transportation failure, heat becomes constrained, phlegm is engendered, blood collects, and food is accumulated. All varieties of blockage and obstruction will occur in the center. It is most essential for the qi and blood of human body to become free, rather than to remain obstructed. And those three methods are the only methods that can free it. Moreover, to eliminate the pathogen is to also tonify the upright. Once the pathogen is eliminated, the upright will recover naturally. Regulate this with normal neutral diet, and the essence-spirit will blossom in just a few days. Women with infertility will conceive just after those methods have been applied. Men's impotence can also be cured in no time. These methods are known to be remarkably effective. The successors do not understand the theory; therefore they do not dare to apply those methods. Instead, they seek a stable effect with warming and tonifying, which kills thousands of millions. What a pity!"

MODERN RESEARCH

Clinical Research

1. PATTERN DIFFERENTIATION AND TREATMENT

Wu Xia divided a group of male infertility patients into five treatment groups based on the following pattern differentiation:

1) Kidney yang deficiency. This pattern is often seen in patients with endocrine disturbances or an infantile uterus. The treatment principle is to supplement the kidney and regulate menstruation.

The formulas *Fù Guì Dì Huáng Wán* (附桂地黄丸) and *Wǔ Zǐ Yǎn Zōng Wán* (五子衍宗丸) are often applied.

Commonly used medicinals include *zǐ hé chē* (Placenta Hominis), *ròu guì* (Cortex Cinnamomi), *shú dì* (Radix Rehmanniae Praeparata), *bái sháo* (Radix Paeoniae Alba), *shān zhū yú* (Fructus Corni), *bā jǐ tiān* (Radix Morindae Officinalis), *dǎng shēn* (Radix Codonopsis), *bái zhú* (Rhizoma Atractylodis Macrocephalae), *fú líng* (Poria), *shān yào* (Rhizoma Dioscoreae), *yín yáng huò* (Herba Epimedii), *hé shǒu wū* (Radix Polygoni Multiflori) and *dù zhòng* (Cortex Eucommiae).

【Modifications】

➤ For severe kidney yang deficiency, add *lù jiǎo shuāng* (Cornu Cervi Degelatinatum) and *suǒ yáng* (Herba Cynomorii).

➤ For cold legs, add *hú lú bā* (Semen Trigonellae) and *xiǎo huí xiāng*

(Fructus Foeniculi).

➢ For aching lower back, add *sāng jì shēng* (Ramus Loranthi seu Visci), *xù duàn* (Radix Dipsaci), *dù zhòng* (Cortex Eucommiae) and *gǒu jǐ* (Rhizoma Cibotii).

➢ For long voidings of clear urine, add *fù pén zǐ* (Fructus Rubi), *yì zhì* (Fructus Alpiniae Oxyphyllae) and *cán jiāng* (Bombyx Bombycis).

➢ For dizziness, add *nǔ zhēn zǐ* (Fructus Ligustri Lucidi), *mò hàn lián* (Herba Ecliptae) and *jú huā* (Flos Chrysanthemi).

➢ For monophase BBT or corpus luteum insufficiency, add *ròu cóng róng* (Herba Cistanches) and *xiān máo* (Rhizoma Curculiginis).

➢ For kidney yin deficiency, add *guī jiǎ* (Carapax et Plastrum Testudinis) and *shú dì* (Radix Rehmanniae Praeparata).

➢ For yin deficiency and internal heat, add *zhī mǔ* (Rhizoma Anemarrhenae) and *huáng bǎi* (Cortex Phellodendri Chinensis).

➢ For infantile uterus, add *zǐ shí yīng* (Fluoritum).

2) Liver depression, qi stagnation and blood stasis. The treatment principle is to course the liver and rectify the qi.

Commonly used formulas are *Kāi Yù Zhòng Yù Tāng* (开郁种玉汤), *Qī Zhì Xiāng Fù Wán* (七制香附丸) and *Jì Shēng Jú Hé Wán* (济生橘核丸).

Medicinals include *dāng guī* (Radix Angelicae Sinensis), *chái hú* (Radix Bupleuri), *xiāng fù* (Rhizoma Cyperi), *bái zhú* (Rhizoma Atractylodis Macrocephalae), *dān pí* (Cortex Moutan), *fú líng* (Poria), *bái sháo* (Radix Paeoniae Alba), *jú yè* (Folium Citri Reticulatae), *jú hé* (Semen Citri Reticulatae), *táo rén* (Semen Persicae), *hóng huā* (Flos Carthami), *tù sī zǐ* (Semen Cuscutae), *yín yáng huò* (Herba Epimedii) and *lù jiǎo shuāng* (Cornu Cervi Degelatinatum).

【Modifications】

➢ For premenstrual breast distention and pain, add *yù jīn* (Radix Curcumae) and *lì zhī hé* (Semen Litchi).

➢ For vexation and disquiet, add *zhī zǐ* (Fructus Gardeniae) and *huáng lián* (Rhizoma Coptidis).

➤ For emotional depression, add *chuān liàn zǐ* (Fructus Toosendan) and *xiǎo mài* (Fructus Tritici Levis).

➤ For kidney deficiency, add *shēng dì* (Radix Rehmanniae Recens), *shān zhū yú* (Fructus Corni), *fù pén zǐ* (Fructus Rubi), and *sāng jì shēng* (Ramus Loranthi seu Visci).

➤ For spleen deficiency, add *shān yào* (Rhizoma Dioscoreae) and *bǎi biǎn dòu* (Semen Lablab Album).

3) *Blood stasis in the uterine vessels*. This pattern is often seen in patients with endometriosis or salpingemphraxis. The treatment principle is to quicken the blood and transform stasis.

Commonly used formulas are *Shào Fù Zhú Yū Tāng* (少腹逐瘀汤), *Xuè Fǔ Zhú Yū Tāng* (血府逐瘀汤) and *Guì Zhī Fú Líng Wán* (桂枝茯苓丸).

Medicinals include *dāng guī* (Radix Angelicae Sinensis), *chuān xiōng* (Rhizoma Chuanxiong), *hóng huā* (Flos Carthami), *niú xī* (Radix Achyranthis Bidentatae), *táo rén* (Semen Persicae), *chì sháo* (Radix Paeoniae Rubra), *dān pí* (Cortex Moutan), *sān léng* (Rhizoma Sparganii), *é zhú* (Rhizoma Curcumae), *xià kū cǎo* (Spica Prunellae), *xiāng fù* (Rhizoma Cyperi), *pú huáng* (Pollen Typhae), *dān shēn* (Radix et Rhizoma Salviae Miltiorrhizae), *jī xuè téng* (Caulis Spatholobi), *guì zhī* (Ramulus Cinnamomi) and *wáng bù liú xíng* (Semen Vaccariae).

【Modifications】

➤ For cold, add *xiǎo huí xiāng* (Fructus Foeniculi), *wū yào* (Radix Linderae) and *pào jiāng* (Rhizoma Zingiberis Praeparatum).

➤ For heat, add *pú gōng yīng* (Herba Taraxaci) and *bài jiàng cǎo* (Herba Patriniae).

➤ For kidney deficiency, add *fù zǐ* (Radix Aconiti Lateralis Praeparata), *dù zhòng* (Cortex Eucommiae), *ròu cóng róng* (Herba Cistanches), and *bǔ gǔ zhī* (Fructus Psoraleae).

➤ For spleen deficiency, add *dǎng shēn* (Radix Codonopsis), *bái zhú*

(Rhizoma Atractylodis Macrocephalae), *fú líng* (Poria), *shān yào* (Rhizoma Dioscoreae), *bǎi biǎn dòu* (Semen Lablab Album), and *yì yǐ rén* (Semen Coicis).

4) Phlegm dampness obstruction. This pattern is often seen in patients with endocrine disturbances or an infantile uterus. The treatment principle is to transform phlegm and dry dampness.

Qǐ Gōng Wán (启宫丸) and *Cāng Fù Dǎo Tán Wán* (苍附导痰丸) are often applied.

Medicinals include *cāng zhú* (Rhizoma Atractylodis), *shí chāng pǔ* (Rhizoma Acori Tatarinowii), *yù jīn* (Radix Curcumae), *jiè zǐ* (Semen Sinapis), *jī nèi jīn* (Endothelium Corneum Gigeriae Galli), *yì mǔ cǎo* (Herba Leonuri), *guì zhī* (Ramulus Cinnamomi) and *qīng méng shí* (Lapis Chloriti). To transform phlegm and soften hardness, select *xià kū cǎo* (Spica Prunellae), *bèi mǔ* (Bulbus Fritillaria), *lóng gǔ* (Os Draconis) and *mǔ lì* (Concha Ostreae).

【Modifications】

➢ For severe dampness, add *hòu pò* (Cortex Magnoliae Officinalis), *yì yǐ rén* (Semen Coicis) and *bái zhú* (Rhizoma Atractylodis Macrocephalae).

➢ For nausea and vomiting, add *zhú rú* (Caulis Bambusae in Taenia) and *shā rén* (Fructus Amomi).

➢ For palpitations, add *yuǎn zhì* (Radix Polygalae), *bǎi zǐ rén* (Semen Platycladi) and *cí shí* (Magnetitum).

5) Dampness and heat brewing and obstructing. This pattern is often seen in patients with pelvic inflammation, trichomonas vaginitis, colpomycosis and cervical erosion. The treatment principle is to clear heat and disinhibit dampness.

The formula *Zhǐ Dài Tāng* (止带汤) is commonly used.

Medicinals include *zhū líng* (Polyporus), *fú líng* (Poria), *bái zhú* (Rhizoma Atractylodis Macrocephalae), *yīn chén* (Herba Artemisiae Scopariae), *chē qián zǐ* (Semen Plantaginis), *zé xiè* (Rhizoma Alismatis), *chì sháo* (Radix Paeoniae Rubra), *dān pí* (Cortex Moutan), *huáng bǎi* (Cortex Phellodendri Chinensis), *zhī zǐ* (Fructus Gardeniae) and *pú gōng yīng* (Herba Taraxaci).

【Modifications】

➤ For genital itching, add *chūn gēn* (Cortex Toonae Radicis) and *bái xiān pí* (Cortex Dictamni).

➤ For severe yin deficiency, add *huáng jīng* (Rhizoma Polygonati), *tiān huā fěn* (Radix Trichosanthis) and *mài dōng* (Radix Ophiopogonis)[1].

Du Ying-han divided subjects into three treatment groups based on the following pattern differentiation.

1) *Kidney yin deficiency*. Modified *Zuǒ Guī Yǐn* was applied.

左归饮 *Zuǒ Guī Yǐn*

熟地	*shú dì*	30g	Radix Rehmanniae Praeparata
山茱萸	*shān zhū yú*	15g	Fructus Corni
枸杞子	*gǒu qǐ zǐ*	10g	Fructus Lycii
山药	*shān yào*	18g	Rhizoma Dioscoreae
杜仲	*dù zhòng*	12g	Cortex Eucommiae
附子	*fù zǐ*	3g	Radix Aconiti Lateralis Praeparata
甘草	*gān cǎo*	6g	Radix et Rhizoma Glycyrrhizae

2) *Dual deficiency of qi and blood*. Modified *Guī Pí Tāng* was applied.

归脾汤 *Guī Pí Tāng*

党参	*dǎng shēn*	15g	Radix Codonopsis
黄芪	*huáng qí*	30g	Radix Astragali
白术	*bái zhú*	15g	Rhizoma Atractylodis Macrocephalae
茯苓	*fú líng*	10g	Poria
酸枣仁	*suān zǎo rén*	15g	Semen Ziziphi Spinosae
龙眼肉	*lóng yǎn ròu*	10g	Arillus Longan
木香	*mù xiāng*	8g	Radix Aucklandiae
当归	*dāng guī*	12g	Radix Angelicae Sinensis
远志	*yuǎn zhì*	12g	Radix Polygalae

阿胶	ē jiāo	12g	Colla Corii Asini
生姜	shēng jiāng	3pieces	Rhizoma Zingiberis Recens
大枣	dà zǎo	6	Fructus Jujubae

3) Blood stasis stagnating. Modified *Shào Fù Zhú Yū Tāng* was applied.

少腹逐瘀汤 Shào Fù Zhú Yū Tāng

小茴香	xiǎo huí xiāng	15g	Fructus Foeniculi
干姜	gān jiāng	12g	Rhizoma Zingiberis
延胡索	yán hú suǒ	12g	Rhizoma Corydalis
没药	mò yào	10g	Myrrha
当归	dāng guī	12g	Radix Angelicae Sinensis
川芎	chuān xiōng	12g	Rhizoma Chuanxiong
肉桂	ròu guì	10g	Cortex Cinnamomi
赤芍	chì sháo	12g	Radix Paeoniae Rubra
蒲黄	pú huáng	19g	Pollen Typhae
五灵脂	wǔ líng zhī	15g	Faeces Togopteri

【Modifications】

➢ For scanty and delayed menstruation, add *dān shēn* (Radix et Rhizoma Salviae Miltiorrhizae), *jī xuè téng* (Caulis Spatholobi) and *ē jiāo* (Colla Corii Asini).

➢ For early menstruation, add *xuán shēn* (Radix Scrophulariae), *mài dōng* (Radix Ophiopogonis), *shēng dì* (Radix Rehmanniae Recens) and *mò hàn lián* (Herba Ecliptae).

➢ For profuse menstruation, add *hǎi piāo xiāo* (Endoconcha Sepiae), *lù hán cǎo* (Herba Evolvuli) and *xiān hè cǎo* (Herba Agrimoniae).

➢ For menstrual pain, add *wú zhū yú* (Fructus Evodiae), *yán hú suǒ* (Rhizoma Corydalis) and *ài yè* (Folium Artemisiae Argyi).

➢ For amenorrhea, add *táo rén* (Semen Persicae), *zé lán* (Herba Lycopi) and *lù jiǎo* (Cornu Cervi).

➢ For salpingemphraxis, apply hydrotubation and the empirical formula *Tōng Guǎn Tāng*.

通管汤 *Tōng Guǎn Tāng*

当归	*dāng guī*	9g	Radix Angelicae Sinensis
香附	*xiāng fù*	10g	Rhizoma Cyperi
延胡索	*yán hú suǒ*	15g	Rhizoma Corydalis
马鞭草	*mǎ biān cǎo*	12g	Herba Verbenae
路路通	*lù lù tōng*	12g	Fructus Liquidambaris
穿山甲	*chuān shān jiǎ*	15g	Squama Manis
丹参	*dān shēn*	15g	Radix et Rhizoma Salviae Miltiorrhizae
茯苓	*fú líng*	15g	Poria
牡丹皮	*mǔ dān pí*	15g	Cortex Moutan

The patients were administered the appropriate formula for 3 months.

Results: In 70 cases of female infertility, 58 subjects achieved a successful pregnancy. The effective rate reached 83%[2].

Liu Xiu-ying states that the main patterns for infertility generally involve qi stagnation, blood stasis, kidney deficiency, blood heat and phlegm-damp. He considers qi stagnation and blood stasis as being common to all kinds of infertility.

1) *Qi stagnation and blood stasis*. The treatment principle is to rectify qi, resolve stasis and free the collaterals.

The prescribed formula contains the following medicinals.

当归	*dāng guī*	15g	Radix Angelicae Sinensis
川芎	*chuān xiōng*	10g	Rhizoma Chuanxiong
赤芍	*chì sháo*	15g	Radix Paeoniae Rubra
丹参	*dān shēn*	20g	Radix et Rhizoma Salviae Miltiorrhizae
香附	*xiāng fù*	15g	Rhizoma Cyperi
青皮	*qīng pí*	10g	Pericarpium Citri Reticulatae Viride
僵蚕	*jiāng cán*	15g	Bombyx Batryticatus
土鳖虫	*tǔ biē chóng*	15g	Eupolyphaga seu Steleophaga
炮山甲	*pào shān jiǎ*	10g	Squama Manis
桃仁	*táo rén*	5g	Semen Persicae
红花	*hóng huā*	5g	Flos Carthami

| 三棱 | sān léng | 10g | Rhizoma Sparganii |
| 莪术 | é zhú | 10g | Rhizoma Curcumae |

2) Kidney deficiency with qi stagnation and blood stasis. The treatment principle is to rectify qi, resolve stasis, supplement the kidney and regulate menstruation.

The prescribed formula contains the following medicinals.

当归	dāng guī	15g	Radix Angelicae Sinensis
川芎	chuān xiōng	10g	Rhizoma Chuanxiong
赤芍	chì sháo	15g	Radix Paeoniae Rubra
丹参	dān shēn	25g	Radix et Rhizoma Salviae Miltiorrhizae
香附	xiāng fù	15g	Rhizoma Cyperi
青皮	qīng pí	15g	Pericarpium Citri Reticulatae Viride
僵蚕	jiāng cán	10g	Bombyx Batryticatus
土鳖虫	tǔ biē chóng	10g	Eupolyphaga seu Steleophaga
乌药	wū yào	10g	Radix Linderae
肉桂	ròu guì	7.5g	Cortex Cinnamomi
小茴香	xiǎo huí xiāng	5g	Fructus Foeniculi
桃仁	táo rén	15g	Semen Persicae
红花	hóng huā	15g	Flos Carthami

3) Blood heat with qi stagnation and blood stasis. The treatment principle is to rectify qi, resolve stasis, clear heat and regulate menstruation.

The prescribed formula contains the following medicinals.

当归	dāng guī	15g	Radix Angelicae Sinensis
生地	shēng dì	15g	Radix Rehmanniae
赤芍	chì sháo	15g	Radix Paeoniae Rubra
川芎	chuān xiōng	10g	Rhizoma Chuanxiong
土鳖虫	tǔ biē chóng	10g	Eupolyphaga seu Steleophaga
槟榔	bīng láng	10g	Semen Arecae
牡丹皮	mǔ dān pí	10g	Cortex Moutan
连翘	lián qiào	15g	Fructus Forsythiae
僵蚕	jiāng cán	15g	Bombyx Batryticatus

4) *Phlegm-damp with qi stagnation and blood stasis*. The treatment is to rectify qi, transform stasis, dry dampness and transform phlegm.

The prescribed formula contains the following medicinals.

当归	*dāng guī*	15g	Radix Angelicae Sinensis
川芎	*chuān xiōng*	10g	Rhizoma Chuanxiong
赤芍	*chì sháo*	15g	Radix Paeoniae Rubra
土鳖虫	*tǔ biē chóng*	10g	Eupolyphaga seu Steleophaga
僵蚕	*jiāng cán*	15g	Bombyx Batryticatus
丹参	*dān shēn*	20g	Radix et Rhizoma Salviae Miltiorrhizae
香附	*xiāng fù*	15g	Rhizoma Cyperi
半夏	*bàn xià*	10g	Rhizoma Pinelliae
苍术	*cāng zhú*	15g	Rhizoma Atractylodis
茯苓	*fú líng*	30g	Poria
益母草	*yì mǔ cǎo*	15g	Herba Leonuri
泽兰	*zé lán*	15g	Herba Lycopi
陈皮	*chén pí*	15g	Pericarpium Citri Reticulatae

Dr. Hu divided 319 cases of infertility into 5 treatment groups based on the following pattern differentiation[3].

1) *Kidney yang deficiency*. The treatment principle is to warm and supplement kidney yang while enriching kidney yin and supplementing spleen qi. The empirical formula *Yì Jīng Èr Fāng* was selected.

益精二方 *Yì Jīng Èr Fāng*

锁阳	*suǒ yáng*	15g	Herba Cynomorii
巴戟天	*bā jǐ*	15g	Radix Morindae Officinalis
枸杞子	*gǒu qǐ zǐ*	15g	Fructus Lycii
白术	*bái zhú*	15g	Rhizoma Atractylodis Macrocephalae
茯苓	*fú líng*	15g	Poria
淫羊藿	*yín yáng huò*	10g	Herba Epimedii
白芍	*bái sháo*	10g	Radix Paeoniae Alba
菟丝子	*tù sī zǐ*	20g	Semen Cuscutae
熟地黄	*shú dì huáng*	20g	Radix Rehmanniae Praeparata
何首乌	*hé shǒu wū*	20g	Radix Polygoni Multiflori

| 党参 | dǎng shēn | 20g | Radix Codonopsis |
| 炙甘草 | zhì gān cǎo | 8g | Radix et Rhizoma Glycyrrhizae Praeparata cum Melle |

2) Kidney yin deficiency. The treatment principle is to enrich kidney yin while warming and supplementing kidney yang. The empirical formula *Yì Jīng Yī Fāng* was selected.

益精一方 *Yì Jīng Yī Fāng*

熟地黄	shú dì huáng	20g	Radix Rehmanniae Praeparata
枸杞子	gǒu qǐ zǐ	20g	Fructus Lycii
何首乌	hé shǒu wū	20g	Radix Polygoni Multiflori
桑寄生	sāng jì shēng	20g	Ramus Loranthi seu Visci
菟丝子	tù sī zǐ	20g	Semen Cuscutae
续断	xù duàn	20g	Radix Dipsaci
山茱萸	shān zhū yú	8g	Fructus Corni
龙眼肉	lóng yǎn ròu	15g	Arillus Longan
山药	shān yào	15g	Rhizoma Dioscoreae
白芍	bái sháo	15g	Radix Paeoniae Alba
旱莲草	hàn lián cǎo	15g	Herba Ecliptae
杜仲	dù zhòng	15g	Cortex Eucommiae

3) Phlegm-damp. The treatment principle is to dry dampness and transform phlegm while supplementing the kidney. Modified *Èr Chén Tāng* was selected.

二陈汤 *Èr Chén Tāng*

半夏	bàn xià	15g	Rhizoma Pinelliae
橘红	jú hóng	15g	Exocarpium Citri Rubrum
白术	bái zhú	15g	Rhizoma Atractylodis Macrocephalae
炙甘草	zhì gān cǎo	10g	Radix et Rhizoma Glycyrrhizae Praeparata cum Melle
浙贝母	zhè bèi mǔ	10g	Bulbus Fritillariae Thunbergii
淫羊藿	yín yáng huò	10g	Herba Epimedii
茯苓	fú líng	30g	Poria
鸡血藤	jī xuè téng	30g	Caulis Spatholobi

何首乌	*hé shǒu wū*	20g	Radix Polygoni Multiflori
续断	*xù duàn*	20g	Radix Dipsaci
白扁豆	*bǎi biǎn dòu*	20g	Semen Lablab Album
远志	*yuǎn zhì*	5g	Radix Polygalae

4) *Liver constraint.* The treatment principle is to course the liver and resolve depression while supplementing the kidney. Modified *Chái Hú Shū Gān Sǎn* was selected.

柴胡疏肝散 *Chái Hú Shū Gān Sǎn*

柴胡	*chái hú*	15g	Radix Bupleuri
白芍	*bái sháo*	15g	Radix Paeoniae Alba
枳壳	*zhǐ qiào*	15g	Fructus Aurantii
香附	*xiāng fù*	15g	Rhizoma Cyperi
郁金	*yù jīn*	15g	Radix Curcumae
牡丹皮	*mǔ dān pí*	15g	Cortex Moutan
陈皮	*chén pí*	10g	Pericarpium Citri Reticulatae
何首乌	*hé shǒu wū*	20g	Radix Polygoni Multiflori
续断	*xù duàn*	20g	Radix Dipsaci
桑寄生	*sāng jì shēng*	20g	Ramus Loranthi seu Visci
薄荷	*bò hé*	5g	Herba Menthae

5) *Blood stasis.* The treatment principle is to resolve stasis and free the collaterals while supplementing the kidney. The formula is *Shào Fù Zhú Yū Tāng* with modifications.

少腹逐瘀汤 *Shào Fù Zhú Yū Tāng*

蒲黄	*pú huáng*	10g	Pollen Typhae
五灵脂	*wǔ líng zhī*	10g	Faeces Togopteri
延胡索	*yán hú suǒ*	10g	Rhizoma Corydalis
赤芍	*chì sháo*	10g	Radix Paeoniae Rubra
路路通	*lù lù tōng*	10g	Fructus Liquidambaris
穿破石	*chuān pò shí*	10g	Radix seu Vanieriae Caulis
威灵仙	*wēi líng xiān*	10g	Radix et Rhizoma Clematidis
益母草	*yì mǔ cǎo*	10g	Herba Leonuri

当归	dāng guī	15g	Radix Angelicae Sinensis
何首乌	hé shǒu wū	20g	Radix Polygoni Multiflori
续断	xù duàn	20g	Radix Dipsaci
杜仲	dù zhòng	20g	Cortex Eucommiae

Results: The recovery rate was 52.35% (167 cases), improved rate was 32.29% (103 cases), and the total effective rate reached 84.64%.

The main cause of infertility is kidney deficiency. However, liver constraint and blood stasis are also involved in many cases. Menstrual irregularities are common to most cases of infertility seen in the clinic. The basic treatment principle for infertility is to supplement the kidney while coursing the liver, quickening the blood, and regulating menstruation[4].

2. SPECIFIC FORMULAS

1) *Jiā Wèi Yù Lín Zhū Tāng* is suitable for infertility due to anovulation. The formula was administered for 3 months as one treatment course, and the effects were evaluated after 3 successive treatment courses. The recovery rate reached 72% (36 cases) and the total effective rate was 94% (47 cases)[5].

加味毓麟珠汤 *Jiā Wèi Yù Lín Zhū Tāng*

熟地黄	shú dì huáng	12g	Radix Rehmanniae Praeparata
当归	dāng guī	12g	Radix Angelicae Sinensis
白芍	bái sháo	12g	Radix Paeoniae Alba
鹿胶	lù jiāo	12g	Colla Cornus Cervi
杜仲	dù zhòng	12g	Cortex Eucommiae
菟丝子	tù sī zǐ	12g	Semen Cuscutae
茯苓	fú líng	12g	Poria
白术	bái zhú	10g	Rhizoma Atractylodis Macrocephalae
川芎	chuān xiōng	10g	Rhizoma Chuanxiong
小茴香	xiǎo huí xiāng	10g	Fructus Foeniculi

2) *Zhù Yùn Hé Jì* is suitable for luteal phase defect infertility and miscarriage resulting from kidney yang deficiency with liver constraint. To be taken in the BBT high temperature phase until the menstrual onset. Treatment was administered for 3 months as one course. The total effective rate reached 94.51%[6].

助孕合剂 *Zhù Yùn Hé Jì*

当归	*dāng guī*	10g	Radix Angelicae Sinensis
赤芍	*chì sháo*	10g	Radix Paeoniae Rubra
白芍	*bái sháo*	10g	Radix Paeoniae Alba
山药	*shān yào*	15g	Rhizoma Dioscoreae
山茱萸	*shān zhū yú*	10g	Fructus Corni
鹿角片	*lù jiǎo piàn*（predecocted）	10g	Sectum Cervi Cornu
菟丝子	*tù sī zǐ*	15g	Semen Cuscutae
柴胡	*chái hú*	6g	Radix Bupleuri

3) *Tōng Rèn Zhòng Zǐ Tāng* is suitable for the treatment of infertility due to obstruction of the fallopian tube. The recovery rate reached 73.2% (52/71)[7].

通任种子汤 *Tōng Rèn Zhòng Zǐ Tāng*

香附	*xiāng fù*	10g	Rhizoma Cyperi
丹参	*dān shēn*	30g	Radix et Rhizoma Salviae Miltiorrhizae
赤芍	*chì sháo*	9g	Radix Paeoniae Rubra
白芍	*bái sháo*	9g	Radix Paeoniae Alba
络石藤	*luò shí téng*	9g	Caulis Trachelospermi
桃仁	*táo rén*	9g	Semen Persicae
红花	*hóng huā*	9g	Flos Carthami
当归	*dāng guī*	12g	Radix Angelicae Sinensis
连翘	*lián qiào*	12g	Fructus Forsythiae
川芎	*chuān xiōng*	6g	Rhizoma Chuanxiong
小茴香	*xiǎo huí xiāng*	6g	Fructus Foeniculi
炙甘草	*zhì gān cǎo*	6g	Radix et Rhizoma Glycyrrhizae Praeparata cum Melle
蜈蚣	*wú gōng*	1piece	Scolopendra

淫羊藿	yín yáng huò	20g	Herba Epimedii
紫石英	zǐ shí yīng	20g	Fluoritum

4) *Bǔ Shèn Xiè Zhuó Tāng*. To be taken from 6 to 15 days before menstruation.

In 47 cases of immune infertility after 10 months of treatment, results showed 36 cases recovered, 10 cases with some effect, and 1 case with no effect[8].

补肾泻浊汤 *Bǔ Shèn Xiè Zhuó Tāng*

菟丝子	tù sī zǐ	10g	Semen Cuscutae
枸杞子	gǒu qǐ zǐ	10g	Fructus Lycii
淫羊藿	yín yáng huò	10g	Herba Epimedii
金银花	jīn yín huā	10g	Flos Lonicerae Japonicae
紫花地丁	zǐ huā dì dīng	10g	Herba Violae
车前子	chē qián zǐ	10g	Semen Plantaginis
牡丹皮	mǔ dān pí	10g	Cortex Moutan
泽泻	zé xiè	10g	Rhizoma Alismatis
川牛膝	chuān niú xī	10g	Radix Cyathulae
牛膝	niú xī	20g	Radix Achyranthis Bidentatae
薏苡仁	yì yǐ rén	20g	Semen Coicis
黄柏	huáng bǎi	5g	Cortex Phellodendri Chinensis
甘草	gān cǎo	9g	Radix et Rhizoma Glycyrrhizae

5) *Yì Shèn Huó Xuè Fāng*. Taken once daily for 30 days as one treatment course.

The formula was administered to 36 infertility cases testing positive for antisperm antibodies. After one course of daily treatment for 30 days, AsAb turned negative in 35 cases. The effective rate was 97%. Antisperm antibodies remained negative in 20 cases after half a year. 11 subjects became pregnant within 2 years, with an overall pregnancy rate of 30.5%[9].

益肾活血方 *Yì Shèn Huó Xuè Fāng*

地黄	dì huáng	15g	Radix Rehmanniae
山茱萸	shān zhū yú	10g	Fructus Corni
山药	shān yào	15g	Rhizoma Dioscoreae

菟丝子	tù sī zǐ	10g	Semen Cuscutae
黄芪	huáng qí	15g	Radix Astragali
茯苓	fú líng	15g	Poria
当归	dāng guī	10g	Radix Angelicae Sinensis
川芎	chuān xiōng	10g	Rhizoma Chuanxiong
丹参	dān shēn	10g	Radix et Rhizoma Salviae Miltiorrhizae
泽兰	zé lán	15g	Herba Lycopi
鹿角片	lù jiǎo piàn	10g	Sectum Cervi Cornu

6) *Xuān Yù Tōng Jīng Tāng* was used in the treatment of 51 cases of infertility due to endometriosis. The pregnancy rate reached 80%[10].

宣郁通经汤 *Xuān Yù Tōng Jīng Tāng*

白芍（stir-fried with wine）	bái sháo	15g	Radix Paeoniae Alba
当归（washed with wine）	dāng guī	15g	Radix Angelicae Sinensis
牡丹皮	mǔ dān pí	15g	Cortex Moutan
炒栀子（stir-fried）	chǎo zhī zǐ	9g	Fructus Gardeniae Praeparatus
芥子（stir-fried and ground）	jiè zǐ	6g	Semen Sinapis
柴胡	chái hú	3g	Radix Bupleuri
香附（stir-fried with wine）	xiāng fù	3g	Rhizoma Cyperi
郁金（stir-fried with vinegar）	yù jīn	3g	Radix Curcumae
黄芩	huáng qín	3g	Radix Scutellariae
甘草	gān cǎo	3g	Radix et Rhizoma Glycyrrhizae

3. Acupuncture and Moxibustion

1) *Acupuncture*

a. *Infertility resulting from ovulation failure*

Kou Jin-mao treated 50 cases of anovulatory infertility with acupuncture. Points were selected according to the following patterns.

For liver constraint and kidney deficiency, SP 6 (*sān yīn jiāo*), RN 6 (*qì hǎi*), LV 3 (*tài chōng*) and RN 4 (*guān yuán*) were selected.

For qi stagnation and blood stasis, SP 6, RN 6, ST 29 (*guī lái*), SP 10 (*xuè hǎi*) and RN 3 (*zhōng jí*) were selected.

For liver and kidney yin deficiency, SP 6, RN 4, KI 12 (dà hè) and RN 12 (zhōng wǎn) were selected.

For spleen and kidney yang deficiency, SP 6, BL 23 (shèn shù) DU 4 (mìng mén) and ST 36 (zú sān lǐ) were selected.

Stimulate with neutral supplementation and drainage. Retain the needles for 30 minutes. Treat once every other day from the 5th day after menstruation for 1 month as one treatment course. Withdraw treatment during menstruation. After 1 to 6 treatment courses, 40 cases were recovered and treatment was shown ineffective in 10 cases[11].

Mo Xiao-ming treated 34 cases of anovulatory infertility with acupuncture.

Points in the first group were RN 4, RN 3, zǐ gōng and SP 6.

The second group included BL 18 (gān shù), BL 23, shí qī zhuī xià and SP 6.

The 2 groups of points were alternated each session. All points were needled with even supplementation and drainage, and retained for 20 to 30 minutes. Treatments were administered 3 times per week for three months, as one treatment course.

Results showed 12 cases with excellent effect, 16 cases with some effect, and 6 cases with no effect[12].

Pu Yun-xing used acupuncture to treat 63 cases of infertility that had not responded well to Chinese medicinal therapy.

The first group of points includes RN 4, KI 12, zǐ gōng and SP 6.

The second group includes BL 23, BL 18, shí qī zhuī xià, BL 32 (cì liáo) and KI 3 (tài xī). The 2 groups of points are alternated each session. Stimulate with medium intensity using rotating, lifting and thrusting manipulations. Retain the needles for 20 minutes after the obtaining of qi. Treat every day for one month, but stop treatment during menstruation. In cases of amenorrhea, treat continuously for 3 months.

The effective rate reached 65% (41/63) with 5 cases becoming pregnant. Follicles developed and ovulated in 20 cases. Abnormal diphasic BBT became normal in 7 cases. 8 cases of monophasic BBT became abnormal diphasic. 2 cases menstruated for 1 cycle. The ineffective rate was 8% (5/63)[13].

Yan Ming applied electroacupuncture in the treatment of 83 cases of infertility due to follicular formation with anovulation.

The main points include RN 4, RN 3, *zĭ gōng*, ST 36 and SP 6. Modifications were made to the point prescription according to pattern identification.

Method: Stimulate RN 4, RN 3 and *zĭ gōng* strongly, needling downward and obliquely. Apply even supplementation and drainage to ST 36, SP 6 and any other points used. After obtaining qi, apply electro acupuncture for 30 minutes using sparse dense wave, at a speed of 16 to 18 times per minute.

The effective rate reached 78.31% (65/83)[14].

Tu Guo-chun treated 36 cases of anovulatory infertility with injecting gonadotropic hormone (HMG) acupuncture point injection. A control group of 26 subjects were used as the control group. The patients in the treatment group took 50mg of clomiphene per day from the 2nd day to the 6th day of the menstrual cycle. HMG was injected into RN 4, RN 6, RN 3, *zĭ gōng*, SP 6 and BL 23 on the 7th, 9th, 11th and 13th day, with one point selected each time. Injection was given to produce distention or downward radiating sensation. Patients in the control group recieved clomiphene from the 2nd day of menstruation, as well as HMG intramuscular injections from the 5th day to 11th day.

The pregnancy rate of the treatment group was 61.1% and 57.7% in the control[15].

b. Tubal infertility

Wang Fang treated 82 cases of with acupuncture and moxibustion with the following method.

The main points include KI 3, SP 10, and RN 4 through to RN 3.

For damp heat, add BL 40 (*wěi zhōng*) and GB 34 (*yáng líng quán*).

For qi stagnation and blood stasis, add ST 36 and LV 3.

For yin deficiency, add SP 6.

For yang deficiency, moxa RN 4 and SP 10.

Subjects were treated once every other day. 61 cases recovered, 4 cases improved, and 17 cases recieved no effect[16].

Ding Hui-jun treated a group of tubal infertility patients with the following points.

The main points include RN 3, *zǐ gōng*, ST 29 and SP 6.

For liver qi stagnation, add LV 3 and PC 6 (*nèi guān*).

For qi and blood deficiency and obstruction of the uterine vessels, add ST 36 and SP 1 (*yǐn bái*).

For cold damp obstruction, select RN 4 and ST 36.

For damp heat obstruction, select SP 9 (*yīn líng quán*) and LV 2 (*xíng jiān*).

For liver and kidney deficiency, select RN 4 and KI 3.

Apply drainage for excess patterns, and supplementation for deficiency patterns. Moxa RN 4 and ST 36 as well. 10 times constitutes one treatment course.

25 cases recovered, 3 cases improved, and 3 cases recieved no effect. The recovery rate was 80.6% and total effective rate 90.3%[17].

2) Moxibustion

Chen Qiong[18] treated 72 cases of infertility due to endometriosis with acupuncture and moxbustion. The selected points were divided into 2 groups.

The first group includes RN 4, RN 3, *zǐ gōng* and SP 10.

The second group includes BL 31 to BL 34 (*bā liáo*) and SP 6.

Needle RN 4, RN 3 and *zǐ gōng* 1.5 to 2.5 cun perpendicularly, and supplement with rotation. Retain the needles for 15 to 20 minutes, stimulating the needles once every 5 minutes. Cover these points with a moxa box after removing the needles, and apply gentle moxibustion with a moxa stick for 20 to 30 minutes.

Needle SP 10 upwards and obliquely 1.5 to 2 *cun*. Lift, thrust and rotate to drain. After obtaining qi, apply shaking to enlarge the point. Remove the needles quickly without pressing the hole.

Also cover BL 31 to BL 34 with a moxa box for 20 to 30 minutes. Then use a three-edged needle to pierce the skin.

Needle SP 6 1.5 to 2.5 *cun* perpendicularly, and apply even supplementation and drainage. Retain the needles for 15 to 20 minutes, stimulating once every 5 minutes.

Treat with both groups of points alternately, with no treatment applied during menstruation.

The pregnancy rate was 58.33% (42/72), significantly effective rate 11.11% (8/72), effective rate 23.61% (17/72), ineffective rate 6.95% (5/72), with the total effective rate reaching 93.05%. Acupuncture and moxbustion significantly improves microcirculation, and also effectively relieves many of the associated symptoms.

Experimental Studies

1. SINGLE HERBS

A. Xiān máo (Rhizoma Curculiginis)

Wang Ben-xiang studied the effect of water extracted *xiān máo* (Rhizoma Curculiginis) on the endocrine system of rats. 10g/kg of *xiān máo* (Rhizoma Curculiginis) was given to female rats by intragastric administration twice a day for 5 days. It increased the weight of the antehypophysis, ovaries, and uterus but had no effect on the level of plasmic LH. It also increased the number of HCG/LH receptors in the ovaries. Deovarian rats were given the same intragastric administration for 5 days. The rats were anesthetized and injected with D-3-LRH intravenously on the 6th day. The secretory reaction of LH in the antehypophysis was improved after injections of LRH. The level of plasmic LH rose 241.58% within 90 minutes.

This indicates that *xiān máo* (Rhizoma Curculiginis) can improve the luteotrophic function of hypothalamus-hypophysis-ovaries axis by improving hypophysis reactivity towards LRH and not by stimulating the secretion of LH[19].

B. Yín yáng huò (Herba Epimedii)

Li Fang-fang observed a culture of icariine, follicular cells and adrenocortical cell for three hours. The hormone content of the culture fluid was also evaluated.

Results: Icariine (30-1000μg/L) could cause follicular cells to secrete E_2. Certain densities of icariine also could cause adrenocortical cells to secrete 11-dehydro-17-hydroxycorticosterone.

Study also shows that 10g/kg to 20g/kg of *yín yáng huò* (Herba Epimedii) can relieve signs resulting from hydrocortisone in yang deficient rat models; increase the weight of the prostate sperm reservoir, levator ani muscle-sponge, uterus, adrenal and thymus gland; and also raise the levels of testosterone and E_2[20].

C. Zǐ hé chē (Placenta Hominis)

Cai Yong-min found that a decoction of *zǐ hé chē* (Placenta Hominis) could combat allergies and regulate immune function. It acts to increase the ratio of T-cells in normal mice without affecting the total lymphocyte count. It resists the immunosuppressive action of prednisone and improves immune function in stressed mouse models. It was also found that *zǐ hé chē* (Placenta Hominis) displays estrogen-like effects. Injections administered to lactating rabbits were shown to promote growth. It can also promote the growth of thymus, spleen, uterus, vagina and the lacteal gland significantly; as well as effecting the thyroid and testicles[21].

D. Tù sī zǐ (Semen Cuscutae)

Cai Yong-min applied water extracted *tù sī zǐ* (Semen Cuscutae) to mice models by intragastric administration. It was found that *tù sī zǐ* (Semen Cuscutae) could promote the cornification of vaginal epithelial cells, and increase the weight of the uterus while also displaying estrogen-like effects. Water extracts of *tù sī zǐ* (Semen Cuscutae) can increase the weight of the antehypophysis, ovaries and uterus. It also increased HCG/LH receptors in the ovaries of rats and improved the secretory reaction of LH in the hypophysis of deovarian rats after LRH injection. Plasmic LH reached the highest level 90 minutes after injection.

This suggests that *tù sī zǐ* (Semen Cuscutae) can improve the luteotrophic function of the hypothalamus-hypophysis-ovarian axis, hypophysis reactivity towards LRH, and ovarian reactivity to LH[21].

2. HERBAL FORMULAS

A. Regulating the hypothalamus-hypophysis-ovarian axis

It has been confirmed by clinical and animal studies that kidney supplementing medicinals can regulate the hypothalamus-hypophysis-ovarian axis.

Luo Yuan-kai administered the empirical formula *Cù Pái Luǎn Tāng* (促排卵汤) to female rabbits. It was found that the corpus luteum was abundant in the ovaries of the rabbits in the medication group. The endometrial glands also increased with obvious secretion. Increased sexual behavior was seen as well. This indicates that kidney supplementing medicinals may increase estrogen levels and also stimulate the hypothalamus and hypophysis[22].

Zhang Ting-ting found that *Wēn Jīng Tāng* (温经汤) could improve the activity of LH-RH by affecting the hypothalamus, reduce PRL by affecting the hypophysis, promote the secretion of LH and FSH, stimulate the ovaries, and induce ovulation. It may cure infertility by affecting the hypophysis, hypothalamus and ovaries directly[23].

Chen Jin-xiu found that *Bǎo Kūn Dān* (保坤丹 , composed of *dāng guī, hóng huā, táo rén, xiāng fù, shēng dì huáng* and *fú líng*) could increase the weight of the uterus and ovaries, promote the growth of follicles, and induce ovulation in mice. There was a significant deviation as compared to a control group. A certain dose of *Bǎo Kūn Dān* can inhibit uterine contractions from hypophysin in vitro and also strengthen rhythmic contraction of the oviduct[24].

Liu Jin-xing found that *Yǎng Jīng Tāng* (养精汤 , composed of *nǚ zhēn zǐ, shēng dì huáng, shān zhū yú, zǐ hé chē, ròu cóng róng, huáng jīng* and *zhì hé shǒu wū*) could promote the release of GnRH in anovulatory rats, increase the weight of the ovaries and uterus, raise the plasmic level of E2 and P, and increase the mass of the corpus luteum. The endometria were thickened and the amount of gland secretions also increased[25].

Gui Sui-qi studied the effects on morphology and immune function of the hypophysis, ovaries and adrenals in infertile rats resulting from androgen (ASR) before and after administration of kidney supplementing medicinals (*fù zǐ, ròu guì, yín yáng huò, tù sī zǐ, huáng jīng, bǔ gǔ zhī* and *shú dì huáng*)[26].

Results: Lipid droplets, vacuole, crinophage and autophagosome were present in the cytoplasm of adenopituicytes. Anovulatory ovaries and zona reticularis hyperplasia of the adrenal cortex could be found. The levels of FSH and LH decreased significantly ($p<0.05$-0.005). The levels of T and DHA increased significantly ($p<0.01$-0.001). Morphology and immune function of ASR recovered after treatment.

Conclusion: Exogenous androgens in 9 day old female SD mice can affect the gonadal and adrenal axis. Kidney supplementing medicinals can decrease androgen and induce ovulation through the regulation of the gonadal axis and adrenals.

Sun Fei administered water extracted *Tiān Guǐ Fāng* (天癸方 , composed of *shēng dì huáng, tù sī zǐ, yín yáng huò, bǔ gǔ zhī* and *nǚ zhēn zǐ*) to ASR. The weight of ASR decreased. Obviously increased leptin decreased the levels of FSH/LH and reproductive function recovered, and ovulation emerged. This suggests that kidney supplementing medicinals may induce ovulation by regulating the function of both center (hypothalamus-hypophysis) and periphery (metabolic-genital axis)[27].

Zhou Hui-fang found that *Zhù Yùn Hé Jì* (助孕合剂 , composed of 10g of *dāng guī, chì sháo, bái sháo, shān zhū yú* and predecocted *lù jiǎo piàn*, 15g of *shān yào* and *tù sī zǐ*, and 6g of vinegar-processed *chái hú*) could resist the increase of PRL resulting from metoclopramide in rats. Meanwhile, it could cure luteal phase defects due to kidney deficiency and liver constraint by increasing serum E_2 and decreasing the organ coefficient of the uterus in rats[6].

Zhang Si-jia found that *Xiān Jiǎ Chōng Jì* (仙甲冲剂 , composed of *chái hú, bái sháo, dāng guī, yín yáng huò* and *chuān shān jiǎ*) had estrogen-like effects similar to clomiphene. It could increase the weight of the ovaries and induce ovulation in rabbits. It could also decrease the level of PRL similar to ergolactin with prolonged action and no side-effects[28].

B. Regulating regulatory factors in the ovaries

Types of PGIs, IGF-1 and Ins have similar structures and consensual reactions. IGF-1 can stimulate the target glands to produce high levels of androgen through the Ins receptors, thus resulting in infertility. ASR presents with descending levels of IGF-1R. IGF-1 plays an important role in regulating its receptors.

Li Gui-ling studied the effect of kidney supplementing medicinals on IGF-1 and IGF-1R in ASR. It was considered that kidney supplementing medicinals could regulate high levels of IGF-1 in the blood and low levels of IGF-1R in the major target organs. It was supposed that kidney supplementing medicinals could induce ovulation in ASR through IGF-1/IGF-1R[29].

C. Effect on uterus estrogen receptor (ER) and progesterone receptor (PR)

Qian Zu-qi found that *Bǔ Shèn Yù Gōng Chōng Jì* (补肾育宫冲剂) could increase the content of ER in the endometria, and promote the effect of estrogen and uterine growth[30].

Xiao Dong-hong applied radioreceptor assay to detect the content of ER, PR and protein in uterine kytoplasm, and the weight of uterus of spayed mice after administration of *Zī Yīn Bǔ Shèn Yù Yīn Líng* (滋阴补肾育阴灵). It was found that *Zī Yīn Bǔ Shèn Yù Yīn Líng* could increase the weight of uterus ($p<0.01$) and content of ER and PR in uterine kytoplasm ($p<0.01$) and promote uterine protein synthesis in spayed mice[31].

D. Effect on trace elements such as Zn, Cu, Fe and Ca

It has been found that kidney supplementing medicinals have an extensive physiological effect on body organization and can induce ovulation by regulating and supplementing the content of trace elements such as Zn, Cu, Fe and Ca.

Kidney supplementing and menstruation regulating medicinals that can improve Zn deficiency and improve sexual function include *dāng guī, dān shēn, chuān xiōng, zǐ hé chē, bā jǐ tiān, yín yáng huò, fù zǐ, shé chuáng zǐ, tù sī zǐ, wǔ wèi zǐ, nǚ zhēn zǐ, dǎng shēn, huáng qí* and *bái zhú*. Some medicinals contain high levels of Cu such as *dān shēn, chuān xiōng, zǐ hé chē, ròu guì, bā jǐ tiān, yín yáng huò, fù zǐ, shé chuáng zǐ, gǒu qǐ zǐ, fù pén zǐ, tù sī zǐ, wǔ wèi zǐ, nǚ zhēn zǐ, běi shā shēn, dǎng shēn, huáng qí* and *bái zhú*. Adequate Cu can promote hypophysis to synthetize ACTH and release of LH, FSH and TSH. Deficiency of Cu can result in infertility, also affecting the synthesis of progesterone[32-33].

Li Gui-xian found that *Cù Pái Luǎn Tāng* (促排卵汤 , composed of *chái hú, chì sháo, bái sháo, gǒu qǐ zǐ* and *tù sī zǐ*) could increase the level of blood calcium, the amount of endometrial glands, and also promote the formation of blastocysts in mice. It was concluded that Chinese medicinals can promote the sexual function of mice significantly[34].

E. Making AsAb negative

Zhang Yong-feng studied on the effect of *Zhù Yùn Líng* (助 孕 灵) granules, composed of *zhī mǔ, huáng bǎi, nǚ zhēn zǐ, shān yào, shān zhū yú, gǒu qǐ zǐ, fú ling, huáng qí, dān shēn, yù jīn, mǔ dān pí* and *bái huā shé shé cǎo* on AsAb positive rat models. It was found that the pregnancy rate, negative rate and the weight of the uterus and ovaries of rats in the treatment group was higher than in the control. *Zhù Yùn Líng* can resist AsAb, promote the growth of the uterus and ovaries, and increase the pregnancy rate[35].

Wang Wang-jiu observed immune infertility mouse models administered with *Miǎn Bù Yī Hào* (免不 1 号). It was found that *Miǎn Bù Yī Hào* could decrease ovarian immune complex deposit and serum AsAb levels with low amplitude of rebound. *Miǎn Bù Yī Hào* also increased pregnancy rates. The litter size in the treatment group was markedly higher than that in the model group ($p<0.05$) and biomedical administration groups ($p<0.05$ or $p<0.01$)[36].

F. Antibiosis and antivirus

Qu Yun-zhi found that *Xiāo Zhēng Sǎn Jié Chōng Jì* (消症散结冲剂) could increase the oviducal patency rate and pregnancy rate in patients with tubal anastomosis. There was a significant difference in oviducal patency between the treatment and control groups. It was concluded that *Xiāo Zhēng Sǎn Jié Chōng Jì* has antibacterial and antiviral actions, quickens the blood, transforms stasis, improves microcirculation and hemodynamic responses of genital system, promotes reorganization and recovery, relieves inflammatory reactions, prevents obstruction and adhesions in the fallopian tubes, increases patency and immunologic mechanism, and reduces ovulation[37].

3. New Preparations

A. Xiāo Zhēng Sǎn Jié Chōng Jì (消症散结冲剂)

Qu Yun-zhi induced metritis, volar swelling, writhing response and polycystic ovary to study the effect of *Xiāo Zhēng Sǎn Jié Chōng Jì* on inflammatory stimulation and immune function in animals. It was found that *Xiāo Zhēng Sǎn Jié Chōng Jì* could increase the pregnancy rate, the average weight of fetal mice and the weight of uterus, and decrease the weight of ovaries in mice which had anovulatory polycystic ovaries resulting from endocrine disturbance.

B. Luó Lè Capsule (罗勒胶囊)

Luó lè (Herba Basilici), is a traditional Chinese medicinal. It acts to course wind, move qi, transform phlegm, disperse food accumulation, quicken the blood and resolve toxins. It has been confirmed by vaginal smear that *Luó Lè Capsule* has estrogen-like activities in spayed mice by increasing uterine weight. It can promote the cuticularization of vaginal epithelial cells and stimulate mice to engage in intercourse. It is also found that *Luó Lè Capsule* does not increase the weight of ovaries and has no effect on their growth. It is also possible that it does not influence the hypothalamus or anterior pituitary. It is proven by ovulation experiments that *Luó Lè Capsule* can improve follicular development and reduce ovulation. The level of blood E2 increases suddenly after administration. E2 can make GnRH nerve cells release GnRH, and thus LH or FSH secreted by the anterior pituitary. *Luó Lè Capsule* can induce ovulation by causing GTH and LH release to peak levels[38].

REFERENCES

[1] Wu Xia. A Perspective on the Treatment of Infertility According to Pattern (辨证论治不孕症之我见). *Zhejiang Journal of Traditional Chinese Medicine* (浙江中医杂志), 2005, (6): 256-257.

[2] Du Ying-han. A Clinical Study on the Treatment of Infertility with Integrated Chinese and Biomedicine According to Pattern (辨证分型中西医结合治疗妇科不孕症的临床探讨). *Chinese Journal of*

Practical Chinese and Modern Medicine (中华实用中西医杂志), 2003, 3 (16): 16-17.

[3] Li Xiu-ying, Liu Shuang. Comprehensive Treatment of Infertility According to Pattern (辨证治疗不孕症的体会). *Liaoning Journal of Traditional Chinese Medicine* (辽宁中医杂志), 2002, 29 (2): 86.

[4] Hu Rui-ying. Clinical Observation of 319 Cases of Infertility Treated According to Pattern (辨证治疗不孕症319例疗效观察). *New Journal of Traditional Chinese Medicine* (新中医), 1998, 30 (8): 41-42.

[5] Wang Geng, Lian Xi-cheng. The Treatment of 50 Cases of Anovulatory Infertility with *Jiā Wèi Yù Lín Zhū Tāng* (加味毓麟珠汤治疗无排卵性不孕症50例). *Shanxi Journal of Traditional Chinese Medicine* (陕西中医), 2001, 22 (11): 664.

[6] Zhou Hui-fang. A Clinical and Experimental Study on the Treatment of Infertility and Miscarriage Resulting from Luteal Phase Defect by *Zhù Yùn Hé Jì* (助孕合剂治疗黄体功能不全性不孕流产的临床及实验研究). *Chinese Journal of Information on Traditional Chinese Medicine* (中国中医药信息杂志), 2001, 8 (3): 44-46.

[7] Wang Zhen-qing. Treatment of 71 Cases of Infertility Resulting from Salpingemphraxis with Modifications of *Tōng Rèn Zhòng Zǐ Tāng* (通任种子汤加味治疗输卵管阻塞性不孕症71例). *New Journal of Traditional Chinese Medicine* (新中医), 2000, 32 (10): 46.

[8] Liang Wen-zhen. Treatment of 78 Cases of Immune Infertility with *Bǔ Shèn Xiè Zhuó Tāng* (补肾泻浊汤治疗免疫性不孕症78例). *New Journal of Traditional Chinese Medicine* (新中医), 1998, (4): 44.

[9] Zhou Ya-ping. Clinical Observation of Immune Infertility Treatment by Supplementing the Kidney and Quickening the Blood (益肾活血法治疗免疫性不孕症的临床观察). *Journal of Zhenjiang Medical College* (镇江医学院学报), 1998, 8 (4): 589.

[10] Lin Ying, Miao Yu-ping. Treatment of 51 Cases of Infertility Resulting from Endometriosis with Xuan Yu Tong Jing Tang (宣郁通经汤治疗子宫内膜异位症致不孕症51例). *Study of Chinese Medicine* (中医药研究), 2001, 17 (4): 23-24.

[11] Kou Jin-mao, Kou Zheng. Clinical Observation of 50 Cases of Anovulatory Infertility Treated with Acupuncture (针刺治疗无排卵性不孕症50例临床观察). *Journal of Henan College of Traditional Chinese Medicine* (河南中医药学刊), 1997, 12 (4): 45.

[12] Mo Xiao-ming. Clinical Study of the Mechanism of Inducing ovulation with Acupuncture (针刺促排卵的临床及机理研究). *Shanghai Acupuncture and Moxibustion Journal* (上海针灸杂志), 1990, (3): 8-9.

[13] Pu Yun-xing, Chen Wen-juan. A Clinical Study of 63 Cases of Inducing Ovulation with Acupuncture (针刺促排卵63例临床观察). *Shanghai Journal of Traditional Chinese Medicine* (上海中医药杂志), 1991, (2): 3.

[14] Yan Ming, Huang Yao-jin. Analysis of Electric Acupuncture Clinical Effects in 83 Cases of Inducied Ovulation (电针促排卵83例临床疗效分析). *Chinese Acupuncture and Moxibustion* (中国针灸), 1997, 16 (11): 651-652.

[15] Tu Guo-chun. Clinical Observation of Acupuncture Point Injection Treatment of Infertility Resulting from Ovulation Failure (穴位注射治疗排卵障碍性不孕症临床观察). *Chinese Acupuncture and Moxibustion* (中国针灸), 1999, 19 (6): 333-334.

[16] Wang Fang. 82 Cases of Infertility Resulting from Salpingemphraxis Treated with

Acupuncture and Moxibustion (针灸治疗输卵管阻塞性不孕症82例). *Chinese Naturopathy* (中国民间疗法), 1998, (1): 33.

[17] Ding Hui-jun. 31 Cases of Infertility due to Salpingemphraxis Treated by Acupuncture and Moxibustion (针灸治疗输卵管阻塞性不孕症31例). *Journal of Clinical Acupuncture and Moxibustion* (针灸临床杂志), 1998, 14 (10): 30.

[18] Chen Qiong, Yue Guang-ping, Zhang Wei-min. Clinical Observation in the Treatment of 72 Cases of Endometriosis (针灸治疗子宫内膜异位症72例临床观察). *Chinese Acupuncture and Moxibustion* (中国针灸), 1996, (2): 25-27.

[19] Wang Ben-xiang, Ma Jin-kai, Deng Wen-long, et al. *Modern Chinese Medicinal Pharmacology* (现代中药药理学). Tianjin: Tianjin Science and Technology Press, 1997, 1256.

[20] Li Fang-fang, Li En, Lv Zhan-jun, et al. Icariine and Secretory Function of Follicular and Adrenocortical Cells in Rats (淫羊藿甙对大鼠卵泡颗粒细胞和肾上腺皮质细胞分泌功能的影响). *China Journal of Chinese Materia Medica* (中国中药杂志), 1997, 22 (8): 499-500.

[21] Cai Yong-min, Ren Yu-rang, Wang Li, et al. *Latest Chinese Medicinal Pharmacology and Clinical Application*(最新中药药理与临床应用). Beijing: Huaxia Press, 1999, 458-473.

[22] Luo Yuan-kai. *Luo Yuankai's Discussion of Medicine* (罗元恺论医集). Beijing: People's Medicial Publishing House, 1990, 38-44.

[23] Zhang Ting-ting. Study and Application of Infertility Treatment in Japan with *Wēn Jīng Tāng* (温经汤治疗不孕症在日本的研究及应用). *Journal of Practical Traditional Chinese Medicine* (实用中医药杂志), 1998, 14 (2): 28-29.

[24] Chen Jin-xiu, Wang Di, Ma Pei-zhi, et al. An Experimental Study on the Treatmnt of Primary Infertility by *Bǎo Kūn Dān* (保坤丹治疗原发性不孕症的实验研究). *Chinese Journal of Information on Traditional Chinese Medicine* (中国中医药信息杂志), 1999, 6 (9): 24-25.

[25] Liu Jin-xing, Liu Min-ru, Song Tao, et al. Clinical and Experimental Study on Inducing Ovulation with *Yǎng Jīng Tāng* (养精汤促排卵的临床及实验研究). *Chinese Journal of Integrated Traditional and Western Medicine* (中国中西医结合杂志), 2001, 21 (2): 94-98.

[26] Gui Sui-qi, Yu Jin, Wei Mei-juan, et al. An Experimental Study on the Effect of Kidney-supplementing Medicinals on the Hypophysis, Ovaries and Adrenal in Infertile Rats Resulting from Androgen (补肾中药对雄激素致不孕大鼠垂体、卵巢及肾上腺作用的实验研究). *Chinese Journal of Integrated Traditional and Western Medicine* (中国中西医结合杂志), 1997, 17 (12): 735-738.

[27] Sun Fei. Effects of *Tiān Guǐ Fāng* on Leptin and PGH in Infertile Rats Resulting from Androgen (中药天癸方对雄激素致不孕大鼠leptin及垂体促性腺激素的影响). *Chinese Journal of Integrated Traditional and Western Medicine* (中国中西医结合杂志), 1999, 19 (6): 350-352.

[28] Zhang Si-jia, He Chun-na, Qiao Le-shi, et al. Experimental Animal Study on Inducing Ovulation by *Xiān Jiǎ Chōng Jì* (仙甲冲剂促排卵的动物实验研究). *Chinese Journal of Birth Health and Heredity* (中国优生与遗传杂志), 1998, 6 (4): 65-66.

[29] Li Gui-ling. The Effects ofKidney-supplementing Medicinals on IGF-1 and IGF-1R in Infertile Rats Resulting from Androgen (补肾中药对雄激素致不孕大鼠胰岛素样生长因子-1及胰岛素因子-1受体的影响). *Chinese Journal of Integrated Traditional and Western Medicine* (中国中西医结合杂志),

2000, 20 (9): 677-680.

[30] Qian Zu-qi, Lu Hui-juan, Wu Ping, et al. The Mechanism of *Bǔ Shèn Yù Gōng Chōng Jì* in the Treatment of Infantile Uterus (补肾育宫冲剂治疗子宫发育不良的机理研究). *Chinese Journal of Integrated Traditional and Western Medicine* (中国中西医结合杂志), 1998, 18 (4): 221-223.

[31] Xiao Dong-hong. Effects of Enriching Yin and Supplementing the Kidney on ER and PR of Spayed Mice (滋阴补肾法对去卵巢小鼠雌孕激素受体的影响). *Hubei Journal of Traditional Chinese Medicine* (湖北中医杂志), 1996, 18 (3): 54-55.

[32] Cai Li-rong. Effects of Supplementing the Kidney and Quickening the Blood on Preventing Experimental Premature Ovarian Failure in Mice (补肾活血对小鼠实验性卵巢早衰防治作用的研究). *Chinese Journal of Integrated Traditional and Western Medicine* (中国中西医结合杂志), 2001, 21 (2): 126-129.

[33] Wang Yong-yan. *Chinese Gynecology Today* (今日中医妇科). Beijing: People's Medicial Publishing House, 2000, 397-398.

[34] Li Gui-xian, Zhang Ya-bin, Xu Qing, et al. Effects of Chinese Medicinals for Inducing Ovulation on the Content of Blood Ca^{2+} in Mice (中草药促排卵对小鼠血清Ca^{2+}等含量的影响). *Reproduction and Contraception* (生殖与避孕), 1996,16(5): 383-385.

[35] Zhang Yong-feng. Effects of *Zhù Yùn Líng* on Male Rat Models with AsAb (助孕灵对抗精子抗体阳性大鼠模型的影响). *Pharmacology and Clinical Chinese Materia Medica* (中药药理与临床), 2001, 17 (5): 38-39.

[36] Wang Wang-jiu, Chan Mei-ying, Huang Zhen, et al. An Experimental Study of *Miǎn Bù Yī Hào* on Immune Infertility in Female Mice (免不1号对雌性小鼠免疫性不孕症的实验研究). *Chinese Journal of Basic Medicine in Traditional Chinese Medicine* (中国中医基础医学杂志), 2002, 8 (9): 20-22.

[37] Qu Yun-zhi, Jiao Xiao-lan, Zhi Xiao-dong, et al. Effects of *Xiāo Zhēng Sǎn Jié Chōng Jì* on Inflammation, Pain and Polycystic Ovaries (消症散结冲剂对炎症、疼痛及多囊卵巢的影响). *Chinese Traditional Patent Medicine* (中成药), 1996, 18 (12): 26-28.

[38] Jin Wei-xin, Sun Shao Xia, Shan Yanmei, et al. Clinical Observation of *Luó Lè* Capsules in the Treatment of Infertility Resulting from Ovulation Failure (罗勒胶囊治疗排卵障碍性不孕的临床观察). *Journal of Traditional Chinese Medicine* (中医杂志), 1991, 32 (2): 43.

Index by Disease Names and Symptoms

Index by Chinese Medicinals and Formulas

General Index

Notes

图书在版编目（CIP）数据

中医临床实用系列：男性不育与女性不孕（英文）/ 陈志强
主编 . —北京：人民卫生出版社，2008.4

ISBN 978-7-117-10024-3

Ⅰ.中… Ⅱ.陈… Ⅲ.①男性不育—中医治疗法—英文
②不孕症—中医治疗法—英文 Ⅳ.R271.14 R256.56

中国版本图书馆 CIP 数据核字（2008）第 034669 号

人卫智网	www.ipmph.com	医学教育、学术、考试、健康，购书智慧智能综合服务平台
人卫官网	www.pmph.com	人卫官方资讯发布平台

中医临床实用系列：男性不育与女性不孕（英文）

主　　编：陈志强
出版发行：人民卫生出版社（中继线010-59780011）
地　　址：北京市朝阳区潘家园南里19号
邮　　编：100021
网　　址：http://www.pmph.com
E - mail：pmph @ pmph.com
发　　行：zzg@pmph.com
购书热线：+8610-5978-7340
开　　本：787×1092　1/16
版　　次：2008 年 4 月第 1 版　2017 年 7 月第 1 版第 2 次印刷
标准书号：ISBN 978-7-117-10024-3/R · 10025
打击盗版举报电话：010-59787491　E-mail：WQ @ pmph.com
（凡属印装质量问题请与本社市场营销中心联系退换）